Imaging in Gynecologic Oncology

Editors

DREW A. TORIGIAN
DOMENICO RUBELLO

PET CLINICS

www.pet.theclinics.com

Consulting Editor
ABASS ALAVI

April 2018 • Volume 13 • Number 2

ELSEVIER

1600 John F. Kennedy Boulevard • Suite 1800 • Philadelphia, Pennsylvania, 19103-2899

http://www.pet.theclinics.com

PET CLINICS Volume 13, Number 2
April 2018 ISSN 1556-8598, ISBN-13: 978-0-323-58318-3

Editor: John Vassallo (j.vassallo@elsevier.com)
Developmental Editor: Casey Potter

PET Clinics (ISSN 1556-8598) is published quarterly by Elsevier Inc., 360 Park Avenue South, New York, NY 10010-1710. Months of issue are January, April, July, and October. Periodicals postage paid at New York, NY, and additional mailing offices. Subscription prices per year are $232.00 (US individuals), $396.00 (US institutions), $100.00 (US students), $263.00 (Canadian individuals), $446.00 (Canadian institutions), $140.00 (Canadian students), $268.00 (foreign individuals), $446.00 (foreign institutions), and $140.00 (foreign students). To receive student and resident rate, orders must be accompanied by name of affiliated institution, date of term, and the signature of program/residency coordinator on institution letterhead. Orders will be billed at individual rate until proof of status is received. Foreign air speed delivery is included in all Clinics subscription prices. All prices are subject to change without notice. POSTMASTER: Send address changes to PET Clinics, Elsevier Health Sciences Division, Subscription Customer Service, 3251 Riverport Lane, Maryland Heights, MO 63043. **Customer Service: 1-800-654-2452 (U.S. and Canada); 314-447-8871 (outside U.S. and Canada). Fax: 314-447-8029. E-mail: journalscustomerservice-usa@elsevier.com (for print support); journalsonlinesupport-usa@elsevier.com (for online support).**

Reprints. For copies of 100 or more of articles in this publication, please contact the Commercial Reprints Department, Elsevier Inc., 360 Park Avenue South, New York, NY 10010-1710. Tel.: 212-633-3874; Fax: 212-633-3820; E-mail: reprints@elsevier.com.

PET Clinics is covered in MEDLINE/PubMed (Index Medicus).

Contributors

CONSULTING EDITOR

ABASS ALAVI, MD, MD (Hon), PhD (Hon), DSc (Hon)
Professor of Radiology and Neurology, Division of Nuclear Medicine, Department of Radiology, Hospital of the University of Pennsylvania, University of Pennsylvania Perelman School of Medicine, Philadelphia, Pennsylvania, USA

EDITORS

DREW A. TORIGIAN, MD, MA, FSAR, FACR
Department of Radiology, Hospital of the University of Pennsylvania, Philadelphia, Pennsylvania, USA

DOMENICO RUBELLO, MD
Head of Service of Nuclear Medicine & PET/CT Centre, Head of Department of Molecular and Radiologic Imaging and Clinical Pathology, S. Maria della Misericordia Hospital, Rovigo, Italy

AUTHORS

R. KATHERINE ALPAUGH, PhD
Director, Protocol Support Laboratory, Department of Diagnostic Imaging, Fox Chase Cancer Center, Philadelphia, Pennsylvania, USA

SANDIP BASU, Diplomate N. B
Consultant Physician, Professor and Head, Nuclear Medicine Academic Programme, Radiation Medicine Centre, Bhabha Atomic Research Centre, Tata Memorial Hospital, Homi Bhabha National Institute, Mumbai, India

PRIYA R. BHOSALE, MD
Professor, Department of Diagnostic Radiology, Abdominal Imaging Section, The University of Texas MD Anderson Cancer Center, Houston, Texas, USA

SOTIRIOS CHONDROGIANNIS, MD
Service of Nuclear Medicine & PET/CT Centre, Department of Molecular and Radiologic Imaging and Clinical Pathology, Rovigo, Italy

CATHERINE DEVINE, MD
Associate Professor, Department of Diagnostic Radiology, Abdominal Imaging Section, The University of Texas MD Anderson Cancer Center, Houston, Texas, USA

MOHAN DOSS, PhD, MCCPM
Medical Physicist, Department of Diagnostic Imaging, Fox Chase Cancer Center, Philadelphia, Pennsylvania, USA

SILVANA FARIA, MD, PhD
Associate Professor, Department of Diagnostic
Radiology, Abdominal Imaging Section, The
University of Texas MD Anderson Cancer
Center, Houston, Texas, USA

WENDY F. GENESTINE, MD
Radiology Resident, NewYork-Presbyterian/
Columbia University Medical Center,
New York, New York, USA

PERRY W. GRIGSBY, MD
Department of Radiation Oncology,
Washington University School of Medicine in
St. Louis, St Louis, Missouri, USA

ELIZABETH M. HECHT, MD
Professor, Department of Radiology,
NewYork-Presbyterian/Columbia University
Medical Center, New York, New York, USA

REVATHY B. IYER, MD
Professor, Division of Diagnostic Imaging,
Department of Diagnostic Radiology, The
University of Texas MD Anderson Cancer
Center, Houston, Texas, USA

SANAZ JAVADI, MD
Assistant Professor, Department of Diagnostic
Radiology, Abdominal Imaging Section, The
University of Texas MD Anderson Cancer
Center, Houston, Texas, USA

ASHWINI KALSHETTY, Diplomate N. B
Consultant Physician, Assistant Professor and
SO-D, Radiation Medicine Centre, Bhabha
Atomic Research Centre, Tata Memorial
Hospital, Homi Bhabha National Institute,
Mumbai, India

BRINDA RAO KORIVI, MD, MPH
Assistant Professor, Department of Diagnostic
Radiology, Abdominal Imaging Section, The
University of Texas MD Anderson Cancer
Center, Houston, Texas, USA

RAKESH KUMAR, MD, PhD
Professor and Head, Department of Nuclear
Medicine, Diagnostic Nuclear Medicine
Division, All India Institute of Medical Sciences,
New Delhi, India

CHYONG-HUEY LAI, MD
Division of Gynecologic Oncology,
Department of Obstetrics and Gynecology,

Chang Gung Memorial Hospital, Chang Gung
University College of Medicine, Taoyuan,
Taiwan

SHERELLE L. LAIFER-NARIN, MD
Associate Professor of Radiology,
Director of Ultrasound and Fetal MRI,
NewYork-Presbyterian/Columbia
University Medical Center, New York,
New York, USA

GIGIN LIN, MD, PhD
Department of Medical Imaging and
Intervention, Chang Gung Memorial Hospital,
Chang Gung University College of Medicine,
Taoyuan, Taiwan

MARIA CRISTINA MARZOLA, MD
Service of Nuclear Medicine & PET/CT
Centre, Department of Molecular and
Radiologic Imaging and Clinical Pathology,
Rovigo, Italy

JEFFREY H. NEWHOUSE, MD
Professor of Radiology and Urology,
NewYork-Presbyterian/Columbia
University Medical Center, New York,
New York, USA

NANCY C. OKECHUKWU, MD
Advanced Body Imaging, Quantum Radiology,
Marietta, Georgia, USA

GIRISH KUMAR PARIDA, MD
Department of Nuclear Medicine,
All India Institute of Medical Sciences,
New Delhi, India

MADHAVI PATNANA, MD
Associate Professor, Division of Diagnostic
Imaging, Department of Diagnostic Radiology,
The University of Texas MD Anderson Cancer
Center, Houston, Texas, USA

YUAN JAMES RAO, MD
Department of Radiation Oncology,
Washington University School of Medicine in
St. Louis, St Louis, Missouri, USA

DOMENICO RUBELLO, MD
Head of Service of Nuclear Medicine & PET/CT
Centre, Head of Department of Molecular
and Radiologic Imaging and Clinical Pathology,
S. Maria della Misericordia Hospital, Rovigo,
Italy

TARA SAGEBIEL, MD
Assistant Professor, Division of Diagnostic
Imaging, Department of Diagnostic Radiology,
The University of Texas MD Anderson Cancer
Center, Houston, Texas, USA

SARTHAK TRIPATHY, MBBS
Department of Nuclear Medicine,
All India Institute of Medical Sciences,
New Delhi, India

CHITRA VISWANATHAN, MD
Associate Professor, Department of Diagnostic
Radiology, Abdominal Imaging Section, The
University of Texas MD Anderson Cancer
Center, Houston, Texas, USA

COURTNEY A. WOODFIELD, MD
Section Head, Body MR Imaging, Department
of Radiology, Abington – Jefferson Health,
Abington, Pennsylvania, USA

TZU-CHEN YEN, MD, PhD
Department of Nuclear Medicine,
Chang Gung Memorial Hospital,
Chang Gung University College of
Medicine, Taoyuan, Taiwan

JIAN Q. YU, MD, FRCPC
Chief, Nuclear Medicine and PET Service,
Department of Diagnostic Imaging,
Fox Chase Cancer Center, Philadelphia,
Pennsylvania, USA

Contents

^{18}F-fluorodeoxyglucose PET/CT as a dual-modality imaging plays a key role in the diagnosis, staging, response assessment, and disease surveillance. Uptake by tumor cells offers an opportunity to differentiate viable malignant cells from posttreatment effects. ^{18}F-fluorodeoxyglucose PET/CT-based criteria have been developed to evaluate treatment response. Uptake can reflect the biologic aggressiveness of the tumor, predicting the risk of metastasis and recurrence. The standardized uptake value can be measured as maximum, mean, or peak. Volumetric uptake measurements have shown substantial promise in providing accurate tumor assessment. We discuss these quantitative parameters in the assessment of gynecologic malignancies.

Molecular imaging (mainly PET and MR imaging) has played important roles in gynecologic oncology. Emerging MR-based technologies, including DWI, CEST, DCE–MR imaging, MRS, and DNP, as well as FDG-PET and many novel PET radiotracers, will continuously improve practices. In combination with radiomics analysis, a new era of decision making in personalized medicine and precisely guided radiation treatment planning or real-time surgical interventions is being entered into, which will have a direct impact on patient survival. Prospective trials with well-defined end points are encouraged to evaluate the multiple facets of these emerging imaging tools in the management of gynecologic malignancies.

PET CLINICS

THE CLINICS ARE AVAILABLE ONLINE!
Access your subscription at:
www.theclinics.com

PROGRAM OBJECTIVE

The goal of the *PET Clinics* is to keep practicing radiologists and radiology residents up to date with current clinical practice in positron emission tomography by providing timely articles reviewing the state of the art in patient care.

TARGET AUDIENCE

Practicing radiologists, radiology residents, and other health care professionals who provide patient care utilizing radiologic findings.

LEARNING OBJECTIVES

Upon completion of this activity, participants will be able to:
1. Review the roles of CT, MRI, and the utility of ultrasonography in gynecologic oncology.
2. Discuss emerging molecular imaging techniques in gynecologic oncology.
3. Recognize normal variants and pitfalls encountered in PET assessment of gynecologic malignancies.

ACCREDITATION

The Elsevier Office of Continuing Medical Education (EOCME) is accredited by the Accreditation Council for Continuing Medical Education (ACCME) to provide continuing medical education for physicians.

The EOCME designates this enduring material for a maximum of 15 *AMA PRA Category 1 Credit*(s)™. Physicians should claim only the credit commensurate with the extent of their participation in the activity.

All other health care professionals requesting continuing education credit for this enduring material will be issued a certificate of participation.

DISCLOSURE OF CONFLICTS OF INTEREST

The EOCME assesses conflict of interest with its instructors, faculty, planners, and other individuals who are in a position to control the content of CME activities. All relevant conflicts of interest that are identified are thoroughly vetted by EOCME for fair balance, scientific objectivity, and patient care recommendations. EOCME is committed to providing its learners with CME activities that promote improvements or quality in healthcare and not a specific proprietary business or a commercial interest.

The planning committee, staff, authors and editors listed below have identified no financial relationships or relationships to products or devices they or their spouse/life partner have with commercial interest related to the content of this CME activity:

Abass Alavi; R. Katherine Alpaugh, PhD; Sandip Basu, Diplomate N. B; Priya R. Bhosale, MD; Sotirios Chondrogiannis, MD; Catherine Devine, MD; Mohan Doss, PhD, MCCPM; Silvana Faria, MD, PhD; Wendy F. Genestine, MD; Perry W. Grigsby, MD; Elizabeth M. Hecht, MD; Revathy B. Iyer, MD; Sanaz Javadi, MD; Ashwini Kalshetty, Diplomate N. B; Alison Kemp; Brinda Rao Korivi, MD, MPH; Rakesh Kumar, MD, PhD; Chyong-Huey Lai, MD; Sherelle L. Laifer-Narin, MD; Gigin Lin, MD, PhD; Maria Cristina Marzola, MD; Jeffrey H. Newhouse, MD; Nancy C. Okechukwu, MD; Girish Kumar Parida, MD; Madhavi Patnana, MD; Yuan James Rao, MD; Domenico Rubello, MD; Tara Sagebiel, MD; Drew A. Torigian, MD, MA; Sarthak Tripathy, MBBS; John Vassallo; Rajakumar Venkatesan; Chitra Viswanathan, MD; Courtney A. Woodfield, MD; Tzu-Chen.Yen, MD, PhD; Jian Q. Yu, MD, FRCPC.

UNAPPROVED/OFF-LABEL USE DISCLOSURE

The EOCME requires CME faculty to disclose to the participants:
1. When products or procedures being discussed are off-label, unlabelled, experimental, and/or investigational (not US Food and Drug Administration [FDA] approved); and
2. Any limitations on the information presented, such as data that are preliminary or that represent ongoing research, interim analyses, and/or unsupported opinions. Faculty may discuss information about pharmaceutical agents that is outside of FDA-approved labelling. This information is intended solely for CME and is not intended to promote off-label use of these medications. If you have any questions, contact the medical affairs department of the manufacturer for the most recent prescribing information.

TO ENROLL

To enroll in the *PET Clinics* Continuing Medical Education program, call customer service at 1-800-654-2452 or sign up online at http://www.theclinics.com/home/cme. The CME program is available to subscribers for an additional annual fee of USD 235.

METHOD OF PARTICIPATION

In order to claim credit, participants must complete the following:
1. Complete enrolment as indicated above.
2. Read the activity.
3. Complete the CME Test and Evaluation. Participants must achieve a score of 70% on the test. All CME Tests and Evaluations must be completed online.

CME INQUIRIES/SPECIAL NEEDS

For all CME inquiries or special needs, please contact elsevierCME@elsevier.com.

Preface
Imaging in Gynecologic Oncology

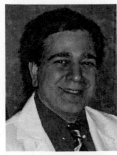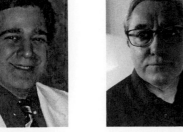

Drew A. Torigian, MD, MA   Domenico Rubello, MD

Editors

Gynecologic malignancies account for a significant proportion of disease-related morbidity and mortality in women throughout the world. Multimodality imaging, predominantly with PET, ultrasonography (US), computed tomography (CT), and MR imaging, plays an essential role in the diagnosis, staging, pretreatment planning, response assessment, and surveillance assessment of patients with such conditions. Therefore, in this issue of *PET Clinics*, we provide a series of state-of-the-art articles regarding the application of multimodality imaging to various gynecologic malignancies.

A review of the role of conventional imaging (namely US, CT, and MR imaging) in patients with gynecologic malignancies is initially provided in two articles, including reviews of the staging assessments for individual tumor types. The role of FDG-PET (including PET/CT and PET/MR imaging) for comprehensive assessment of patients with cervical cancer, ovarian cancer, and other gynecologic cancers (including endometrial cancer, vulvar cancer, vaginal cancer, and uterine sarcoma) is then discussed in three articles. Radiation therapy, which is an important therapeutic option in the management of gynecologic tumors, is discussed in the context of PET imaging. Subsequently, non-FDG-PET radiotracers that may add value for optimizing the management of patients with gynecologic tumors are reviewed. Importantly, PET assessment of gynecologic malignancies may be confounded by normal variants as well as other pitfalls, and so these are highlighted in order to minimize errors in clinical PET study interpretation.

Quantitative imaging is playing an increasingly significant role in the assessment of patients with various disease conditions, and so this important topic is discussed in the context of gynecologic oncology. Last, an article is provided that discusses some emerging molecular imaging techniques in gynecologic oncology, including new MR imaging–based technologies such as chemical exchange saturation transfer imaging and MR spectroscopy with dynamic nuclear polarization, as well as radiomics.

We would like to thank all of the authors who contributed articles to this issue of *PET Clinics*. It is our hope that readers of these articles will utilize the knowledge within to help ameliorate the suffering of women with gynecologic malignancies worldwide by optimizing personalized diagnosis and treatment through the use of multimodality imaging.

Drew A. Torigian, MD, MA
Department of Radiology
Hospital of the University of Pennsylvania
3400 Spruce Street
Philadelphia, PA 19104, USA

Domenico Rubello, MD
Department of Nuclear Medicine PET/CT Centre
S. Maria della Misericordia Hospital
Viale Tre Martiri, 140, 45100 RO, Italy

E-mail addresses:
Drew.Torigian@uphs.upenn.edu (D.A. Torigian)
domenico.rubello@libero.it (D. Rubello)

PET Clin 13 (2018) xiii
https://doi.org/10.1016/j.cpet.2018.01.001
1556-8598/18/© 2018 Published by Elsevier Inc.

pet.theclinics.com

The Role of Computed Tomography and Magnetic Resonance Imaging in Gynecologic Oncology

Sherelle L. Laifer-Narin, MD[a],*, Wendy F. Genestine, MD[a],
Nancy C. Okechukwu, MD[b], Elizabeth M. Hecht, MD[a],
Jeffrey H. Newhouse, MD[a]

KEYWORDS

- Gynecology • Malignancy • Computed tomography (CT) • Magnetic resonance (MR)
- International federation of gynecology and obstetrics (FIGO) classification system
- Endometrial • Cervical • Ovarian

KEY POINTS

- Gynecologic malignancies are staged by clinical, surgical, or histopathological criteria. The most current staging systems for the various gynecologic cancers are reviewed. This includes the new classification of extrauterine pelvic serous carcinoma, postulated to develop from serous tubal intraepithelial carcinomas.
- CT and MR imaging play a crucial role in the preoperative evaluation of the disease and surveillance of patient undergoing treatment. Strengths and weaknesses of CT and MR imaging for staging and monitoring therapy are discussed for the various gynecologic malignancies.
- Accuracy of disease staging is crucial, because this dictates treatment options, including surgical resection, chemotherapy, and/or radiation therapy.

IMAGING RECOMMENDATIONS AND GUIDELINES

Gynecologic malignancies are predominately staged by clinical, surgical, or histopathologic criteria. The American College of Radiology (ACR), National Comprehensive Cancer Network (NCCN), and International Federation of Gynecology and Obstetrics (FIGO) provide recommendations and guidelines on the role of imaging in gynecologic malignancies. CT and MR imaging also play critical roles in patient evaluation and surveillance.

Malignancy may initially be detected at CT for vague symptoms or incidentally, but more commonly CT is used for staging once the diagnosis is suspected. Ideally, CT should be performed with oral and intravenous contrast material during the venous phase of enhancement. Positive oral contrast material is useful for bowel wall implants and negative oral contrast material is useful for calcified tumor implants.[1] Peritoneal tumor implants less than 1 cm in size can be difficult to detect, particularly in the absence of ascites. When lymph nodes measure greater than 1 cm in short axis, or when there are morphologic changes, such as rounded shape or necrosis, tumor involvement is suspected. Disadvantages of CT include radiation exposure, adverse reactions

[a] Department of Radiology, Columbia University Medical Center, New York-Presbyterian Hospital, 622 West 168th Street, Ph1-317, New York, NY 10032, USA; [b] Advanced Body Imaging, Quantum Radiology, Marietta, GA, USA
* Corresponding author. 10 Sutton Place, Englewood, NJ 07631.
E-mail address: sll2122@cumc.columbia.edu

PET Clin 13 (2018) 127–141
https://doi.org/10.1016/j.cpet.2017.11.002

to iodinated contrast material, and lower soft tissue resolution compared with MR imaging.

MR imaging is often used for its superior soft tissue resolution and tissue characterization permitting better assessment of a primary tumor's extent and local invasion of adjacent structures. MR imaging of the abdomen is also helpful for detecting metastatic disease, especially if liver lesions on CT are indeterminate. For routine pelvic MR imaging protocols, it is recommended that patients fast for at least 4 hours prior to the examination to reduce motion artifact from bowel peristalsis, and antiperistaltic agents can also be used. MR imaging assessment of local invasion is best assessed in 2 perpendicular planes, the sagittal and transverse to the long axis of the uterus. Vaginal gel is useful for assessment of vaginal masses and cervical lesions. Additional MR imaging sequences serve as excellent problem-solving tools. Dynamic contrast-enhanced imaging is useful for the detection of hypervascular tumors. Chemical shift or fat-suppressed imaging sequences are ideal for the detection of fat within lesions. Fat-suppressed postcontrast T1-weighted images facilitate detection of peritoneal tumor implants. Diffusion-weighted imaging (DWI) is sensitive to water molecule motion at the cellular level.[2] Malignant tumors, for example, are more likely to demonstrate high signal intensity on high b-value (1000) DWI and appear dark on apparent diffusion coefficient (ADC) maps. DWI combined with dynamic contrast-enhanced MR imaging can improve tumor characterization and staging; assess for distant spread, including detection of subtle peritoneal disease; and assess tumor response and recurrence.[3] DWI and its corresponding ADC maps can improve tumor characterization and staging in patients with endometrial and cervical carcinoma but is less specific when differentiating between benign and malignant myometrial tumors and ovarian masses.[4] When patients are unable to receive intravenous gadolinium chelates due to renal dysfunction, DWI is of particular benefit. Despite its lack of ionizing radiation, disadvantages of MR imaging include its limited availability worldwide, higher cost, long image acquisition times leading to motion artifact, and decreased patient compliance and safety issues related to MR imaging unsafe or conditional devices.

ENDOMETRIAL CANCER
Introduction

Endometrial cancer is the most common gynecologic malignancy and the fourth most common malignancy in women in the United States. It primarily presents in the sixth to seventh decades as postmenopausal bleeding. Due to the early presentation in general, patients have a higher survival rate than that seen in other gynecologic malignancies. Currently, FIGO recommends surgical staging, although the guidelines continue to evolve.[5]

Endometrial carcinomas are subdivided into 2 groups. Type 1 includes grades 1 and 2 endometrioid carcinomas and comprises approximately 80% of endometrial carcinomas. Type 2 includes serous, clear cell, and mucinous carcinomas, carcinosarcoma, and grade 3 endometrioid carcinomas. Due to the poorer prognosis associated with type 2 carcinomas, the NCCN guidelines have separate treatment recommendations.[6] Specific risk factors affecting survival include myometrial invasion, cervical stromal involvement, lymphovascular space invasion, level of lymph node involvement, and distant spread.[7]

Staging and Treatment

Surgical staging currently includes total abdominal hysterectomy (TAH), bilateral salpingo-oophorectomy (BSO), peritoneal washings, and lymph node sampling. Routine lymph node sampling is highly controversial due to the high rate of complications and the surgical skill required. Level of lymph node involvement is especially important for prognosis and survival; therefore, imaging to preselect patients requiring lymph node dissection is helpful for surgical management. Although fewer than 5% of patients with less than 50% myometrial invasion have lymph node involvement, a much higher percentage of patients with greater than 50% myometrial invasion or lymphovascular invasion have lymph node involvement.[8]

For type I endometrial carcinomas, treatment typically includes TAH/BSO with optional radiation therapy confined to the uterus for stages I and II. In stages III and IV, resection plus systemic chemotherapy and/or radiation therapy is recommended. If there is cervical involvement, a radical hysterectomy plus BSO and radiation therapy is indicated. Type II endometrial carcinomas tend to be more aggressive, and therefore systemic chemotherapy is recommended in tumors as early as stage IB.

Imaging

For endometrial carcinoma, the ACR Appropriateness Criteria (ACRAC)[9] and NCCN strongly recommend pelvic MR imaging without and with intravenous contrast material to assess depth of myometrial invasion and tumor extent for treatment planning. In the evaluation of locally advanced disease, MR imaging with contrast is superior to contrast-enhanced CT, ultrasonography, and MR imaging without intravenous contrast. Pelvic CT with contrast may be performed if MR imaging cannot be obtained. CT without contrast is not recommended by the ACR. Both contrast-enhanced CT and MR imaging of the abdomen and pelvis are useful for lymph node evaluation. For high-grade tumors, CT of the chest is also recommended to evaluate for metastatic disease.[10]

Stages I to IIIB

MR imaging of the pelvis is preferred for evaluation of local extent of disease over CT or PET.[11–13] The American Joint Committee on Cancer (AJCC) separates stage 1 tumors into less than 50% or greater than or equal to 50% myometrial invasion (**Fig. 1**, **Table 1**). Stage 2 involves the cervical stroma, which widens the internal os. Stages 3A and 3B comprise local invasion of the serosa, adnexa, vagina, and parametrium. Accuracy of determining myometrial and cervical invasion increases with the addition of dynamic contrast imaging[14,15] and is best performed approximately 2 minutes to 4 minutes after administration of contrast. For patients unable to receive intravenous contrast material, DWI has demonstrated similar sensitivity and specificity to contrast-enhanced imaging in the detection of myometrial invasion.[16,17]

Stages IIIC to IV

To evaluate lymph node involvement and distant spread, MR imaging or CT of the abdomen with contrast is currently recommended for initial treatment planning and to help guide lymph node sampling. Pelvic, para-aortic, or inguinal lymph node involvement affects prognosis. Stage IIIC involves pelvic and para-aortic lymph nodes, and stage IV involves distant spread outside the true pelvis.

Table 1 Endometrial cancer	
FIGO Stage	**Description**
Stage I	Tumor confined to the corpus uteri
IA	<50% myometrial invasion
IB	≥50% myometrial invasion
Stage II	Cervical stroma invasion (DO NOT include endocervical mucosa or glandular elements)
Stage III	
IIIA	Involving serosa or adnexa
IIIB	Involving vagina or parametrium
IIIC1	Involving pelvic lymph nodes
IIIC2	Involving para-aortic lymph nodes
Stage IV	Distant metastases
IVA	Tumor invading bladder or bowel mucosa
IVB	Distant metastasis, including inguinal lymph nodes, intraperitoneal disease, lung, liver, or bone

DWI has similar accuracy to contrast-enhanced imaging for lymph node evaluation[18] (**Fig. 2**).

UTERINE SARCOMA
Introduction

Uterine sarcoma is a rare form of mesenchymal tumor and represents 2% to 3% of uterine cancers.[6] Because leiomyosarcomas can be difficult to distinguish from benign leiomyomas, diagnosis is typically made after hysterectomy. In the most recent AJCC guidelines, endometrial sarcomas are staged separately from endometrial carcinomas. Subtypes include leiomyosarcomas, endometrial stromal sarcoma (ESS), undifferentiated endometrial sarcoma (UES), and adenosarcoma. Leiomyosarcoma and UES are aggressive tumors with a poor prognosis (**Fig. 3**), whereas ESS and adenosarcoma are generally slow growing with a more favorable prognosis.[19]

Staging and Treatment

FIGO staging includes tumor size (greater or <5 cm) as well as local and distant spread (**Table 2**). Treatment of different sarcomas is divided between low-grade and high-grade sarcomas. In the low-grade tumors, hormonal therapy and radiation therapy is considered after surgical

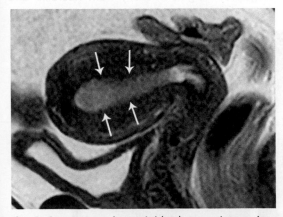

Fig. 1. Stage IA endometrioid adenocarcinoma in a 27-year-old woman with long-standing history of irregular menses. Sagittal T2-weighted image shows hypointense mass (*arrows*) distending the endometrial cavity with disruption of the junctional zone but with less than 50% myometrial invasion.

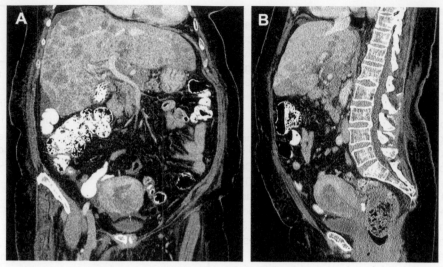

Fig. 2. Stage IVB uterine carcinosarcoma in a 77-year-old woman with abdominal pain and weakness. Coronal (*A*) and sagittal (*B*) contrast-enhanced CT images demonstrate a thickened, expanded endometrial cavity with infiltration of the anterior myometrium (*arrows*). There are multiple hypoenhancing hepatic metastases as well as ascites.

resection. For the high-grade tumors, including UES and leiomyosarcoma, systemic chemotherapy with or without radiation is thought to be better than hormonal therapy.

Imaging

CT or MR imaging of the abdomen and pelvis may be performed, although MR imaging is preferred for local extension or in patients with incidentally found tumors with incomplete resections after myomectomy or morcellation.[20] CT of the chest is also recommended given the frequency of thoracic metastases. For post-therapy monitoring,

CT of the chest, abdomen, and pelvis is recommended. MR imaging of the pelvis is most useful if local recurrence is suspected.

There are significant differences in imaging features among sarcoma subtypes, including tumor location, contour, and hemorrhagic, necrotic, or cystic components.[21] Unless there is extremely rapid growth or visible metastases, leiomyosarcomas are difficult to differentiate from leiomyomas with imaging. Leiomyosarcomas typically appear as infiltrating myometrial masses with irregular or ill-defined margins. On postcontrast imaging, there is peripheral enhancement with central heterogeneous signal intensity from necrosis and

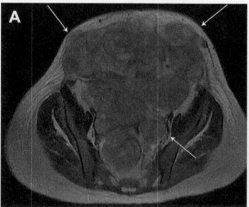
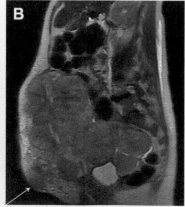

Fig. 3. Recurrent stage IVB leiomyosarcoma in a 32-year-old woman who underwent TAH 2 years ago. Large multilobulated, heterogeneously enhancing, aggressive mass (*arrows*) occupies the pelvis with extension into the anterior abdominal wall. Axial (*A*) and sagittal (*B*) T2-weighted MR images demonstrate tumoral involvement of the colon, bladder, small bowel, retroperitoneum, and pelvic vasculature.

Table 2
Uterine sarcoma

FIGO Stage	Description
Stage I	Tumor confined to the corpus uteri
IA	Tumor ≤5 cm
IB	Tumor >5 cm
Stage II	
IIA	Involves adnexa
IIB	Involves other pelvic tissues
Stage III	Involves abdominal tissues
IIIA	One site
IIIB	More than 1 site
Stage IV	
IVA	Invades bladder/rectum
IVB	Distant metastasis
Adenosarcoma	Stage I is different from other sarcomas
IA	Confined to endometrium/endocervix
IB	<50% myometrial invasion
IC	≥50% myometrial invasion

hemorrhage. ESS and UES more commonly appear as polypoid endometrial masses with wormlike bands of low T2-weighted signal intensity corresponding to regions of preserved myometrium.[8] They can also have more marginal nodularity due to their propensity for lymphovascular invasion. Adenosarcomas are mixed tumors, composed of benign and malignant components, and typically appear as complex, multiseptated, cystic, and solid polypoid endometrial masses. There is considerable overlap of ADC values between benign leiomyomas and sarcomas, which limits the usefulness of DWI; however, it should be used to help aid in diagnosis if patients are unable to receive contrast.[22]

CERVICAL CANCER
Introduction

Cervical cancer is the second most common gynecologic malignancy worldwide.[23] Its incidence and mortality rates have continued to decline in the United States since the introduction of the Papanicolaou test in the mid-twentieth century.[24] There has been no significant improvement, however, in the survival rates for patients who present with advanced disease.

The most common histologic type of cervical cancer is squamous cell carcinoma, which comprises approximately 80% to 90% of cases and arises from the squamocolumnar junction. Additional subtypes include adenocarcinoma, adenosquamous carcinoma, adenocystic carcinoma, small cell carcinoma, and lymphoma.[15,25] Cervical cancer spreads most commonly by direct invasion, followed by lymph node metastasis and rarely by hematogenous spread.

Staging and Treatment

Cervical cancer is staged clinically, using the FIGO classification system. Pretreatment planning with imaging is recommended but is not mandatory. Early-stage disease includes stages IA, IB1, and IIA1 and is usually treated surgically, either with radical hysterectomy or trachelectomy; the latter an option for patients seeking to preserve fertility. Bulky early-stage disease includes stages IB2 and IIA2, with tumors measuring more than 4 cm in size. Locally advanced disease includes stage IIB and higher. The treatment of bulky early-stage disease and locally advanced disease is radiation therapy and concurrent chemotherapy.[26]

MR imaging is the best modality for monitoring treatment response and evaluating for recurrent disease. In the early post-treatment time period, it may be difficult to distinguish residual tumor from post-treatment and inflammatory changes. Tumor recurrence often occurs in the cervix, vaginal cuff, parametrium, or pelvic sidewall. Recurrences in previously nonradiated fields may be treated with radiation therapy. Recurrence in a previously radiated field may require pelvic exenteration as salvage therapy.[25]

Imaging

Diagnostic imaging has not been formally integrated into the revised FIGO staging system, in part due to the limited accessibility of advanced imaging techniques in developing countries where cervical cancer is more prevalent.[15] Imaging is optional in patients with FIGO stage IB1 disease or lower. It is valuable, however, for important prognostic factors, such as tumor size, parametrial spread, and lymph node metastases (**Table 3**). For patients requiring preoperative planning, contrast-enhanced pelvic MR imaging is preferred. For FIGO stage II disease or higher, CT of the chest, abdomen, and pelvis is recommended to search for metastatic disease and contrast-enhanced pelvic MR imaging to assess for local tumor extent.[27]

On MR imaging, T2-weighted large field-of-view sequences as well as the small field-of-view sections obtained perpendicular to the endocervical canal are preferred to evaluate the primary tumor. Vaginal gel is recommended to allow for better evaluation of the vaginal fornices for local spread.

Table 3 Cervical cancer	
FIGO Stage	**Description**
Stage 0	Carcinoma in situ
Stage I	Tumor confined to cervical stroma
IA1	Microscopic invasion depth ≤3 mm and width ≤7 mm
IA2	Microscopic invasion depth 3–5 mm and ≤7 mm in width
IB	Clinically identified stromal tumor ≤4 cm (IB1) or >4 cm (IB2)
Stage II	Tumor extension to upper two-thirds of vagina
IIA	Without parametrial invasion ≤4 cm (IIA1) or >4 cm (IIA2)
IIB	With parametrial invasion
Stage III	Pelvic spread
IIIA	Extension to the lower one-third of vagina
IIIB	Pelvic wall invasion ± hydronephrosis
Stage IV	Distant spread
IVA	Involvement of bladder or rectal mucosa
IVB	Distant metastasis beyond the true pelvis

Contrast improves detection of small tumors, depth of stromal invasion, and bladder or rectal wall invasion.[28] DWI can also assist in tumor detection because cervical cancer normally exhibits lower ADC values than the normal cervix.[29]

Stages 0 to I

Stage I disease is confined to the cervix. Stage IA represents microinvasive disease and cannot be reliably detected with any imaging modality. Microinvasive tumor may appear as a focus of early enhancement on dynamic contrast-enhanced magnetic resonance sequences. Stage IB represents clinically visible tumor and is subdivided based on size greater or less than 4 cm (**Fig. 4**). Imaging with CT and MR imaging is optional in stage IB1 disease and lower but may be used to assess for distant metastatic disease or preoperative planning for fertility-preserving trachelectomy. Requirements for trachelectomy include a tumor smaller than 2 cm, cervical length greater than 2 cm, and tumor distance from the internal cervical os greater than 1 cm.

On MR imaging, the normal cervix has a trilaminar appearance on T2-weighted imaging with a high signal intensity endocervical mucosa, a low signal intensity fibromuscular stroma, and an intermediate signal intensity outer smooth muscle layer. Tumors appear intermediate to high in T2-weighted signal intensity relative to the hypointense middle stromal layer and have variable enhancement pattern on postcontrast sequences. On CT, cervical cancer may appear hypoattenuating or isoattenuating to the normal cervical stroma after the administration of intravenous contrast.[30]

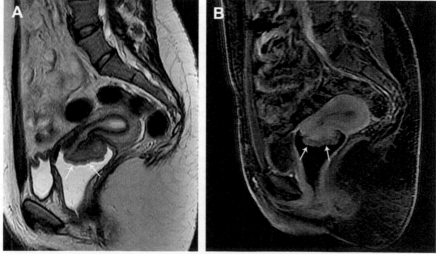

Fig. 4. Stage IB2 cervical squamous cell carcinoma in a 22-year-old woman with irregular vaginal bleeding. Sagittal T2-weighted (*A*) and T1-weighted postcontrast (*B*) images demonstrate an irregular enhancing 4.2 cm cervical mass (*arrows*), which extends into the posterior fornix of vagina (distended with high T2-weighted and low T1-weighted signal intensity gel).

Stage II

Stage II disease extends beyond the uterus but does not involve the pelvic sidewalls or the lower one-third of the vagina. Stage IIA disease extends into the upper two-thirds of the vagina and is subdivided by tumor size greater or less 4 cm. Parametrial invasion indicates stage IIB disease. MR imaging findings highly indicative of parametrial invasion include disruption of the low T2-weighted signal intensity inner cervical stromal ring and/or presence of nodular or irregular tumor extending into the parametrium. If the inner cervical stromal rim is thicker than 3 mm, parametrial invasion may be confidently excluded, a finding known as the hypointense rim sign. CT findings suggestive of parametrial invasion include encasement of the ureters and/or vasculature as well as thickening of the uterosacral ligaments. DWI with ADC sequences may be helpful to distinguish benign reactive changes or stromal edema from true tumor invasion (**Fig. 5**).

Stage III

Stage III disease includes invasion of the pelvic sidewall, lower one-third of the vagina, or associated hydronephrosis. In stage IIIA, the tumor extends to the lower one-third of the vagina. Stage IIIB disease involves extension to the pelvic sidewall or involvement of the ureters. Pelvic sidewall involvement is suggested when the tumor is within 3 mm of the pelvic sidewall musculature, by enlargement of the pelvic sidewall musculature with an enhancing soft tissue mass, and by encasement or narrowing of the iliac vasculature by tumor.

Stage IV

Stage IV disease includes invasion of the urinary bladder, rectum, or tumor extension beyond the true pelvis. Stage IVA is invasion of the bladder or rectum. Invasion is suggested by loss of the perivesical or perirectal fat plane, disruption of the normal muscle low T2-weighted signal intensity, asymmetric nodular wall thickening, intraluminal mass, or fistula. Stage IVB disease involves tumor extension beyond the pelvis.

Lymph node involvement

Lymph node metastasis is an important prognostic factor in cervical cancer staging because it is associated with a reduction in survival, but it is not currently included in the FIGO classification system. Cervical lymph nodes initially drain to the parametrial nodes and later spread to involve the external iliac, internal iliac, presacral, common iliac, and para-aortic lymph nodes. CT and MR imaging demonstrate greater than 90% specificity in the detection of lymph node metastasis but less than 60% sensitivity.[29] Surgical lymphadenectomy remains the standard for the diagnosis of lymph node metastasis. A short-axis diameter greater than 1 cm is the main imaging criterion used to identify abnormal lymph nodes. CT or MR imaging, however, cannot reliably detect micrometastases. Additional imaging features suggesting nodal metastasis include a rounded shape, irregular margins, clusters of multiple small lymph nodes, signal intensity similar to the primary tumor, and necrosis.

OVARIAN/FALLOPIAN TUBE/PRIMARY PERITONEAL CANCER
Introduction

Ovarian cancer represents 1% to 2% of all new cancer cases in the United States but is the fifth

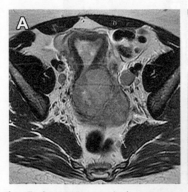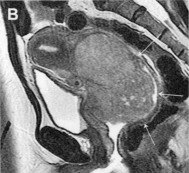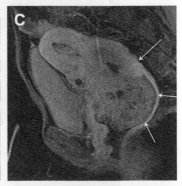

Fig. 5. Stage IIB cervical squamous cell carcinoma in a 60-year-old woman with postcoital bleeding. Axial T2-weighted (*A*) MR image shows a large enhancing cervical mass extending into the upper half of the vagina with loss of the low signal intensity inner cervical stroma consistent with left parametrial invasion (*arrows*). Also note presence of bilateral pelvic sidewall lymphadenopathy. Sagittal T2-weighted (*B*) and T1-weighted post-contrast (*C*) MR images demonstrate a large 9 cm enhancing cervical mass (*arrows*) extending into the upper vagina.

most common cause of death from cancer in women. It has the highest mortality rate of the gynecologic malignancies, which is often attributed to the advanced stage of disease at initial presentation.[31,32] Currently, the US Preventive Services Task Force does not recommend routine screening of asymptomatic women for ovarian cancer because transvaginal ultrasonography and serum cancer antigen 125 (CA-125) testing do not reduce mortality.[24,33] Although most ovarian cancers are sporadic, inherited familial syndromes, including BRCA1/2 genes and hereditary nonpolyposis colorectal cancer, increase risk and are the only reason for which annual transvaginal ultrasonography is recommended.[34]

Recent advances postulate that malignant cells derived from the epithelium of the fallopian tube fimbri, known as serous tubal intraepithelial carcinoma (STIC), are the precursor for the majority of high-grade serous carcinomas, primary peritoneal serous carcinomas, and primary fallopian tube carcinomas.[35,36] Ovarian serous carcinomas develop from STIC that implants on the ovarian surface, primary peritoneal serous carcinoma arises from spillage of STIC into the peritoneum, and fallopian tube carcinoma arises from STIC retained in the fallopian tube. Primary peritoneal serous carcinoma is indistinguishable from ovarian serous carcinoma both clinically and histopathologically, with the exception of relative lack of involvement of the ovaries[37] (**Fig. 6**). Ovarian tumors are classified into 3 major categories: epithelial-stromal tumors, sex cord–stromal tumors, and germ cell tumors. Most ovarian tumors are of epithelial origin and include serous, endometrioid, clear cell, transitional cell, mucinous, and carcinosarcomas. Ovarian cancer spreads most commonly by intraperitoneal dissemination, but also via lymph nodes, direct extension, and hematogenous spread.

Staging and Treatment

Advancements in the STIC theory led to the 2014 FIGO staging classification, which unified the staging of extrauterine pelvic serous carcinomas, that is, ovarian, primary fallopian, and primary peritoneal cancers.[38] Stage I disease no longer distinguishes between cancers of ovarian or fallopian tube origin whereas stage II disease now also includes primary peritoneal cancers. The standard treatment of ovarian cancer is primary cytoreductive surgery (tumor debulking) followed by adjuvant chemotherapy. Optimal cytoreduction, defined as removal of all tumors greater than 1 cm, is an important prognostic factor for patient survival.[39] When preoperative imaging suggests that optimal cytoreduction cannot be obtained, neoadjuvant chemotherapy followed by cytoreductive surgery is recommended. Adjuvant chemotherapy is recommended in all patients, except in those with stage IA-B disease.[40]

CT and MR imaging are both recommended in the evaluation of ovarian cancer recurrence, but accuracy is limited due to a combination of distortion from primary treatment and non-visualization of microscopic disease. Patients are monitored for recurrence with serial CA-125 levels. DWI can assist in distinguishing post-treatment changes from tumor recurrence.[3]

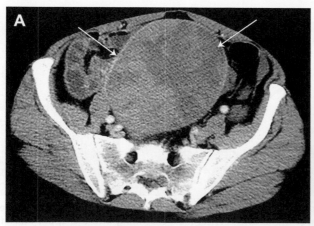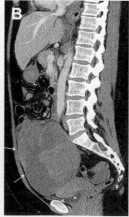

Fig. 6. Stage IC ovarian endometrioid adenocarcinoma in a 58-year-old woman who presented with shortness of breath and pulmonary emboli. Axial (*A*) and sagittal (*B*) contrast-enhanced CT images demonstrate a large, complex, heterogeneous adnexal mass (*arrows*). The uterus (*arrowheads*) appeared normal and there was no ascites. Tumor involved the right ovary with capsular rupture and surface adhesions but without tumor deposits.

Imaging

For ovarian cancer, NCCN guidelines recommend contrast-enhanced CT of the chest, abdomen, and pelvis or abdominal and pelvic MR imaging for initial work-up and surveillance. The ACRAC gives contrast-enhanced CT of the abdomen and pelvis the highest rating for both pretreatment staging and surveillance.[41]

Stage I

Although difficult to differentiate benign from malignant ovarian tumors by imaging, certain imaging findings are useful (**Table 4**). Wall irregularity or thickening greater than 3 mm, enhancing solid components, mural nodules, and papillary projections strongly suggest malignancy. Serous cystadenocarcinomas may contain microcalcifications. Serous cystadenomas are usually small and unilocular whereas mucinous cystadenomas are larger multilocular masses. Mucinous tumors demonstrate high attenuation on CT and heterogeneous signal intensity on T1-weighted and T2-weighted MR images resulting in a stained glass appearance.[12] Primary fallopian tube malignancies may appear as solid masses, mixed solid/cystic masses, or as papillary projections within dilated fallopian tubes, which enhance less than myometrium on CT and MR imaging. The appearance of a sausage-like adnexal mass with associated hydrosalpinx and intrauterine fluid is highly suggestive for fallopian tube malignancy.

Stages II to III

MR imaging with both dynamic contrast enhancement and DWI improves detection of pelvic and peritoneal tumor implants. Tumor may spread by direct invasion of adjacent pelvic structures. Findings suggestive of local spread include loss of fat planes between the tumor and adjacent pelvic structures, irregularity of the interface between the tumor and adjacent structures, less than 3-mm distance between the tumor and the pelvic sidewall, ureteral obstruction, and displacement/encasement of the iliac vessels.[1] MR imaging is superior to CT for identifying direct invasion. Imaging findings suggesting bowel involvement include bowel wall thickening and irregularity. Lymphatic metastasis to retroperitoneal, pelvic, and inguinal lymph nodes is possible. CT lacks accuracy in identifying metastatic lymph nodes because microscopic disease and reactive lymphadenopathy can confound findings (**Fig. 7**).

Peritoneal carcinomatosis manifests as peritoneal thickening and enhancement, peritoneal/omental/mesenteric nodularity, omental caking, and/or mesenteric infiltration. The presence of ascites should raise suspicion for peritoneal disease. Oral contrast material also may improve detection. CT has limited detection of peritoneal implants less than 1 cm, particularly in the absence of

Table 4
Ovarian/fallopian tube/primary peritoneal cancer

FIGO Stage	Description
Stage I	
IA	Tumor confined to 1 ovary or fallopian tube
IB	Tumor confined to both ovaries or fallopian tubes
IC	Tumor confined to 1 or both ovaries or fallopian tubes with surgical spill (IC1), capsule rupture (IC2), or tumor cells in peritoneal fluid/washings (IC3)
Stage II	Involves pelvic extension or implants
IIA	To uterus and/or fallopian tubes and/or ovaries
IIB	To other pelvic intraperitoneal tissues
Stage III	Involves extrapelvic peritoneal spread and/or retroperitoneal (pelvic and para-aortic) lymph node involvement
IIIA1	Retroperitoneal lymph nodes ≤10 mm (IIIA1i) or >10 mm (IIIA1ii)
IIIA2	Microscopic peritoneal involvement ± retroperitoneal nodes
IIIB	Macroscopic peritoneal metastasis ≤2 cm ± retroperitoneal nodes
IIIC	Macroscopic peritoneal metastasis >2 cm ± retroperitoneal nodes
IV	Distant spread
IVA	Pleural effusion
IVB	Parenchymal metastases, or metastases to inguinal nodes or other nodes outside of the abdomen or pelvis

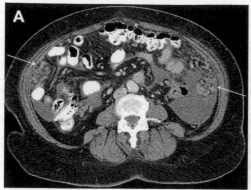
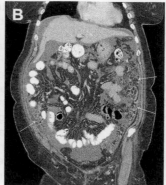
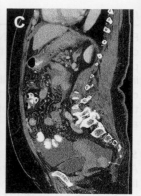

Fig. 7. Stage IIIC ovarian papillary serous adenocarcinoma in a 73-year-old woman with abdominal pain. Axial (*A*) and coronal (*B*) contrast-enhanced CT images demonstrate extensive peritoneal carcinomatosis (*arrows*) and ascites. Sagittal (*C*) contrast-enhanced CT image shows a large cul-de-sac nodule (*arrow*). Surgical exploration demonstrated tumoral involvement of the uterus, ovaries, peritoneum, omentum, lymph nodes, and bowel.

ascites. The normal route of peritoneal fluid circulation involves the dependent pelvis to the paracolic gutters and eventually to the diaphragms (**Fig. 8**).

Stage IV

Direct extension, transperitoneal, lymphatic, or hematogenous spread are possible routes of dissemination; the most common sites of involvement are the liver and lungs. Although cytologic evaluation is necessary to definitely confirm a malignant pleural effusion, presence of pleural thickening, nodularity, or masses suggests a malignant pleural effusion. Imaging is particularly helpful to differentiate capsular tumor implants from true parenchymal metastases because capsular tumor implants are considered resectable disease whereas parenchymal metastases are not resectable. Capsular tumor implants are well-defined, smooth-bordered,

and biconvex in appearance; parenchymal metastases are less well defined and are surrounded by organ parenchyma.[1]

Ovarian metastases

Metastatic disease to the ovary may be seen with gastrointestinal, genitourinary, lung, or breast primary malignancies. Additionally, lymphoma or leukemia may secondarily involve the ovaries. Krukenberg tumors by strict definition only refer to ovarian metastases with microscopic features of diffuse signet ring cell infiltration and are often bilateral.[42] Appearances of ovarian metastases vary according to the origin of the primary malignancy. Because an ovarian metastatic lesion may be confused with a primary tumor, accurate and timely diagnosis is essential for proper management and prognosis (**Fig. 9**).

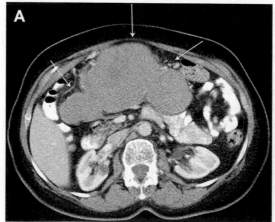
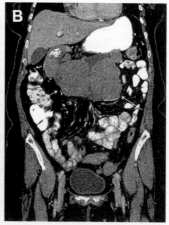

Fig. 8. Stage IIIC primary peritoneal carcinoma in a 77-year-old woman with left lower quadrant abdominal pain. Axial (*A*) and coronal (*B*) contrast-enhanced CT images demonstrate large, lobulated solid upper abdominal mass (*arrows*) exerting mass effect on the stomach, duodenum, and colon. There was tumoral involvement of stomach and mesentery, with normal ovaries, uterus, and colon and absence of disease in the lymph nodes.

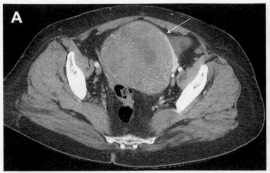
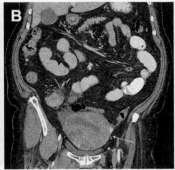
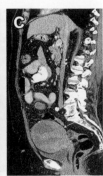

Fig. 9. Krukenberg tumor (metastatic colon adenocarcinoma) in a 73-year-old woman with remote past history of TAH and newly diagnosed colon cancer. Axial (*A*), coronal (*B*), and sagittal (*C*) contrast-enhanced CT images demonstrate a large heterogeneous complex pelvic mass (*arrows*). The left ovary was extensively replaced and enlarged by metastatic mucinous adenocarcinoma with signet ring cell features.

VULVAR CANCER

Vulvar cancers comprise approximately 5% of gynecologic malignancies, and more than 90% are squamous cell carcinomas. The most important prognostic factor is presence of nodal disease.[43–45] Treatment predominantly includes surgical resection with lymph node dissection. Radiation therapy is recommended for local spread combined with chemotherapy for lymph node or distant spread.[46] The pattern of growth of vulvar tumors is direct extension to adjacent organs, including the vagina, urethra, perineum, and/or anus. Inguinal and femoral lymph nodes are generally affected (**Table 5**). Physical examination is used for local staging. MR imaging is valuable for assessing regional disease, specifically degree of infiltration into surrounding tissues. CT is used for assessment of distant spread including pelvic lymph nodes, peritoneal carcinomatosis, and distant metastases. MR imaging is best performed with a pelvic coil to allow for a small field-of-view and thinner sections. This may help visualize the primary tumor, which is typically small. T2-weighted images are best for tumor size and local invasion; and contrast-enhanced imaging improves staging accuracy. T1-weighted images are helpful to assess the surrounding fat and lymph nodes.[47,48]

VAGINAL CANCER

Vaginal malignancies are extremely rare, comprising only 1% to 2% of all gynecologic malignancies.[49] Primary tumors are usually squamous cell carcinomas, but the majority of vaginal cancers have invaded from a primary tumor elsewhere within the pelvis, including endometrial, cervical, rectal, colon, ovarian, vulvar, and urinary tract cancers.[50] Given the rarity of primary vaginal malignancy, there has been little investigation of the role of imaging for guidance of management. A majority of recommendations have been extrapolated from cervical and anal cancers. MR imaging is superior to CT for evaluation of the primary lesion.[51] Either may be

Table 5 Vulvar cancer	
FIGO Stage	**Description**
Stage I	Tumor confined to vulva and/or perineum
IA	Lesion ≤2 cm with stromal invasion ≤1 mm
IB	Lesions >2 cm or with stromal invasion >1 mm
Stage II	Involving local pelvic structures: perineum, distal 1/3 urethra, distal 1/3 vagina, anus
Stage III	Involving inguinal or femoral lymph nodes
Stage IV	Distant spread
IVA	Involves upper 2/3 urethra, upper 2/3 vagina, bladder mucosa, rectal mucosa, or fixed to bone (IVAi) Fixed or ulcerated inguinal or femoral lymph nodes (IVAii)
IVB	Involves distant organs, including pelvic lymph nodes

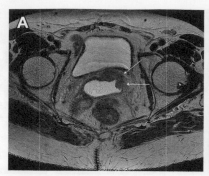

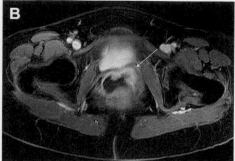

Fig. 10. Stage III vaginal squamous cell carcinoma in a 74-year-old woman with remote history of TAH/BSO for fibroids, now with vaginal bleeding. Axial T2-weighted (A) and T1-weighted postcontrast (B) MR images demonstrate thickened left anterolateral vaginal wall with extension into surrounding parametrium (arrows).

used for nodal evaluation.[52] The recommended imaging sequences are similar to those used for uterine carcinomas. Intravenous contrast material is of limited use in patients whose vaginal mucosa has been inflamed by chemotherapy or radiation therapy. The typical morphologic patterns seen on MR imaging include ulcerating, fungating, and annular constrictive types. In primary malignancies, the tumor is typically low in signal intensity on T1-weighted images and intermediate in signal intensity on T2-weighted images (**Fig. 10**). If high in T2-signal intensity, the tumor may be poorly differentiated or an alternative diagnosis, including metastatic disease, should be considered. The role of DWI in primary vaginal tumors has not been explored, but DWI has been shown helpful in detecting vaginal recurrence in other gynecologic malignancies.

Further study is needed to ascertain the role of DWI in primary vaginal cancers.

MUCOSAL MELANOMA

Melanoma of the reproductive organs comprises less than 1% of all gynecologic malignancies and may involve the vulva, vagina, or cervix. There are no AJCC guidelines for mucosal melanomas.[53] Multiple different staging systems have been proposed, and currently AJCC's cutaneous melanoma guidelines using the Breslow method are suggested for staging.[54,55] Pelvic MR imaging is recommended for local staging and surgical planning. Melanoma typically appears high in signal intensity on T1-weighted images due to the paramagnetic effect of melanin and low to intermediate in signal intensity on T2-weighted images[56] (**Fig. 11**).

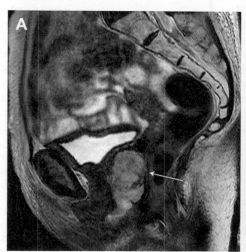

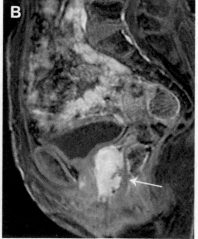

Fig. 11. Vaginal melanoma in a 79-year-old woman with intermittent vaginal bleeding. Sagittal T2-weighted (A) and T1-weighted postcontrast (B) MR images demonstrate an avidly enhancing vaginal mass extending from the external cervical os to the introitus, consistent with melanoma (arrows).

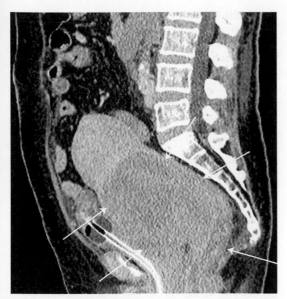

Fig. 12. Cervical lymphoma in a 70-year-old woman with urinary tract obstruction. Sagittal contrast-enhanced CT image shows a marked expansile cervical mass (*arrows*) inseparable from bladder, urethra, and rectum resulting in bilateral hydroureteronephrosis. Note Foley catheter within the decompressed urinary bladder more anteriorly. Pathology demonstrated atypical B-cell lymphocytic proliferation with extensive necrosis, consistent with a lymphoid neoplasm. The patient was subsequently diagnosed with systemic diffuse large B-cell lymphoma.

LYMPHOMA

Primary uterine lymphoma is rare, with involvement of the myometrium and preservation of the endometrium, with primary cervical lymphoma an even more uncommon occurrence. More often, there is secondary involvement of the female genital tract localized to the ovaries, uterus, and fallopian tubes, with established primary extrauterine disease elsewhere (**Fig. 12**).

GESTATIONAL TROPHOBLASTIC NEOPLASM
Introduction

Gestational trophoblastic neoplasms (GTNs) encompass a spectrum of diseases, including hydatidiform mole, invasive mole, choriocarcinoma, placental site trophoblastic tumors, and epithelioid trophoblastic tumors. GTNs develop due to aberrant fertilization of an empty ovum with 2 sperm (complete mole) or a normal ovum with 2 sperm (partial mole) and have varying malignant potential.

Staging and Treatment

Approximately 80% to 85% of molar pregnancies are benign, 15% to 20% develop locally invasive disease, and 3% to 5% develop metastatic disease. The initial evaluation for suspected GTNs includes beta human chorionic gonadotropin (β-hCG) levels, transvaginal ultrasonography, and chest radiography. Treatment of local disease is suction and curettage, and chemotherapy is administered for invasive and metastatic disease. β-hCG is used as a tumor marker for surveillance and recurrence. Hysterectomy may be indicated for recurrent or persistent disease.

Imaging

Complete moles lack an embryo and demonstrate a heterogeneous, expansile endometrial mass containing numerous cystic spaces, which represent diffusely hyperplastic and hydropic villi. A partial mole is associated with a triploid fetus, which may appear anomalous, growth-restricted, or nonviable. The ovaries may be large and multicystic due to the presence of theca lutein cysts. Contrast-enhanced MR imaging can depict tumor invasion into the myometrium and extension to the parametrium, adnexa, and vagina (**Fig. 13**). CT of the abdomen and pelvis and brain MR imaging depict distant metastatic disease.[57,58]

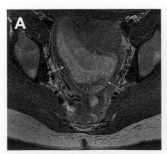
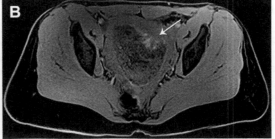

Fig. 13. Invasive molar pregnancy in a 23-year-old woman G1P0 with β-hCG greater than 300,000. Axial T2-weighted (*A*) MR image demonstrates a large mass with multiple tiny cystic lesions expanding the endometrial cavity (*arrows*) consistent with a hydatidiform mole. Axial T1-weighted postcontrast (*B*) MR image demonstrates penetration of tumor into the anterior myometrium (*arrow*).

REFERENCES

1. Woodward PJ, Hosseinzadeh K, Saenger JS. From the archives of the AFIP: radiologic staging of ovarian carcinoma with pathologic correlation. Radiographics 2004;24:225–46.

2. Kyriazi S, Collins DJ, Morgan VA, et al. Diffusion-weighted imaging of peritoneal disease for noninvasive staging of advanced ovarian cancer. Radiographics 2010;30:1269–85.

3. Fischerova D, Burgetova A. Imaging techniques for the evaluation of ovarian cancer. Best Pract Res Clin Obstet Gynaecol 2014;28:697–720.

4. Levy A, Medjhoul A, Caramella C, et al. Interest of diffusion-weighted echo-planar MR imaging and apparent diffusion coefficient mapping in gynecological malignancies: a review. J Magn Reson Imaging 2011;33:1020–7.

5. Creasman W. Revised FIGO staging for carcinoma of the endometrium. Int J Gynaecol Obstet 2009; 105:109.

6. National Comprehensive Cancer Network. Uterine neoplasms (version 1.2017). 2017. Available at: https://www.nccn.org/professionals/physician_gls/pdf/uterine.pdf. Accessed December18, 2017.

7. Erickson BA, Olawaiye AB, Bermudez A, et al. AJCC Cancer Staging Manual: Cervix Uteri. New York: Springer; 2017.

8. Leursen G, Gardner CS, Sagebiel T, et al. Magnetic resonance imaging of benign and malignant uterine neoplasms. Semin Ultrasound CT MR 2015;36:348–60.

9. Lalwani N, Dubinsky T, Javitt MC, et al. ACR appropriateness criteria® pretreatment evaluation and follow-up of endometrial cancer. Ultrasound Q 2014;30:21–8.

10. Haldorsen IS, Salvesen HB. What is the best preoperative imaging for endometrial cancer? Curr Oncol Rep 2016;18:25.

11. Kinkel K, Kaji Y, Yu KK, et al. Radiologic staging in patients with endometrial cancer: a meta-analysis. Radiology 1999;212:711–8.

12. Grossman J, Ricci ZJ, Rozenblit A, et al. Efficacy of contrast-enhanced CT in assessing the endometrium. AJR Am J Roentgenol 2008;191:664–9.

13. Park JY, Kim EN, Kim DY, et al. Comparison of the validity of magnetic resonance imaging and positron emission tomography/computed tomography in the preoperative evaluation of patients with uterine corpus cancer. Gynecol Oncol 2008;108:486–92.

14. Haldorsen IS, Salvesen HB. Staging of endometrial carcinomas with MRI using traditional and novel MRI techniques. Clin Radiol 2012;67:2–12.

15. Freeman SJ, Aly AM, Kataoka MY, et al. The revised FIGO staging system for uterine malignancies: implications for MR imaging. Radiographics 2012;32:1805–27.

16. Beddy P, Moyle P, Kataoka M, et al. Evaluation of depth of myometrial invasion and overall staging in endometrial cancer: comparison of diffusion-weighted and dynamic contrast-enhanced MR imaging. Radiology 2012;262:530–7.

17. Das SK, Niu XK, Wang JL, et al. Usefulness of DWI in preoperative assessment of deep myometrial invasion in patients with endometrial carcinoma: a systematic review and meta-analysis. Cancer Imaging 2014;14:32.

18. Rechichi G, Galimberti S, Oriani M, et al. ADC maps in the prediction of pelvic lymph nodal metastatic regions in endometrial cancer. Eur Radiol 2013;23:65–74.

19. Santos P, Cunha TM. Uterine sarcomas: clinical presentation and MRI features. Diagn Interv Radiol 2015;21:4–9.

20. Dizon DS, Olawaiye AB, Brookland RK, et al. AJCC Cancer Staging Manual: Corpus Uteri - Sarcoma. New York: Springer; 2017.

21. Sumi A, Terasaki H, Sanada S, et al. Assessment of MR imaging as a tool to differentiate between the major histological types of uterine sarcomas. Magn Reson Med Sci 2015;14:295–304.

22. Lin G, Yang LY, Huang YT, et al. Comparison of the diagnostic accuracy of contrast-enhanced MRI and diffusion-weighted MRI in the differentiation between uterine leiomyosarcoma/smooth muscle tumor with uncertain malignant potential and benign leiomyoma. J Magn Reson Imaging 2016;43:333–42.

23. Bourgioti C, Chatoupis K, Moulopoulos LA. Current imaging strategies for the evaluation of uterine cervical cancer. World J Radiol 2016;8:342–54.

24. Smith RA, Andrews KS, Brooks D, et al. Cancer screening in the United States, 2017: a review of current American Cancer Society guidelines and current issues in cancer screening. CA Cancer J Clin 2017;67:100–21.

25. Devine C, Gardner C, Sagebiel T, et al. Magnetic resonance imaging in the diagnosis, staging, and surveillance of cervical carcinoma. Semin Ultrasound CT MR 2015;36:361–8.

26. National Comprehensive Cancer Network. Cervical cancer (version 1.2017). 2017.Available at: https://www.nccn.org/professionals/physician_gls/pdf/cervical.pdf. Accessed December 18, 2017.

27. Siegel CL, Andreotti RF, Cardenes HR, et al. ACR appropriateness criteria® pretreatment planning of invasive cancer of the cervix. J Am Coll Radiol 2012;9:395–402.

28. Nicolet V, Carignan L, Bourdon F, et al. MR imaging of cervical carcinoma: a practical staging approach. Radiographics 2000;20:1539–49.

29. Liu B, Gao S, Li S. A comprehensive comparison of CT, MRI, positron emission tomography or positron emission tomography/CT, and diffusion weighted

imaging-MRI for detecting the lymph nodes metastases in patients with cervical cancer: a meta-analysis based on 67 studies. Gynecol Obstet Invest 2017;82:209–22.

30. Pannu HK, Corl FM, Fishman EK. CT evaluation of cervical cancer: spectrum of disease. Radiographics 2001;21:1155–68.

31. Togashi K. Ovarian cancer: the clinical role of US, CT, and MRI. Eur Radiol 2003;13(Suppl 4):L87–104.

32. Nougaret S, Addley HC, Colombo PE, et al. Ovarian carcinomatosis: how the radiologist can help plan the surgical approach. Radiographics 2012;32: 1775–800 [discussion: 1800–3].

33. Moyer VA, U.S. Preventive Services Task Force. Screening for ovarian cancer: U.S. Preventive Services Task Force reaffirmation recommendation statement. Ann Intern Med 2012;157:900–4.

34. Javadi S, Ganeshan DM, Qayyum A, et al. Ovarian cancer, the revised FIGO Staging system, and the role of imaging. AJR Am J Roentgenol 2016;206: 1351–60.

35. Saida T, Tanaka YO, Matsumoto K, et al. Revised FIGO staging system for cancer of the ovary, fallopian tube, and peritoneum: important implications for radiologists. Jpn J Radiol 2016;34: 117–24.

36. Katabathina VS, Amanullah FS, Menias CO, et al. Extrauterine pelvic serous carcinomas: current update on pathology and cross-sectional imaging findings. Radiographics 2016;36:918–32.

37. Tanaka YO, Okada S, Satoh T, et al. Differentiation of epithelial ovarian cancer subtypes by use of imaging and clinical data: a detailed analysis. Cancer Imaging 2016;16:3.

38. Prat J, Olawaiye AB, Bermudez A, et al. AJCC Cancer Staging Manual: Ovary, Fallopian Tube, and Primary Peritoneal Carcinoma. New York: Springer; 2017.

39. Zeppernick F, Meinhold-Heerlein I. The new FIGO staging system for ovarian, fallopian tube, and primary peritoneal cancer. Arch Gynecol Obstet 2014;290:839–42.

40. National Comprehensive Cancer Network. Ovarian cancer including fallopian tube cancer and primary peritoneal cancer (Verison 1.2017). 2017.Available at: https://www.nccn.org/professionals/physician_gls/pdf/ovarian.pdf. Accessed December 18, 2017.

41. Mitchell DG, Javitt MC, Glanc P, et al. ACR appropriateness criteria staging and follow-up of ovarian cancer. J Am Coll Radiol 2013;10: 822–7.

42. Koyama T, Mikami Y, Saga T, et al. Secondary ovarian tumors: spectrum of CT and MR features with pathologic correlation. Abdom Imaging 2007; 32:784–95.

43. Homesley HD, Bundy BN, Sedlis A, et al. Prognostic factors for groin node metastasis in squamous cell carcinoma of the vulva (a Gynecologic Oncology Group study). Gynecol Oncol 1993;49: 279–83.

44. Burger MP, Hollema H, Emanuels AG, et al. The importance of the groin node status for the survival of T1 and T2 vulval carcinoma patients. Gynecol Oncol 1995;57:327–34.

45. Gibb RK, Olawaiye AB, Chen L, et al. AJCC Cancer Staging Manual: Vulva. New York: Springer; 2017.

46. National Comprehensive Cancer Network. Vulvar cancer (squamous cell carcinoma) (version 1.2017). 2017.Available at: https://www.nccn.org/professionals/physician_gls/pdf/vulvar.pdf. Accessed December 18, 2017.

47. Sohaib SA, Richards PS, Ind T, et al. MR imaging of carcinoma of the vulva. AJR Am J Roentgenol 2002; 178:373–7.

48. Kataoka MY, Sala E, Baldwin P, et al. The accuracy of magnetic resonance imaging in staging of vulvar cancer: a retrospective multi-centre study. Gynecol Oncol 2010;117:82–7.

49. Gibb RK, Olawaiye AB, Chen L, et al. AJCC Cancer Staging Manual: Vagina. New York: Springer; 2017.

50. Grant LA, Sala E, Griffin N. Congenital and acquired conditions of the vulva and vagina on magnetic resonance imaging: a pictorial review. Semin Ultrasound CT MR 2010;31:347–62.

51. Kim KW, Shinagare AB, Krajewski KM, et al. Update on imaging of vulvar squamous cell carcinoma. AJR Am J Roentgenol 2013;201:W147–57.

52. Parikh JH, Barton DP, Ind TE, et al. MR imaging features of vaginal malignancies. Radiographics 2008; 28:49–63 [quiz: 322].

53. Mihajlovic M, Vlajkovic S, Jovanovic P, et al. Primary mucosal melanomas: a comprehensive review. Int J Clin Exp Pathol 2012;5:739–53.

54. Breslow A. Thickness, cross-sectional areas and depth of invasion in the prognosis of cutaneous melanoma. Ann Surg 1970;172:902–8.

55. Piura B. Management of primary melanoma of the female urogenital tract. Lancet Oncol 2008;9:973–81.

56. Leitao MM Jr, Cheng X, Hamilton AL, et al. Gynecologic Cancer InterGroup (GCIG) consensus review for vulvovaginal melanomas. Int J Gynecol Cancer 2014;24:S117–22.

57. Micco M, Sala E, Lakhman Y, et al. Imaging features of uncommon gynecologic cancers. AJR Am J Roentgenol 2015;205:1346–59.

58. Goldstein DP, Berkowitz RS. Current management of gestational trophoblastic neoplasia. Hematol Oncol Clin North Am 2012;26:111–31.

The Usefulness of Ultrasound Imaging in Gynecologic Oncology

Courtney A. Woodfield, MD

KEYWORDS

- Pelvic ultrasound • Uterine sarcoma • Endometrial carcinoma • Cervical carcinoma
- Ovarian carcinoma • Fallopian tube carcinoma • Gestational trophoblastic disease

KEY POINTS

- Ultrasound examination is the primary imaging modality for evaluating pelvic symptomatology in female patients, and is often the first study to detect a gynecologic neoplasm.
- Myometrial masses are readily visualized and monitored, but there is imaging overlap in the appearance of large, degenerated benign leiomyomas and more aggressive leiomyoma variants and uterine sarcomas.
- The thickness and appearance of the endometrium is readily amenable to evaluation by transvaginal ultrasound imaging.
- Ovarian cysts are routinely encountered on pelvic ultrasound examination; many cysts can be fully characterized and managed based predominantly on their sonographic appearance.
- Gestational trophoblastic disease encompasses a spectrum of placental origin tumors with a variety of manifestations at pelvic ultrasound examination.

INTRODUCTION

Pelvic ultrasound (US) examination is the primary imaging modality for evaluating female patients with a wide range of pelvic symptomatology including abnormal vaginal bleeding, endocrine abnormalities, pelvic pain, pelvic infection, and pelvic masses. US imaging can identify the primary site of origin for a wide range of pelvic pathologies, and in many cases render a specific diagnosis that immediately directs patient management. Included in this role of pelvic US examination as a first-line gynecologic imaging modality is the ability to detect or suggest the presence of a gynecologic neoplasm. Familiarity with the varied sonographic appearance of gynecologic neoplasms and potential neoplasm mimics facilitates the timely diagnosis and management of patients. This article reviews the US appearance of gynecologic neoplasms grouped by anatomic site of origin, the US appearance of select benign pelvic pathology not to be misinterpreted as malignancy, as well as available US-based guidelines for managing potential gynecologic neoplasms.

IMAGING TECHNIQUE AND NORMAL ANATOMY

Imaging Technique

Pelvic US examination to evaluate the uterus, ovaries, and adnexa is routinely performed using a combination of transabdominal (TA) and transvaginal (TV) imaging approaches (**Table 1**). As an imaging modality in general, US examination has the

Disclosure Statement: The author has no disclosures. The author has no relationship with a commercial company that has a direct financial interest in subject matter or materials discussed in article or with a company making a competing product.
Body MR Imaging, Department of Radiology, Abington Hospital, Jefferson Health, 1200 Old York Road, Abington, PA 19001, USA
E-mail address: Courtney.woodfield@jefferson.edu

PET Clin 13 (2018) 143–163
https://doi.org/10.1016/j.cpet.2017.11.003
1556-8598/18/

Table 1
Components of the female pelvis ultrasound examination

Component	Purpose
Transabdominal imaging	Pelvic overview; screen for large masses and free fluid
Transvaginal imaging	Close visualization of the uterus, ovaries, and adnexa
Gray-scale imaging	Differentiate normal anatomy and pathology; assess cystic vs solid nature and complexity
Color and spectral Doppler imaging	Detect and differentiate true vascularity and solid elements in structures
Sonohysterography	Detect and localize endometrial lesions

advantages of being widely available, portable, free of ionizing radiation, not requiring the use of oral or intravenous contrast material, and being relatively inexpensive. Limitations inherent to US imaging include a relatively small field of view, reliance on operator performance and experience, dependence on the patient's body habitus and mobility, and the presence of overlying structures, such as an air-filled bowel, which may obscure anatomy and pathology. Patient information that should be available at the time of performing and interpreting pelvic US examinations includes the examination indication, any relevant laboratory test results such as serum cancer antigen 125 level or serum β-human chorionic gonadotropin (β-hCG) level, date of last menstrual period, any prior pelvic surgeries, and any hormonal replacement therapy.

Gray scale ultrasound imaging

A complete US examination of the female pelvis usually begins with TA imaging to obtain an overall view of the pelvis, and to screen for and evaluate larger pelvic masses and free fluid that might otherwise be overlooked or incompletely evaluated on smaller field of view TV imaging. TA imaging is typically performed with a 2.5- to 5.0-MHz transducer and a full bladder. A full bladder serves as an acoustic window to the pelvic organs and can help to displace potentially overlying bowel out of the pelvis. After emptying the bladder, TV imaging is then performed with a higher frequency transducer (5–8 MHz) that has a smaller

field of view, but allows for closer and higher resolution visualization of the uterus, ovaries, and adnexa.[1] In cases where TV imaging cannot be performed owing to patient preference or contraindications, that is, premenarchal, a transperineal US approach may be used to further visualize the vaginal canal and cervix. Many US machines are also now equipped with 3-dimensional software that can further demonstrate the overall size and orientation of pelvic anatomy and pathology. Other US techniques under investigation for use in pelvic imaging include US elastography, contrast-enhanced US, and specialized transcervical US transducers.[2–5]

Spectral Doppler ultrasound imaging

Color and power spectral Doppler imaging techniques are routinely used during a pelvic US examination to evaluate both anatomic and pathologic vascularity. Color and power Doppler imaging are especially useful for detecting and confirming solid components and vascularity in pelvic pathology and structures. Spectral Doppler interrogation of apparent areas of power and color Doppler vascularity helps to further differentiate true vascularity from artifactual color flashes of random motion. The use of a spectral Doppler pulsatility index (peak systolic velocity – end diastolic velocity/mean velocity) or resistive index ([peak systolic velocity – end diastolic velocity]/peak systolic velocity) as a means of differentiating between benign and malignant vascularity in ovarian and adnexal pathology is not currently in widespread used owing to overlap in the index values for both benign and malignant masses.[6] Originally, detection of lower resistance, higher diastolic vascular flow in a mass was thought to be more indicative of malignant neovascularity than benign vascularity.[7,8] More helpful than a discriminatory vascularity index may be the subjective assessment and location of vascularity in a mass, with greater overall vascularity and more central vascularity being more suspect for malignancy than minimal or peripheral vascularity.[9]

Sonohysterography

Saline-infused sonohysterography (SIS) is a specialized pelvic US examination that can be performed to further evaluate the endometrium for pathology following a routine pelvic US examination. In particular, it can detect focal endometrial pathology such as polyps, focal hyperplasia, and polypoid carcinomas that might otherwise be occult with routine TV imaging or missed with random endometrial biopsies. SIS involves placement of a thin (5 or 7 Fr) catheter into the endometrial cavity, catheter retraction to the level of the internal cervical os, and saline balloon inflation to secure the catheter. Sterile saline is then hand injected through the catheter to distend the endometrial cavity and reveal the presence, size, and location of potential endometrial masses. The ideal timing of a SIS examination is between days 7 and 10 of the menstrual cycle to image the endometrium at its thinnest level and to avoid complicating a potential early pregnancy. Contraindications to SIS include pregnancy and active pelvic inflammatory disease.[10]

Normal Anatomy

Uterus

The uterus is composed of 2 major portions, the uterine body (corpus) and cervix, and is most commonly anteverted and anteflexed. The size of the adult uterus is variable, depending on both parity and menopausal status. The average nulliparous adult uterus is 6.0 to 8.5 cm longitudinal × 2.0 to 4.0 cm anterior posterior × 3.0 to 5.0 cm transverse in size, including the length of the cervix, which is normally 2.5 to 3.0 cm.[11] Uterine size then increases by approximately 1 cm in each direction with increasing parity. The approximate ratio of the uterine body (corpus) length to cervical length is 1:1 for the adult nulliparous uterus, 2:1 for the adult multiparous uterus, and 1:1 for the postmenopausal uterus.[12]

On US examination, the myometrium is normally homogeneously low to intermediate in echogenicity with a thinner, more hypoechoic and hypovascular layer immediately surrounding the endometrium, corresponding with the junctional zone. In postmenopausal women, a peripheral rim of increased echogenicity may also be seen in the myometrium corresponding to calcified arcuate vessels.[13]

The US appearance and thickness of the normal endometrium varies throughout the menstrual cycle. As imaged and measured in the midsagittal plane on TVUS, during the menstrual phase, the endometrium is a thin, 1- to 4-mm, echogenic line. During the subsequent proliferative phase, the endometrium remains echogenic and gradually increases to 4 to 8 mm in thickness. At the time of midcycle ovulation, the endometrium has a trilaminar appearance composed of a central thin echogenic line surrounded by middle hypoechoic layers and outer thin echogenic layers, with an overall thickness of 6 to 10 mm (**Fig. 1**). During the late secretory phase, the endometrium again becomes more uniformly echogenic and thickens up to a maximal diameter of 16 mm. The postmenopausal endometrium is normally a thin echogenic line by US examination, typically measuring less than 5 mm in thickness.[14] A small amount of

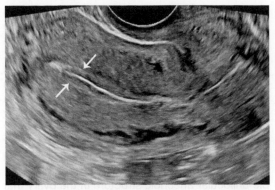

Fig. 1. Normal midcycle endometrium. Gray-scale sagittal transvaginal ultrasound image of the uterus shows the characteristic trilaminar appearance of the endometrium (*arrows*) at the time of midcycle ovulation.

simple anechoic fluid may be seen in the endometrial cavity by US examination, in which case the endometrial thickness is determined by separating, measuring, and adding together the thickness of the 2 individual endometrial walls.

The normal cervix has a layered ultrasonographic appearance consisting of a thin central echogenic line, representing the collapsed endocervical canal, surrounded by a variable hypoechoic, 2- to 4-mm thick, submucosal layer, and a more uniformly hypoechoic outer stromal layer with echogenicity similar to the myometrium. A small amount of anechoic to hypoechoic fluid may distend the endocervical canal during the periovulatory period. In some cases, the serpentine endocervical folds or mucosal serrations of the cervix may be visible by US examination. On color or power Doppler US examination, the normal cervix has little or no vascularity.[15]

Ovary

The size and appearance of the normal adult ovary by US examination also varies with both patient age and the phase of the menstrual cycle. The normal premenopausal adult ovary has an average volume of 9 mL, but can be as large as 22 mL. The postmenopausal ovary then decreases in size to a mean volume of 2 to 3 mL by US examination.[16] The premenopausal adult ovary has a central slightly echogenic medulla and multiple, subcentimeter, peripheral anechoic follicles that vary in size with patient age and the menstrual cycle. During the early proliferative phase, these subcentimeter follicles form and increase in size through days 8 to 9, at which time a dominant follicle develops and reaches a maximum size of typically 2.0 to 2.5 cm. Just before ovulation, a thin peripheral circular echogenic structure may be seen in the dominant follicle, the cumulus oophorus, which is a cellular layer encompassing the unreleased ovum within the dominant follicle (**Fig. 2**). After ovulation, the dominant follicle becomes the corpus luteum, developing a thicker, more vascularized, and crenulated appearing wall as well as internal echoes. If ovulation does not occur, the dominant follicle persists as a 2.5 cm or larger simple cyst before spontaneously resolving. If the corpus luteum fails to resolve after ovulation, it can also persist as a 2.5 cm or greater corpus luteal cyst before spontaneously resolving by the time of menstruation.[17,18] In general, a simple unilocular anechoic structure in the ovary that measures less than or equal to 2.5 cm in size is referred to as a follicle, whereas one that is greater than 2.5 cm in size is referred to as a cyst.

The smaller postmenopausal ovary is more uniformly homogeneous and hypoechoic in echotexture with occasional 1 cm and smaller simple remnant follicles.[19] Peripheral, 1 to 3 mm in size, echogenic foci representing the sequela of previously involved follicles or cysts may also be seen in the walls of ovaries.[20]

IMAGING FINDINGS AND PATHOLOGY
Uterus

Myometrial pathology
Leiomyoma The most common uterine neoplasm is a benign leiomyoma (fibroid).[21] US examination is commonly used to screen for leiomyomas as a source of a pelvic symptomatology as well as to follow-up the size and appearance of known leiomyomas. Sonographically, a benign leiomyoma usually appears as a round or oval, well-circumscribed, hypoechoic mass with posterior acoustic shadowing owing to calcifications and/or edge shadowing at the leiomyoma–myometrial

interface. Leiomyomas that have undergone degeneration can develop internal areas of variable echogenicity owing to cystic, hemorrhagic, or rarely fatty change.[22]

Uterine sarcoma There are no ultrasonographic features that definitively differentiate a benign leiomyoma from a leiomyoma variant (mitotically active, cellular, atypical, smooth muscle tumors of uncertain malignant potential), or uterine sarcoma.[23,24] Uterine sarcomas are rare gynecologic malignancies accounting for 2% to 3% of all uterine malignancies. Risk factors for a uterine sarcoma include prior pelvic radiation, advancing patient age, long-term (>5 years) tamoxifen use, African American ethnicity, and hereditary syndromes. Uterine sarcomas are classified based on the cell type of origin as low- or high-grade endometrial stromal sarcoma, undifferentiated uterine sarcoma, uterine leiomyosarcoma, and other extremely rare uterine mesenchymal sarcoma subtypes including adenosarcoma, perivascular epithelioid cell tumor, and rhabdomyosarcoma.[24–26] US examination also does not reliably differentiate between the uterine sarcoma subtypes.

There can be overlap in the ultrasonographic appearance of a large, degenerated benign leiomyoma and a uterine sarcoma. However, in general a uterine sarcoma on US examination manifests as a large (>10 cm, but can range from 4 to 40 cm), heterogeneous in echotexture mass with marked central vascularity (**Fig. 3**).[27,28] In contrast, a large benign leiomyoma with heterogeneous echotexture owing to degeneration does not typically maintain prominent internal vascularity. Rapid growth of a uterine mass in a

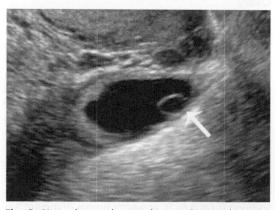

Fig. 2. Normal cumulus oophorus. Gray-scale transverse transvaginal ultrasound image of the ovary demonstrates a thin, circular structure, the cumulus oophorus (*arrow*) within the periphery of a dominant ovarian follicle.

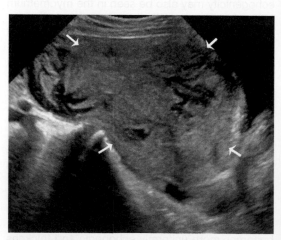

Fig. 3. Uterine leiomyosarcoma. Gray-scale sagittal transabdominal ultrasound image of the uterus reveals a heterogeneously echogenic mass (*arrows*) with irregular margins almost completely replacing the uterus.

postmenopausal patient, as well as a mass with irregular margins, extensive internal hemorrhage, and ascites are additional findings suggesting the possibility of a uterine sarcoma rather than a degenerated benign leiomyoma (**Box 1**).[22]

Endometrial pathology

Most endometrial pathology presents with abnormal uterine bleeding. Pelvic TVUS imaging is the first imaging test of choice for evaluating abnormal premenopausal and postmenopausal uterine bleeding. In the premenopausal setting, abnormal uterine bleeding is most often secondary to hormonal imbalance, leiomyomas, or adenomyosis. In the postmenopausal setting, abnormal uterine bleeding is more likely to be due to endometrial atrophy, hyperplasia, polyps, or carcinoma (**Table 2**).[29] The endometrium is usually well-visualized by TVUS examination, allowing for accurate measurement and detection of focal or diffuse endometrial thickening or a more discrete endometrial mass that should be targeted for biopsy.[30] There is imaging overlap in the appearance and thickness of the endometrium owing to endometrial hyperplasia versus polyp(s) versus carcinoma on TVUS examination. Therefore, there is a low threshold to perform endometrial biopsy in a patient with abnormal bleeding and a slightly thickened endometrium by US examination (**Table 3**).

In a patient with abnormal bleeding, the endometrium is most often considered abnormally thickened if it measures 16 mm or greater in thickness in a premenopausal patient and 5 mm or greater in thickness in a postmenopausal patient by TVUS.[31] In both instances, the endometrium warrants further evaluation with endometrial biopsy if the endometrial thickness is at or above the threshold normal thickness for menopausal status.[30] The risk of endometrial cancer is approximately 7% if the endometrium is greater than 5 mm and 0.07% if the endometrium is less

than 5 mm in a postmenopausal patient with bleeding.[31]

The endometrial threshold thickness by TVUS examination for determining the need for endometrial biopsy in a postmenopausal patient without bleeding is more variable, with recommended thickness thresholds ranging from 8 to 11 mm. The risk of cancer in a postmenopausal woman without bleeding and an endometrial thickness of greater than 11 mm is 6.7%, and 0.002% if the endometrium is less than 11 mm.[31] The threshold normal endometrial thickness for a premenopausal patient without bleeding is also less defined, but in general the endometrium is abnormally thickened if it measures greater than 16 mm in thickness premenopausal. Sonohysterography can also be performed for further evaluation of a potential endometrial lesion for targeted biopsy in the setting of persistent abnormal uterine bleeding, especially if a prior TVUS examination was normal or if a prior endometrial biopsy was benign.[32]

Tamoxifen acts as an estrogen antagonist in the breast, but as an estrogen agonist in the uterus, where it increases the rate of endometrial hyperplasia, polyps, and cancer. Patients on tamoxifen commonly develop subcentimeter cystic spaces

---

Table 2
Common causes of uterine bleeding

Premenopausal	Postmenopausal
Hormonal imbalance	Endometrial atrophy
Leiomyomas	Endometrial hyperplasia
Adenomyosis	Endometrial polyps
	Endometrial carcinoma

Table 3
Threshold endometrial thickness by transvaginal ultrasound imaging for recommending endometrial biopsy

	Endometrial Thickness (mm)
Premenopausal	
Asymptomatic	>16
Abnormal uterine bleeding	≥16
Postmenopausal	
Asymptomatic	>8–11
Abnormal uterine bleeding	≥5
Tamoxifen use	
Asymptomatic	≥9
Abnormal uterine bleeding	≥5

Box 1
Ultrasound features associated with uterine sarcomas

Large size, >10 cm

Irregular margins

Heterogeneous echotexture

Extensive internal hemorrhage

Marked vascularity

Rapid postmenopausal growth

Ascites

within the endometrium and subendometrium by US examination. Patients on tamoxifen with vaginal bleeding should also undergo an endometrial biopsy if the endometrial thickness is 5 mm or greater by TVUS examination. There is no consensus on the management of asymptomatic patients on tamoxifen with a thickened endometrium, but most guidelines suggest endometrial biopsy of asymptomatic patients on tamoxifen when the endometrium measures 9 mm or greater by TVUS examination.[33]

Hyperplasia Endometrial hyperplasia is the result of endometrial gland proliferation with an associated increase in the gland to stromal endometrial ratio. Hyperplasia can be focal or diffuse and associated with or without atypia. Up to 25% of endometrial hyperplasia with atypia may progress to carcinoma versus less than 2% of endometrial hyperplasia without atypia.[34] Hyperplasia develops in the setting of unopposed estrogen stimulation of the endometrium with risk factors including unopposed estrogen hormone replacement therapy, obesity, anovulatory cycles, and estrogen-secreting ovarian tumors. On US examination, hyperplasia usually manifests as a diffusely thickened and echogenic endometrium with well-defined margins and, in some cases, subcentimeter cystic spaces.[35]

Polyps Endometrial polyps develop from a localized proliferation of endometrial glands and stroma with a central vascular core, and can be single, multiple, sessile, or pedunculated. On US examination, individual polyps are most commonly seen as round or oval, well-circumscribed, hyperechoic masses with a central feeding vessel, and often with cystic spaces. Multiple or sessile polyps may manifest as more diffuse echogenic endometrial thickening with or without cystic spaces along the endometrial cavity. Color Doppler imaging is useful for detecting the central vascular core of a polyp.[36] Sonohysterography can also be performed to better detect and localize an endometrial polyp that might otherwise be obscured by more diffuse generalized endometrial thickening (**Fig. 4**). Most endometrial polyps are benign, with only 5.4% of polyps in postmenopausal women and 1.7% of polyps in premenopausal women being premalignant or malignant in nature.[37]

Carcinoma Endometrial carcinoma is the most common gynecologic malignancy in developed countries, accounting for 6% of all cancers in women with a peak age at diagnosis between 55 and 65 years.[38] The most common risk factors for endometrial carcinoma are unopposed estrogen replacement, obesity, diabetes mellitus, polycystic ovarian syndrome, nulliparity, and tamoxifen use. Most patients with endometrial carcinoma present with postmenopausal or intermenstrual bleeding. There are 2 predominant types of endometrial cancer: endometrioid adenocarcinoma (type 1), graded from 1 (well-differentiated) to 3 (poorly differentiated), and clear cell and serous adenocarcinomas (type 2). Both high-grade type 1 carcinomas and all type 2 carcinomas have a poor prognosis.[39]

In addition to the thickness of the endometrium by TVUS (≥5 mm postmenopausal, ≥16 mm premenopausal), other ultrasonographic features that suggest endometrial cancer include a heterogeneous endometrial echotexture, prominent vascularity in the endometrium on color or power Doppler imaging, and an indistinct endometrial–myometrial interface (**Fig. 5**).[40,41] Subcentimeter cystic spaces along the endometrium can also be seen with endometrial carcinoma.[35]

Although TVUS can readily detect an abnormally thickened endometrium, the reliability of US

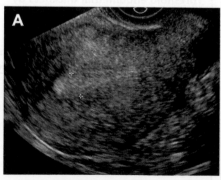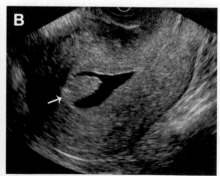

Fig. 4. Endometrial polyp. (*A*) Gray-scale sagittal transvaginal ultrasound image of the uterus demonstrates near uniform echogenicity of the endometrium (calipers [+]). (*B*) Subsequent sagittal transvaginal sonohysterogram image further reveals an ovoid, echogenic, polypoid mass (*arrow*) arising from the fundal wall of the endometrial cavity, outlined by saline within the endometrial cavity.

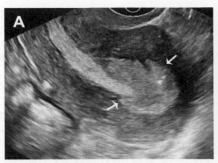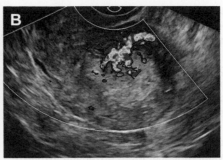

Fig. 5. Endometrial carcinoma, grade 2 endometrial adenocarcinoma with superficial invasion. (*A*) Gray-scale sagittal transvaginal ultrasound (US) image of the uterus shows abnormal thickening (endometrial thickness measures 18 mm) and heterogeneous echogenicity of the endometrium, particularly toward the fundus, with irregularity of the endometrium–myometrium border (*arrows*). (*B*) Color Doppler sagittal transvaginal US image of the uterus demonstrates prominent increased vascularity within the abnormally thickened endometrium.

examination for determining the presence and depth of myometrial invasion of endometrial carcinoma is more variable. The reported sensitivities, specificities, and accuracies of TVUS for detecting myometrial invasion by endometrial carcinoma range from 71% to 85%, 72% to 90%, and 72% to 84%, respectively, and those for detecting cervical invasion by endometrial carcinoma are 29% to 93%, 92% to 94%, and 78% to 92%, respectively.[42–46] Sonohysterography has a reported greater accuracy for evaluating the depth of myometrial invasion, which is up to 96.4%.[47] However, there is a risk of disseminating malignant cells with sonohysterography.[48] Sonographic features associated with a higher grade and more deeply invasive endometrial carcinoma include larger tumor size, mixed echogenicity or hypoechoic endometrial echotexture, an irregular endometrium–myometrium border, and a greater degree of endometrial vascularity (**Box 2**; see **Fig. 5**).[42–46] MR imaging is the preferred modality for accurately determining the presence and degree of myometrial invasion. However, several studies have also shown that TVUS performed by an experienced imager may be as accurate as MR imaging for correctly identifying 50% or greater depth of myometrial invasion as well as cervical stromal invasion, both of which characterize the cancer as higher risk.[42,49,50]

Box 2
Ultrasound features of higher grade and invasive endometrial carcinoma

Larger tumor size

Mixed or hypoechoic echotexture

Irregular endometrial–myometrial border

Prominent endometrial vascularity

Cervical pathology

Polyps Cervical polyps are the most common benign cervical lesion, and are most often found in multiparous women of 30 to 50 years of age. Polyps may be detected on routine physical examination or manifest as a cause of intermenstrual bleeding.[51] Up to 25% of cervical polyps coexist with endometrial polyps,[52] and most cervical polyps are benign in nature. The rate of malignancy or dysplasia in a cervical polyp is reportedly 1.5% or less, and more common in perimenopausal patients.[53] Similar to endometrial polyps, cervical polyps typically appear on US examination as an ovoid, hyperechoic mass lesion with a central vascular stalk. Polyps may be mobile during real-time imaging, and it is important for patient management planning to determine the exact location of a polyp as arising directly from the cervix versus arising from the endometrial cavity and protruding downward into the endocervical canal.

Carcinoma Cervical carcinoma is the third most common gynecologic malignancy in the United States, and the leading gynecologic cancer worldwide. Risk factors for cervical carcinoma include multiple sexual partners, early age at first intercourse, multiparity, lower socioeconomic standing, cigarette smoking, immunosuppression, oral contraceptive use, and human papilloma virus subtypes 16, 18, 31, 33, and 56.[54] Cervical carcinoma is usually detected on physical examination and with Papanicolaou testing, and is traditionally staged clinically. However, the most recent International Federation of Gynecologic Oncology (FIGO) staging system also recommends the use of imaging, especially computed tomography and MR imaging, for pretreatment planning via detection of disease in local and distant sites.[55] US examination is not recommended for the screening or staging of cervical carcinoma, but as a common first test for evaluating a wide range of pelvic symptomatology, US imaging may be the first examination to detect a cervical lesion.

Cervical carcinomas most commonly arise at the junction where squamous and columnar epithelium meet, and up to 80% to 90% are squamous cell carcinomas and 5% to 20% are adenocarcinomas.[56] Early cervical carcinomas may be difficult to visualize on US examination owing to a small size and an echogenicity similar to the normal cervical mucosa. More advanced invasive cervical carcinomas are more likely to be visible sonographically and can have a variety of appearances, ranging from a subtle area of altered echotexture and loss of the normal cervical zonal anatomy to distortion of the cervical shape and complete replacement of the cervix with an isoechoic to hypoechoic mass (**Fig. 6**). Most cervical carcinomas by US examination are also hypervascular with irregular margins. A large amount of simple or complicated fluid in the endometrial and/or endocervical canal can be a secondary sign of a potentially more distal obstructing cervical lesion. Invasive features of cervical carcinoma that may manifest on US examination include mass extension into the vaginal fornices and parametrium, loss of cervical mobility or compressibility, and direct bladder and/or rectal invasion. When a cervical carcinoma is suspected on pelvic US examination, the retroperitoneum can also be surveyed sonographically for enlarged lymph nodes, hydroureter, and hydronephrosis.[15,57]

Ovary

US examination is the primary imaging examination for detecting, characterizing, and directing the management of ovarian cysts and masses. Many ovarian lesions have specific sonographic features that enable a definitive diagnosis by US examination alone. In addition, many different prediction models have been developed and tested to combine the US features of an ovarian lesion with additional biochemical and patient features to risk stratify an ovarian lesion as more likely benign or malignant. One of the first prediction models in use is the risk of malignancy index, which combines the US features of an ovarian lesion with the serum cancer antigen 125 level and the menopausal status of the patient to provide a quantitative assessment of the risk of malignancy.[58,59] Subsequent additional risk stratification models include logistic regression models, US-based simple rules, and most recently The Assessment of Different NEoplasias in the adneXa (ADNEX) model created by the International Ovarian Tumor Analysis group.[60] The ADNEX model consists of 3 clinical predictors (age, serum cancer antigen 125, type of referred imaging center) and 6 US predictors (maximal lesion diameter, proportion of solid tissue, number of papillary projections, presence of >10 cyst locules, acoustic shadows, and presence of ascites; **Table 4**). The ADNEX model is the first risk model designed to differentiate between benign, borderline, stage I invasive, stage II to IV invasive ovarian cancers, and secondary metastasis.[61]

Correct classification of an ovarian lesion as more likely benign or malignant aids in directing lesion management to observation alone versus resection with a minimally invasive surgical approach without a surgical staging procedure versus gynecologic oncologist management of a lesion with resection and a surgical staging procedure. There are also several US technologies under investigation for potential use in further characterizing ovarian lesions, including contrast-enhanced TVUS and Doppler US examination to evaluate tumor microvasculature, and molecular US imaging using microbubbles coupled with various antibodies.[62,63]

Ovarian cysts

Ovarian cysts are common incidental findings on pelvic US examination in both premenopausal

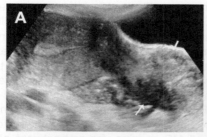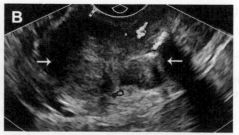

Fig. 6. Cervical carcinoma. (*A*) Gray-scale sagittal transabdominal ultrasound (US) image of the uterus shows an enlarged, heterogeneous, ill-defined appearance of the cervix (*arrows*). (*B*) Color Doppler sagittal transvaginal US image of the cervix further reveals a hypoechoic mass (*arrows*) with internal vascularity and lobulated margins replacing the cervix.

Table 4
ADNEX model's clinical and ultrasound predictors for risk stratifying ovarian lesions

Clinical Predictors	Ultrasound Predictors
Patient age	Maximal lesion diameter
Serum cancer antigen 125	Proportion of solid tissue
	Number of papillary projections
Type of referred imaging center	Presence of >10 cyst locules
	Acoustic shadows
	Presence of ascites

and postmenopausal patients. Familiarity with both the characteristically benign and suspicious features of ovarian cysts on US examination can help direct patient management. The Society of Radiologists in Ultrasound (SRU) have developed guidelines to help with the management of incidental asymptomatic ovarian cysts as detected by US examination (**Table 5**).[64] The SRU guidelines help to direct which asymptomatic ovarian and adnexal cysts can be left alone and which may need additional imaging or surgical evaluation.

Simple and probably benign cysts Simple cysts on US imaging are characterized by a round or

Table 5
Society of Radiologists in Ultrasound recommendations for management of asymptomatic ovarian and adnexal cysts on pelvic US imaging (in nonpregnant adult women)

US Appearance	Follow-up Recommendation
Simple cyst Thin-walled cyst with single thin septation Thin-walled cyst with focal wall calcification	Reproductive age: • ≤5 cm, no follow-up • >5 cm to ≤7 cm, yearly US follow-up • >7 cm, further imaging (MR imaging) or surgical evaluation Postmenopausal: • ≤1 cm, no follow-up • >1 cm to ≤7 cm, yearly US follow-up • >7 cm, further imaging (MR imaging) or surgical evaluation
Hemorrhagic cyst	Reproductive age: • ≤5 cm, no follow-up • >5 cm, 6–12 wk US follow-up Early postmenopausal: • Any size, 6–12 wk US follow-up Late postmenopausal: • Consider surgical evaluation
Endometrioma	Any age: • 6–12 wk US follow-up, then yearly US follow-up if not resected
Dermoid	Any age: • Yearly US follow-up if not resected
Cyst suggestive of, but not classic for, hemorrhagic cyst, endometrioma, or dermoid	Reproductive age: • 6–12 wk US follow-up • If unchanged at first US follow-up, then additional follow-up with US or MR imaging • If not confirmed as endometrioma or dermoid after second follow-up, consider surgical evaluation Postmenopausal: • Consider surgical evaluation
Cyst with multiple thin (<3 mm) septations	Any age: • Consider surgical evaluation
Cyst with nodule (nonhyperechoic) without blood flow	Any age: • Consider further evaluation with MR imaging or surgical evaluation
Cyst with thick (>3 mm) irregular septations	Any age: • Consider surgical evaluation
Cyst with nodule with blood flow	Any age: • Consider surgical evaluation

Data from Levine D, Brown DL, Andreotti RF, et al. Management of asymptomatic ovarian and other adnexal cysts imaged at US. Society of Radiologists in Ultrasound consensus conference statement. Ultrasound Q 2010;26(3):121–31.

oval shape, well-circumscribed margins, thin and smooth walls, posterior acoustic enhancement, and the absence of septations, solid component, or internal vascularity. Simple cysts, especially when less than 7 cm in size, are most commonly physiologic, paraovarian, or benign neoplastic cysts (cystadenomas).[65] The SRU guidelines recommend that in women of reproductive age, asymptomatic simple cysts of 5 cm or less do not require follow-up imaging, cysts greater than 5 cm and 7 cm or less in size can be followed up with yearly US examination, and cysts greater than 7 cm in size can be further evaluated with MR imaging (because small mural nodules in cysts >7 cm may not be visible on US examination) and/or surgical evaluation. In postmenopausal women, simple cysts 1 cm or smaller do not need follow-up imaging, simple cysts greater than 1 cm to 7 cm or smaller can be followed up with yearly US examination, and cysts greater than 7 cm in size can be further evaluated with MR imaging and/or surgical evaluation.[64] The risk of malignancy in a simple unilocular cyst smaller than 5 cm has been reported as less than 1% in premenopausal women and 1.6% in postmenopausal women.[65] Cysts greater than 10 cm in size have a reported 13% chance of malignancy.[66]

Minimally complicated, but still probably benign cysts, that is, cysts with a single thin (<3 mm thickness) internal septation or a single focal wall calcification, can be managed using the same size and menopausal status algorithm as simple cysts. Cysts with features suggestive of, but not definitive for, a hemorrhagic cyst, endometrioma, or mature cystic teratoma can be followed up with pelvic US examination in 6 to 12 weeks in a premenopausal woman, and if unchanged then additional follow-up with US or MR imaging can be performed in another 6 to 12 weeks. If still indeterminate at the time of second follow-up imaging,

surgical evaluation can be considered for definitive management. In contrast, cysts suggestive of, but not classic for, a hemorrhagic cyst, endometrioma, or mature cystic teratoma in postmenopausal women can proceed directly to consideration for surgical evaluation. In both premenopausal and postmenopausal women, even more indeterminate cysts with multiple thin internal septations and/or a nonhyperechoic nodule without detectable flow at Doppler US examination, can proceed directly to surgical consultation and/or MR imaging for further evaluation.[64]

Hemorrhagic cyst Hemorrhagic cysts are commonly encountered in premenopausal women secondary to hemorrhage within a corpus luteum. The US appearance of a hemorrhagic cyst varies with the age of the cyst. In the acute setting, a hemorrhagic cyst is predominantly hyperechoic to heterogeneous in echotexture without internal vascularity. In the subacute setting, the blood products in the cyst become more organized and visible as retracting, variable echogenicity, concave avascular material from the cyst wall. In the more chronic setting, the blood products further resorb into the appearance of thin strands and lacelike reticulation in the cyst (**Fig. 7**).[64,67] The fibrin strands of a hemorrhagic cyst are very thin, numerous, and do not extend across the entire cyst lumen. In contrast, true septations in cysts are thicker, less numerous, and extend across the entire cyst lumen.[68]

For premenopausal women, similar to simple cysts, no follow-up imaging is required for hemorrhagic cysts 5 cm or smaller in size, and hemorrhagic cysts greater than 5 cm in size can be managed with follow-up US examination in 6 to 12 weeks (premenopausal hemorrhagic cysts usually resolve in 8 weeks). In the early postmenopausal period, all hemorrhagic cysts, regardless

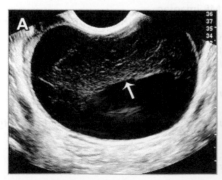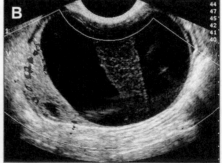

Fig. 7. Hemorrhagic ovarian cyst. (*A*) Gray-scale transverse transvaginal ultrasound (US) image of the ovary shows the characteristic appearance of a chronic hemorrhagic cyst with reticular, lacelike, retracting echoes with concave margins (*arrow*). (*B*) Color Doppler transverse transvaginal US image demonstrates absence of internal vascularity in the cyst contents.

of size, should be followed up with US examination in 6 to 12 weeks. In the late postmenopausal period, a physiologic hemorrhagic cyst should not develop and the appearance of a hemorrhagic cyst in a postmenopausal ovary is suspect for an ovarian neoplasm, such that surgical evaluation should be considered directly.[64]

Endometrioma The classic US appearance of endometriomas is that of a round or oval, well-circumscribed, smooth-walled cyst with homogeneous low to intermediate level internal echoes (**Fig. 8**).[22,64] The US appearance of an endometrioma can overlap with that of an acute hemorrhagic cyst. For this reason, a follow-up US examination in 6 to 12 weeks in premenopausal women can help to differentiate between acute hemorrhagic cysts and endometriomas, because hemorrhagic cysts would be expected to evolve and decrease in size during this time, whereas endometriomas typically persist without appreciable change over a short follow-up time interval. Multiplicity, bilaterality, and the presence of echogenic foci in the walls of endometriomas are additional features that can help to primarily differentiate an endometrioma from a hemorrhagic cyst.[69] Once a lesion is characterized as an endometrioma, yearly follow-up US imaging is recommended to screen for malignant degeneration. Rarely, there can be malignant degeneration of an endometrioma into, most commonly, a clear cell or endometrioid carcinoma. Malignant degeneration of an endometrioma should be suspected if an endometrioma rapidly increases in size (especially to >9 cm in size in a woman >40 years of age)

and/or develops solid mural nodularity with vascularity.[70]

Ovarian neoplasms
Ovarian carcinoma is the seventh most common cancer among women worldwide. The FIGO classification system for staging ovarian cancer was updated in 2014 and now unifies the staging of ovarian, fallopian tube, and peritoneal carcinoma, and reflects that tubal carcinomas may be the site of origin of some high-grade serous carcinomas of the ovary and peritoneum.[71,72]

Risk factors for ovarian carcinoma include family history, BRCA 1 or 2, hereditary nonpolyposis colorectal cancer (Lynch II syndrome), infertility, multiparity, late menopause, and early menarche. The role of US examination in screening for ovarian cancer has been limited to variable screening of high-risk patients and is still under investigation.[60] Primary ovarian neoplasms are classified into 3 subtypes: epithelial, germ cell, and sex cord-stromal cell (**Box 3**). In general, the US features of an ovarian malignancy regardless of

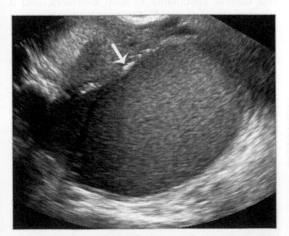

Fig. 8. Ovarian endometrioma. Gray-scale sagittal transvaginal ultrasound image of the ovary illustrates the characteristic appearance of an endometrioma with uniform low level internal echoes and several peripheral echogenic foci (*arrow*) in the wall.

Box 3
Classification of ovarian neoplasms

Epithelial (60%–70% overall, 90% of malignant neoplasms)

Serous

Mucinous

Endometrioid

Clear cell

Brenner

Germ cell (15%–20%)

Mature cystic teratoma

Immature teratoma

Struma ovarii

Dysgerminoma

Endodermal sinus tumor

Embryonal cell carcinoma

Sex cord-stromal cell (5%–10%)

Fibroma

Thecoma

Fibrothecoma

Granulosa cell tumor

Sclerosing stromal cell tumor

Sertoli-Leydig tumor

Sertoli cell tumor

Leydig tumor

subtype are a solid component (papillary projection, nodule, wall irregularity) with vascularity, thick septations (≥3 mm thickness), peritoneal or omental implants, and moderate to large ascites.[68,73]

Epithelial neoplasm Epithelial ovarian neoplasms account for up to 60% to 70% of all ovarian neoplasms and 90% of malignant ovarian neoplasms. They are further subclassified as serous, mucinous, endometrioid, clear cell, and Brenner tumors, and can be benign, borderline, or malignant.[74] Serous tumors are the most common epithelial tumor of the ovary and are bilateral in up to 20% of cases. Most persistent large simple cysts in postmenopausal women are serous cystadenomas.[75] Serous cystadenocarcinomas are more complex in appearance, having solid components, most commonly papillary projections, and areas of internal vascularity (**Fig. 9**).[22,74]

Mucinous epithelial tumors in comparison to serous tumors by US examination are more commonly larger (>6 cm), unilateral, and multilocular with numerous, smooth, thin internal septations in the setting of a benign cystadenoma, and with thicker internal septations and mural nodularity in the setting of a borderline or malignant cystadenocarcinoma (**Fig. 10**). Locule echogenicity in a mucinous neoplasm on US examination is often variable with low-level echoes in various locules reflecting varying degrees of mucin content[22] (**Table 6**).

Clear cell and endometrioid neoplasms are associated with endometriosis and appear as complex cystic masses on US examination. Brenner tumors are often associated with another epithelial tumor, a serous or mucinous cystadenoma. Brenner tumors are otherwise usually seen as small, solid, hypoechoic ovarian masses by US examination.[76]

Germ cell neoplasms Germ cell neoplasms comprise 15% to 20% of all ovarian tumors and 3% to 7% of malignant ovarian tumors. Germ cell neoplasms are further classified by the dominant cell type, with the most common germ cell neoplasm being a mature cystic teratoma (dermoid cyst). Mature cystic teratomas are bilateral up to 10% to 15% of the time. The US appearance of a mature cystic teratoma is quite variable, but there are several classic US features including echogenic areas with posterior acoustic shadowing ("tip of the iceberg" sign; **Fig. 11**), fat–fluid levels, hyperechoic lines and dots ("dot-dash," dermoid mesh; **Fig. 12**), floating spheres (hair balls), and a small, highly echogenic, avascular mass[77,78] (**Box 4**).

Mature cystic teratomas can be complicated by ovarian torsion, rupture, and rarely malignant degeneration (0.17%–2.00%, into squamous cell carcinoma). A characteristic mature cystic teratoma less than 4 to 5 cm in size may be managed with yearly follow-up US examination. Clinical and US features that raise the possibility of a malignant teratoma, either malignant degeneration of a mature cystic teratoma or a malignant immature teratoma, include a larger size (especially if >10 cm), patient age greater than 50 years, a predominantly solid mass with minimal fatty component, solid areas with color Doppler flow (especially if centrally), and an invasive appearance.[79,80]

Other rare germ cell neoplasms are struma ovarii, dysgerminoma, endodermal sinus tumor, and embryonal cell carcinoma. Struma ovarii is a rare teratoma (2%–3% of teratomas) composed mainly of thyroid tissue and on US examination has central vascularity in solid elements, and a greater size (>6 cm).[81] Dysgerminoma is a rare malignant germ cell tumor (1%–2% of primary ovarian malignancies) that is composed of undifferentiated germ cells, most often occurs in

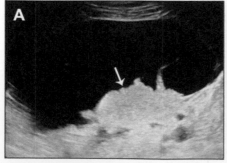 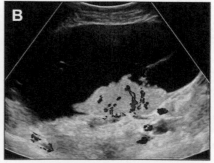

Fig. 9. Ovarian serous borderline neoplasm. (*A*) Gray-scale transverse transvaginal ultrasound (US) image shows an ovarian cyst with a prominent irregular mural nodule (*arrow*). (*B*) Color Doppler transverse transvaginal US image of the ovarian cyst demonstrates prominent vascularity within the solid mural nodule.

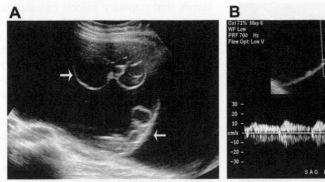

Fig. 10. Ovarian mucinous cystadenocarcinoma. (*A*) Gray-scale sagittal transabdominal ultrasound (US) image reveals an ovarian cyst (measuring up to 19 cm) with multiple variable thickness internal septations (*arrows*). (*B*) Color Doppler sagittal transabdominal US image of the cyst demonstrates vascularity in one of the nodular, thickened septations with a low resistance arterial waveform.

women under the age of 30, can be bilateral in up to 15%, and appears on US examination as a solid, predominantly echogenic mass with occasional areas of hemorrhage or necrosis. Endodermal sinus tumor is also a rare malignant germ cell tumor with a poor prognosis that is most commonly encountered under the age of 20 years, has an association with elevated serum alpha-fetoprotein levels, and most often appears as a solid mass on US examination.[82]

Sex cord-stromal cell tumors Sex cord-stromal ovarian neoplasms comprise 5% to 10% of ovarian neoplasms and include fibromas, thecomas, fibrothecomas, Sertoli-Leydig cell, Sertoli cell, Leydig, sclerosing stromal cell, and granulosa cell tumors. Fibromas, thecomas, and fibrothecomas are all benign neoplasms that typically appear on US examination as round or oval, solid, homogenous to mildly heterogeneous hypoechoic masses with associated posterior acoustic shadowing and minimal detectable vascularity (**Fig. 13**). Occasionally, the masses can have

internal areas of cystic degeneration. The thecoma element is associated with estrogen activity, which can promote associated endometrial thickening and pathology. Thecomas and fibrothecomas are more commonly found in postmenopausal women (mean age, 59 years) who may present with postmenopausal bleeding owing to the thecoma estrogen effect on the endometrium.[22,74]

Sertoli-Leydig cell tumors and associated subtypes are rare (<0.5% of ovarian tumors) benign or malignant neoplasms associated with androgen excess, less commonly estrogen production, which most often present clinically with amenorrhea and virilization. These tumors may be difficult to detect on US examination, but are most often, small, unilateral, solid, hypoechoic masses in women less than 30 years of age (75%).[83]

Granulosa cell tumors have a more variable US appearance, ranging from a solid mass to a

Table 6 Ultrasound features of serous versus mucinous ovarian neoplasms		
Feature	**Serous**	**Mucinous**
Bilateral	20%	Rare
Size	Smaller (<6 cm)	Larger (>6 cm)
Septations	None to few	Multiple, multilocular, thin
Echogenicity	Predominantly anechoic	Variable low-level echoes

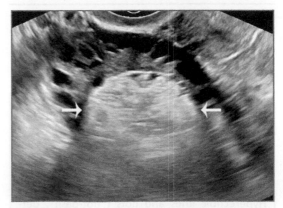

Fig. 11. Ovarian mature cystic teratoma. Gray-scale sagittal transvaginal ultrasound image of the ovary illustrates a markedly hyperechoic lesion (*arrows*) with posterior acoustic shadowing, the "tip of the iceberg" appearance of a mature teratoma.

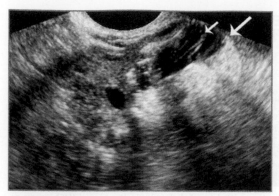

Fig. 12. Ovarian mature cystic teratoma. Gray-scale sagittal transvaginal ultrasound image of the ovary shows a variable echogenicity lesion with a fat–fluid level (*long arrows*) and hyperechoic lines (*short arrow*).

complex multiloculated cystic mass owing variable areas of internal hemorrhage (**Fig. 14**).[22] Granulosa cell tumors have adult (>30 years of age) and juvenile (<30 years of age) subtypes with the adult type peaking between the ages of 50 and 55 years. Granulosa cell tumors may also produce estrogen and result in abnormal thickening and pathology of the endometrium.[84]

Metastasis Ovarian metastasis can be secondary to lymphoma or, more commonly, primary tumors of the stomach, breast, or uterus. In most cases, ovarian metastasis manifest as a solid mass of the ovary on US examination with ovarian enlargement and maintained ovoid shape. In contrast, metastases from the colon, rectum, and biliary tree are more often multicystic with irregular margins.[85]

Fallopian Tube

Primary fallopian tube carcinoma was traditionally believed to be the least common gynecologic malignancy, accounting for 0.5% of gynecologic tumors.[86] However, more recent investigation now favors that papillary serous carcinoma, the most common subtype of epithelial ovarian carcinoma and the most common type of fallopian tube carcinoma, arises from the lining of the fallopian tube with subsequent involvement of the ovaries and peritoneum.[87,88] The entity of a serous carcinoma primarily originating in the fallopian tube is referred to as a serous tubal intraepithelial carcinoma (STIC), and was incidentally discovered within the fallopian tubes of patients with BRCA mutations who underwent prophylactic salpingo-oophorectomies. The STIC theory of origin is that most high-grade serous carcinomas originate from STIC in the distal fallopian tube with subsequent implantation and involvement of the ovary and peritoneum.[72] In particular, an STIC lesion located in the fimbriated end of the fallopian tube can grow outward to implant on the ovary and ultimately develop into an invasive high-grade serous carcinoma.[89]

Most fallopian tube cancers are unilateral, located in the distal two-thirds of the tube, have an average size of 5 cm at time of detection, and often have some degree of tumor necrosis and hemorrhage.[90] US examination can typically differentiate between tubal enlargement owing to benign hydrosalpinx and a neoplasm. The sonographic appearance of benign hydrosalpinx is that of a dilated, elongated, cystic structure with incomplete septations, and indentation of opposing walls (the "waist" sign; **Fig. 15**). In the setting of benign acute inflammation, the wall of the tube may also seem to be thickened with a "cogwheel" appearance (**Fig. 16**), and in the setting of more chronic dilation, small (<3 mm) mural nodules representing endosalpingeal folds may be seen within the tube.[91]

The sonographic appearance of fallopian tube carcinoma varies with the presence or absence of associated hydrosalpinx. In the presence of hydrosalpinx, fallopian tube carcinoma can manifest as a papillary projection or solid mural nodule projecting into the lumen of the dilated tube. It can also appear as a completely solid ovoid or oblong adnexal mass. Color spectral Doppler imaging is useful for confirming vascularity within the solid elements of a tubal neoplasm and for differentiating it from tubal luminal echogenicity owing to avascular blood products or debris.[92,93]

Gestational Trophoblastic Disease

Gestational trophoblastic disease (GTD) is a term encompassing a spectrum of placental origin tumors including benign (but premalignant) complete and partial moles, invasive mole, choriocarcinoma, placental site trophoblastic tumor

---

Box 4
Various ultrasound features of a mature cystic teratoma

Echogenic area with posterior acoustic shadowing ("tip of the iceberg" sign)

Fat–fluid level

Hyperechoic lines and dots ("dot-dash", dermoid mesh)

Floating spheres (hair balls)

Small, highly echogenic avascular mass

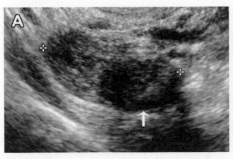
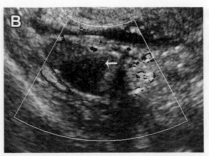

Fig. 13. Ovarian fibroma. (*A*) Gray-scale sagittal transvaginal ultrasound (US) image of the ovary shows an ovoid, well-circumscribed hypoechoic mass (*arrow*) with posterior acoustic shadowing. (*B*) Color Doppler transverse transvaginal US image demonstrates minimal internal vascularity (*arrow*) in the mass.

(PSTT), and epithelioid trophoblastic tumor (ETT). Invasive mole, choriocarcinoma, PSTT, and ETT are further classified as gestational trophoblastic neoplasia (GTN; **Box 5**). Risk factors for GTD include extremes of maternal age (<20 years and >40 years), a history of prior molar pregnancy, and a history of oral contraceptive use.[94] US examination is the first imaging study of choice for evaluating the female pelvis during and after pregnancy, and is usually the first imaging study to detect GTD.

Complete and partial moles

Complete and partial moles are benign, but premalignant, subtypes of GTD resulting from fertilization error, and account for up to 80% of GTD (0.6–1.1 of 1000 pregnancies in North America).[95] A complete mole results from fertilization of an empty ovum without maternal chromosomes by a sperm with paternal chromosomes and subsequent duplication of paternal DNA to a diploid, most commonly 46,XX, karyotype. A partial mole results from fertilization of a normal ovum with maternal chromosomes by 2 sperms with a resulting triploid, most commonly 69,XXY,

karyotype.[95,96] Complete moles have no fetal tissue, only hydropic villi, and trophoblastic hyperplasia. Partial moles have an embryo or fetus with variable viability into the second trimester. Complete moles typically present in the first trimester with vaginal bleeding, uterine enlargement, and an abnormally increased serum β-hCG (>100,000 IU/L). In contrast, partial moles more often manifest as a missed or incomplete abortion without uterine enlargement or an abnormally increased serum β-hCG.[97]

The classic US appearance of a complete mole is that of an enlarged uterus with a vascular, heterogeneously echogenic mass in the endometrium with numerous predominantly subcentimeter hypoechoic spaces ("snowstorm" appearance) or more cystic appearing spaces ("cluster of grapes" appearance), corresponding with dilated hydropic placental villi (**Fig. 17**). No gestational sac or embryo is seen with a complete mole. The ovaries may also be enlarged with simple theca lutein cysts in response to the increased β-hCG level.[98] Partial moles have less extensive echogenic and cystic changes of the abnormal placental tissue (**Fig. 18**), and have a more variable US

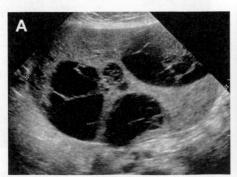
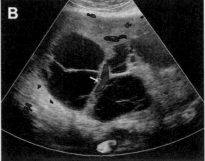

Fig. 14. Granulosa cell tumor. (*A*) Gray-scale sagittal transabdominal ultrasound (US) image of the ovary demonstrates an ovoid, partly cystic and partly solid ovoid mass (calipers [+]). (*B*) Color Doppler sagittal transabdominal US image demonstrates vascularity (*arrow*) within a solid area in the mass.

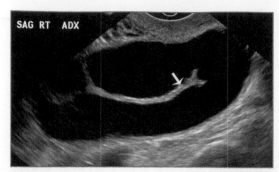

Fig. 15. Simple hydrosalpinx. Gray-scale sagittal transvaginal ultrasound image illustrates a serpentine, cystic structure with an incomplete septation (*arrow*).

presentation ranging from an empty gestational sac, a gestational sac with indistinct echoes, an elongated gestational sac, fetal demise with anomalies and/or growth restriction, oligohydramnios, and placental size greater than expected for uterine size[99] (**Table 7**).

In part owing to the earlier and more widespread use of US examination in the first trimester for purposes of pregnancy dating and viability, molar pregnancies are now more often imaged before developing the characteristic multicystic appearance, and instead may less specifically manifest as an irregular gestational sac without an embryo. In addition, it can be difficult to differentiate a partial mole from retained products of conception. Overall, the US diagnosis of a molar pregnancy (both complete and partial) has a sensitivity of 44%, specificity of 74%, positive predictive value of 88%, and negative predictive value of 23%.[100] For this reason, correlating and serially following the β-hCG level in addition to the US findings is essential for not overlooking a molar pregnancy as a simple failed pregnancy. Complete and partial

Box 5
Spectrum of gestational trophoblastic disease
Complete mole
Partial mole
Gestational trophoblastic neoplasia
Invasive mole
Choriocarcinoma
Placental site trophoblastic tumor
Epithelioid trophoblastic tumor

moles are both managed with curettage followed by surveillance weekly β-hCG testing through 3 negative levels, and then monthly β-hCG testing for 6 months to detect recurrent neoplasm. Patients are also advised to delay any subsequent pregnancy for 12 months and to have an early screening US examination with any subsequent pregnancies.[101]

Gestational trophoblastic neoplasia
Even after the evacuation of a complete or partial molar pregnancy, a more aggressive GTN can persist as an invasive mole or choriocarcinoma. Up to 15% to 20% of complete moles and 5% of partial moles can progress to an invasive mole or choriocarcinoma.[101] In the setting of a persistently increased β-hCG levels after curettage for a molar pregnancy, pelvic US examination is the imaging test of choice to evaluate for a potential new

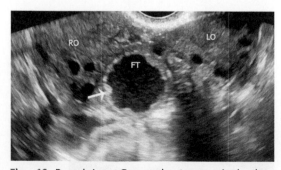

Fig. 16. Pyosalpinx. Gray-scale transvaginal ultrasound image of the fallopian tube (FT) illustrates acute tubal inflammation with nodular inner tubal wall thickening (*arrow*), the "cogwheel" sign, and low level echoes in the tube. LO, left ovary; RO, right ovary.

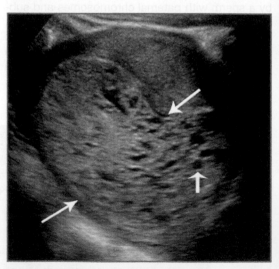

Fig. 17. Complete mole. Gray-scale sagittal transabdominal ultrasound image of the uterus demonstrates an echogenic mass (*long arrows*) centered in the endometrial cavity with multiple cystic spaces (*short arrow*).

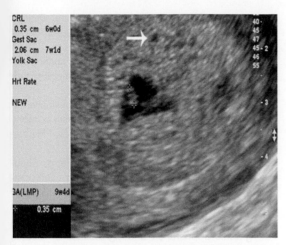

CRL
0.35 cm 6w0d
Gest Sac
2.06 cm 7w1d
Yolk Sac
Hrt Rate
NEW
3A(LMP) 9w4d
0.35 cm

Fig. 18. Partial mole. Gray-scale sagittal transvaginal ultrasound image of the uterus demonstrates an intrauterine gestation with an embryo (calipers [+]) and subtle cystic spaces (*arrow*) in surrounding echogenic tissue.

pregnancy, assess for residual disease, and measure uterine volume as a prognostic factor. On US examination, an irregular margin or asymmetric extension of the echogenic endometrial tissue of a complete or partial mole into the myometrium suggests myometrial invasion by the mole. In addition, an enlarged uterus, irregular bleeding, and bilaterally enlarged ovaries after evacuation of a molar pregnancy are signs of a persistent post molar GTN.[98,102] FIGO defines a post molar GTN as persistently plateaued or rising serum β-hCG over 2 to 3 weeks, a persistent detectable β-hCG 6 months after evacuation of a mole, a histologic diagnosis of choriocarcinoma, and/or metastasis.[103] Choriocarcinoma, PSTT, and ETT can also present months to years after a normal term pregnancy with an elevated β-hCG helping to confirm the diagnosis.[99]

Choriocarcinoma is a rare (1 in 20,000 to 1 in 40,000 pregnancies) aggressive neoplasm with a propensity for local pelvic invasion and distant metastasis, most commonly to the lungs (in 80% of cases), vagina, liver, and brain. Up to 50% of choriocarcinomas occur after a molar pregnancy with the remainder occurring after an abortion (25%) or term gestation (25%).[99,104] PSTT and ETT more commonly occur after a full-term pregnancy, and represent neoplastic growth of trophoblasts at the site of prior placental implantation. In contrast with choriocarcinoma, PSTT and ETT tend to be slower growing with local spread and lymphatic metastasis before hematogenous metastasis.[105]

The general appearance of an invasive mole, choriocarcinoma, PSTT, and ETT in the uterus on pelvic US examination is that of hypervascular mass centered in the myometrium with variable endometrial extent and variable echogenicity owing to hemorrhage and necrosis. The marked vascularity of the neoplasm is well-depicted with color Doppler imaging and parametrial invasion may also be visible sonographically.[102,106] MR imaging and computed tomography scans then typically follow the diagnosis of GTN for further staging of any local pelvic invasion as well as screening and detection of distant metastasis. Invasive moles and choriocarcinoma are treated with chemotherapy, PSTT and ETT are managed with hysterectomy, and all are further monitored with β-hCG surveillance for at least 12 months after treatment. There is no set imaging follow-up interval guidelines once treatment has begun, and imaging is not performed routinely unless complications are suspected, including pelvic and pulmonary arteriovenous malformations.[99]

SUMMARY

Pelvic US examination is used to evaluate a wide range of pelvic symptomatology, and is often the first examination to suggest a gynecologic neoplasm. Pelvic US examination is particularly useful for evaluating the appearance and thickness of the endometrium in patients with abnormal uterine bleeding, helping to direct the need and

Table 7	
Various ultrasound features of complete and partial moles	

	US Feature
Complete mole	Enlarged uterus
	Echogenic endometrial mass with subcentimeter hypoechoic/cystic spaces ("snowstorm"/"cluster of grapes")
	No gestational sac
	No embryo
	Enlarged ovaries with theca lutein cysts
Partial mole	Less echogenic and cystic placental tissue compared with complete mole
	Placenta size greater than expected for uterine size
	Empty gestational sac
	Gestational sac with indistinct echoes
	Elongated gestational sac
	Fetal demise with anomalies with or without growth restriction
	Oligohydramnios

location for any subsequent endometrial biopsy. Ovarian cysts are also routinely encountered and characterized on pelvic US examination, and through the application of current guidelines and risk stratification models, the management of such cysts is largely determined by the imaging features on US examination. Through the combined use of TA and TV imaging, color and spectral Doppler imaging, and in some cases SIS, pelvic US examination can detect, localize, and in many cases fully characterize pelvic pathology as benign or likely malignant, facilitating patient management.

REFERENCES

1. American College of Radiology (ACR). ACR-ACOG-AIUM SRU Practice parameter for the performance of ultrasound of the female pelvis. 2014. Available at: https://www.acr.org/~/media/ACR/Documents/PGTS/guidelines/US_Pelvic.pdf. Accessed July 2, 2017.

2. Dutta S, Wang F, Fleischer AC, et al. New frontiers for ovarian cancer risk evaluation: proteomics and contrast-enhanced ultrasound. AJR Am J Roentgenol 2010;194:349–54.

3. Lu R, Xiao Y, Liu M, et al. Ultrasound elastography in the differential diagnosis of benign and malignant cervical lesions. J Ultrasound Med 2014;33:667–71.

4. Wu Y, Peng H, Zhao X. Diagnostic performance of contrast-enhanced ultrasound for ovarian cancer: a meta-analysis. Ultrasound Med Biol 2015;41:967–74.

5. Dubinsky TJ, Reed SD, Grieco V, et al. Intra-cervical sonographic-pathologic correlation: preliminary results. J Ultrasound Med 2003;22:61–7.

6. Valentin L. Gray scale sonography, subjective evaluation of the color Doppler image and measurement of blood flow velocity for distinguishing benign and malignant tumors of suspected adnexal origin. Eur J Obstet Gynecol Reprod Biol 1997;72:63–72.

7. Stein SM, Laifer-Narin S, Johnson MB, et al. Differentiation of benign and malignant adnexal masses: relative value of gray-scale, color Doppler, and spectral Doppler sonography. AJR Am J Roentgenol 1995;164:381–6.

8. Buy JN, Ghossain MA, Hugol D, et al. Characterization of adnexal masses: combination of color Doppler and conventional sonography compared with spectral Doppler analysis alone and conventional sonography alone. AJR Am J Roentgenol 1996;166:385–93.

9. Timmerman D, Valentin L, Bourne TH, et al. Terms, definitions and measurements to describe the sonographic features of adnexal tumors: a consensus opinion from the International Ovarian Tumor Analysis (IOTA) group. Ultrasound Obstet Gynecol 2000;16:500–5.

10. Berridge DL, Winter TC. Saline infusion sonohysterography: technique, indications, and imaging findings. J Ultrasound Med 2004;23:97–112.

11. Cheerer LJ, Bartolucci L. Ultrasound evaluation of the cervix. In: Callen PW, editor. Ultrasonography in obstetrics and gynecology. 5th edition. Philadelphia: WB Saunders; 2007. p. 479–85.

12. Merz E, Miric-Tesanic D, Bahlmann F, et al. Sonographic size of uterus and ovaries in pre- and postmenopausal women. Ultrasound Obstet Gynecol 1996;7:38–42.

13. Occhipinti K, Kutcher R, Rosenblatt R. Sonographic appearance and significance of arcuate artery calcification. J Ultrasound Med 1991;10:97–100.

14. Fleischer AC, Kalermeri GC, Entmann SS. Sonographic depiction of the endometrium during normal cycles. Ultrasound Med Biol 1986;12:271–7.

15. Wildenberg JC, Yam BI, Langer JE, et al. US of the nongravid cervix with multimodality imaging correlation: normal appearance, pathologic conditions, and diagnostic pitfalls. Radiographics 2016;36:596–617.

16. Cohen HL, Tice HM, Mandel FS. Ovarian volumes measured by US: bigger than we think. Radiology 1990;177:189–92.

17. Hall DA, Hann LE, Ferrucci JT Jr, et al. Sconographic morpology of the normal menstrual cycle. Radiology 1979;133:185–8.

18. Baerwald AR, Adams GP, Pierson RA. Form and function of the corpus luteum during the human menstrual cycle. Ultrasound Obstet Gynecol 2005;25:498–507.

19. Healy DL, Bell R, Robertson DM, et al. Ovarian status in healthy postmenopausal women. Menopause 2008;15:1109–14.

20. Muradlai D, Colgin T, Hayeems E, et al. Echogenic ovarian foci without shadowing: are they caused by psammomatous calcifications? Radiology 2002;224:429–35.

21. Lune S, Piper I, Woliovitch I, et al. Age-related prevalence of sonographicaly confirmed uterine myomas. J Obstet Gynaecol 2005;25:42–4.

22. Chu LC, Coquia SF, Hamper UM. Ultrasonography evaluation of pelvic masses. Radiol Clin North Am 2014;52:1237–52.

23. Arleo EK, Schwartz PE, Hui P, et al. Review of leiomyoma variants. AJR Am J Roentgenol 2015;205:912–21.

24. Miccò M, Sala E, Lakhman Y, et al. Imaging features of uncommon gynecologic cancers. AJR Am J Roentgenol 2015;205:1346–59.

25. D'Angelo E, Prat J. Uterine sarcomas: a review. Gynecol Oncol 2010;116:131–9.

26. Meinhold-Heerlein I, Fotopoulou C, Harter P, et al. The new WHO classification of ovarian, fallopian tube, and primary peritoneal cancer and its clinical implications. Arch Gynecol Obstet 2016;293(4):695–700.

27. Kurjak A, Kupesic S, Shalan H, et al. Uterine sarcoma: a report of 10 cases studied by transvaginal color and pulsed Doppler sonography. Gynecol Oncol 1995;59:342–6.

28. Exacoustos C, Romanini ME, Amadio A, et al. Can gray-scale and color Doppler sonography differentiate between uterine leiomyosarcoma and leiomyoma? J Clin Ultrasound 2007;35:449–57.

29. Goldstein RB, Bree RL, Benson CB, et al. Evaluation of the woman with postmenopausal bleeding. Society of Radiologist in Ultrasound-sponsored consensus conference statement. J Ultrasound Med 2001;20:1025–36.

30. Lee SI. An imaging algorithm for evaluation of abnormal uterine bleeding: does sonohysterography play a role? Menopause 2017;14:823–5.

31. Smith-Bindman R, Weiss E, Feldstein V. How thick is too thick? When endometrial thickness should prompt biopsy in postmenopausal women without vaginal bleeding. Ultrasound Obstet Gynecol 2004;24:558–65.

32. Erdem M, Bilgin U, Bozkurt N, et al. Comparison of transvaginal ultrasonography and saline infusion sonohysterography in evaluating the endometrial cavity in pre- and postmenopausal women with abnormal uterine bleeding. Menopause 2007;14:846–52.

33. Shi AA, Lee SI. Algorithmic workup of abnormal vaginal bleeding with endovaginal sonography and sonohysterography: self-assessment nodule. AJR Am J Roentgenol 2008;191:S74–8.

34. Kurman RJ. Blaustein's pathology of the female genital tract. 4th edition. New York: Springer-Verlag; 1994.

35. Nalahoff KM, Pellerito JS, Ben-Levi E. Imaging the endometrium: disease and normal variants. Radiographics 2001;21:1409–24.

36. Shia S, Wilson SR. Gynecologic ultrasound. In: Rumcak CM, Wilson SR, Charboneau WJ, et al, editors. Diagnostic ultrasound. 3rd edition. Philadelphia: Elsevier Mosby; 2005. p. 527–87.

37. Cruz Lee S, Kaunitz AM, Sanchez-Ramos L, et al. The oncogenic potential of endometrial polyps. A systematic review and meta-analysis. Obstet Gynecol 2010;116:1197–205.

38. Siegel R, Naishadham D, Memal A. Cancer statistics, 2012. CA Cancer J Clin 2012;62:10–29.

39. Tirumani SF, Shanghogue AKP, Prasa SR. Current concepts in the diagnosis and management of endometrial and cervical carcinomas. Radiol Clin North Am 2016;51:1087–110.

40. Epstein E, Skoog L, Isberg PE, et al. An algorithm including results of gray-scale and power Doppler ultrasound examination to predict endometrial malignancy in women with postmenopausal bleeding. Ultrasound Obstet Gynecol 2002;20:370–6.

41. Opolskiene G, Sladkevicius P, Valentin L. Prediction of endometrial malignancy in women with postmenopausal bleeding and sonographic endometrial thickness ≥4.5mm. Ultrasound Obstet Gynecol 2011;37:232–40.

42. Savelli L, Ceccarini M, Ludovisi M, et al. Preoperative local staging of endometrial cancer: transvaginal sonography vs. magnetic resonance imaging. Ultrasound Obstet Gynecol 2008;31:560–6.

43. Antonsen SL, Jensen LN, Loft A, et al. MRI, PET/CT and ultrasound in the preoperative staging of endometrial cancer—a multicenter prospective comparative study. Gynecol Oncol 2013;128:300–8.

44. Fischerova D, Fruhauf F, Zikan M, et al. Factors affecting sonographic preoperative local staging of endometrial cancer. Ultrasound Obstet Gynecol 2014;4:575–85.

45. Alcazar JL, Pineda L, Martinez-Astorquiza CT, et al. Transvaginal/transrectal ultrasound for assessing myometrial invasion in endometrial cancer: a comparison of six different approaches. J Gynecol Oncol 2015;26:201–7.

46. Alcazar JL, Orozco R, Martinez-Astorquiza CT, et al. Transvaginal ultrasound for preoperative assessment of myometrial invasion in patients with endometrial cancer: a systematic review and meta-analysis. Ultrasound Obstet Gynecol 2015;46:405–13.

47. Takac I. Transvaginal ultrasonography with and without saline infusion in assessment of myometrial invasion of endometrial cancer. J Ultrasound Med 2007;26:949–55.

48. Alcazar JL, Errasti T, Zornoza A. Saline infusion sonohysterography in endometrial cancer: assessment of malignant cells dissemination risk. Acta Obstet Gynecol Scand 2000;79:321–2.

49. Akbayir O, Corbacioglu A, Numanoglu C, et al. Preoperative assessment of myometrial and cervical invasion in endometrial carcinoma by transvaginal ultrasound. Gynecol Oncol 2011;122:600–3.

50. Jantarasaengaram S, Praditphol N, Tansathit T, et al. Three-dimensional ultrasound with volume contrast imaging for preoperative assessment of myometrial invasion and cervical involvement in women with endometrial cancer. Ultrasound Obstet Gynecol 2014;43:569–74.

51. Katz VL. Benign gynecological lesions. In: Lentz GM, Lobo RA, Gershenson M, et al, editors. Comprehensive gynecology. 6th edition. Philadelphia: Elsevier Mosby; 2012. p. 383–432.

52. Stamatellos I, Stamatopoulos P, Bontis J. The role of hysteroscopy in the current management of the cervical polyps. Arch Gynecol Obstet 2017;276:299–303.

53. Esim Buyukbayrak E, Karageyim Karisday AY, Kars B, et al. Cervical polyps: evaluation of routine removal and need for accompanying D&C. Arch Gynecol Obstet 2011;283:581–4.

54. Jhingran A, Russell AH, Seiden MV, et al. Cancers of the cervix, vulva, and vagina. In: Niederhuber JE, Armitage JO, Doroshow JH, et al, editors. Abeloff's clinical oncology. 5th edition. Philadelphia: Elsevier Saunders; 2014. p. 1534–74.

55. Freeman SJ, Aly AM, Kataoka MY, et al. The revised FIGO staging system for uterine malignancies: implications for MR imaging. Radiographics 2012;32:1805–27.

56. Okamoto Y, Tanaka YO, Nishida M, et al. MR imaging of the uterine cervix: imaging-pathology correlation. Radiographics 2003;23:425–46.

57. Testa AC, Ludovisi M, Manfredi R, et al. Transvaginal ultrasonography and magnetic resonance imaging for assessment of presence, size and extent of invasive cervical cancer. Ultrasound Obstet Gynecol 2009;34:335–44.

58. Jacobs I, Oram D, Fairbanks J, et al. A risk of malignancy index incorporating CA 125, ultrasound and menopausal status for the accurate preoperative diagnosis of ovarian cancer. Br J Obstet Gynaecol 1990;97:922–9.

59. Tingulstad S, Hagen B, Skjeldestad FE, et al. Evaluation of a risk of malignancy index based on serum CA125, ultrasound findings and menopausal status in the pre-operative diagnosis of pelvic masses. Br J Obstet Gynaecol 1996;103:826–31.

60. Twickler DM, Moschos E. Ultrasound and assessment of ovarian cancer risk. AJR Am J Roentgenol 2010;194:322–9.

61. International Ovarian Tumor Analysis (IOTA). 2017 ADNEX model. 2017. Available at: http://www.iotagroup.org/adnexmodel/. Accessed July 2, 2017.

62. Deshpande N, Ren Y, Foygel K, et al. Tumor angiogenic marker expression levels during tumor growth: longitudinal assessment with molecularly targeted microbubbles and US imaging. Radiology 2011;258:804–11.

63. Ohman AW, Hasan N, Dinulescu DM. Advances in tumor screening, imaging, and avatar technologies for high-grade serous ovarian cancer. Front Oncol 2014;4:322.

64. Levine D, Brown DL, Andreotti RF, et al. Management of asymptomatic ovarian and other adnexal cysts imaged at US. Society of Radiologists in Ultrasound consensus conference statement. Ultrasound Q 2010;26:121–31.

65. Ekerhovd E, Wienerroith H, Staudach A, et al. Preoperative assessment of unilocular adnexal cysts by transvaginal ultrasonography: a comparison between ultrasonographic morphologic imaging and histopathologic diagnosis. Am J Obstet Gynecol 2001;184:48–54.

66. Ghezzi F, Cromi A, Bergamini V, et al. Should adnexal mass size influence surgical approach? A series of 186 laparoscopically managed large adnexal masses. BJOG 2008;115:1020–7.

67. Laing FC, Allison SJ. US of the ovary and adnexa: to worry of not to worry? Radiographics 2012;32: 1621–39.

68. Patel MD. Practical approach to the adnexal mass. Radiol Clin North Am 2006;44:879–99.

69. Sokalska A, Timmerman D, Testa AC, et al. Diagnostic accuracy of transvaginal ultrasound examination for assigning a specific diagnosis to adnexal masses. Ultrasound Obstet Gynecol 2009;34:462–70.

70. Kobayashi H, Sumimoto K, Kitanaka T, et al. Ovarian endometrioma: risk factors of ovarian cancer development. Eur J Obstet Gynecol Reprod Biol 2008;138:187–93.

71. Prat J, FIGO Committee on Gynecologic Oncology. Staging classification for cancer of the ovary, fallopian tube, and peritoneum. Int J Gynaecol Obstet 2014;124:1–5.

72. Javadi S, Ganeshan DM, Qayyum A, et al. Ovarian cancer, the revised FIGO staging system, and the role of imaging. AJR Am J Roentgenol 2016;206: 1351–60.

73. Brown DL, Doubilet PM, Miller FH, et al. Benign and malignant ovarian masses: selection of the most discriminating gray scale and Doppler sonographic features. Radiology 1998;208:103–10.

74. Ackerman S, Irshad A, Lew M, et al. Ovarian cystic lesions: a current approach to diagnosis and management. Radiol Clin North Am 2013; 51:1067–85.

75. Castillo G, Alcázar JL, Jurado M. Natural history of sonographically detected simple unilocular adnexal cysts in asymptomatic postmenopausal women. Gynecol Oncol 2004;92:965–9.

76. Green GE, Mortele KJ, Glickman JN, et al. Brenner tumors of the ovary: sonographic and computed tomographic imaging features. J Ultrasound Med 2006;25:1245–51.

77. Caspi B, Appelman Z, Rabinerson D, et al. Pathognomonic echo patterns of benign cystic teratomas of the ovary: classification, incidence and accuracy rate of sonographic diagnosis. Ultrasound Obstet Gynecol 1996;7:275–9.

78. Patel MD, Feldstein VA, Lipson SD, et al. Cystic teratomas of the ovary: diagnostic value of sonography. AJR Am J Roentgenol 1998;171:1061–5.

79. Rim SY, Kim SM, Choi HS. Malignant transformation of ovarian mature cystic teratoma. Int J Gynecol Cancer 2006;16:140–4.

80. Yamanaka Y, Tateiwa Y, Miyamoto H, et al. Preoperative diagnosis of malignant transformation in mature cystic teratoma of the ovary. Eur J Gynaecol Oncol 2005;26:391–2.

81. Talerman A. Germ cell tumors of the ovary. In: Kurman RJ, editor. Blaustein's pathology of the female genital tract. 5th edition. New York: Springer-Verlag; 2002. p. 967–1033.

82. Kim SH, Kang SB. Ovarian dysgerminoma: color Doppler ultrasonographic findings and comparison with CT and MR imaging findings. J Ultrasound Med 1995;14:843–8.

83. Demidov VN, Lipatenkova J, Vikhareva O, et al. Imaging of gynecological disease (2): clinical and ultrasound characteristics of Sertoli cell tumors, Sertoli-Leydig cell tumors and Leydig cell tumors. Ultrasound Obstet Gynecol 2008;31:85–91.

84. Van Holsbeke C, Domali E, Holland TK, et al. Imaging of gynecological disease (3): clinical and ultrasound characteristics of granulosa cell tumors of the ovary. Ultrasound Obstet Gynecol 2008;31:450–6.

85. Testa AC, Ferrandina G, Timmerman D, et al. Imaging in gynecologic disease (1): ultrasound features of metastases in the ovaries differ depending on the origin of the primary tumor. Ultrasound Obstet Gynecol 2007;29:505–11.

86. Schneider C, Wight E, Perucchini D, et al. Primary carcinoma of the fallopian tube. A report of 19 cases with literature review. Eur J Gynaecol Oncol 2000;21:578–82.

87. Callahan MJ, Crum CP, Medeiros F, et al. Primary fallopian tube malignancies in BRCA-positive women undergoing surgery for ovarian cancer risk reduction. J Clin Oncol 2007;25:3985–90.

88. Kurman RJ, Shih Ie M. The origin and pathogenesis of epithelial ovarian cancer: a proposed unifying theory. Am J Surg Pathol 2010;34:433–43.

89. Vang R, Shih Le M, Kurman RJ. Fallopian tube precursors of ovarian low- and high-grade serous neoplasms. Histopathology 2013;16:44–58.

90. Vang R, Wheeler JE. Diseases of the fallopian tube and paratubal region. In: Kurman RJ, Ellenson LH, Ronnett BM, editors. Blaustein's pathology of the female genital tract. 6th edition. New York: Springer-Verlag; 2011. p. 554–69.

91. Patel MD, Acord DL, Young SW. Likelihood ratio of sonographic findings in discriminating hydrosalpinx from other adnexal masses. AJR Am J Roentgenol 2006;186:1033–8.

92. Ko ML, Jeng CJ, Chen SC, et al. Sonographic appearance of fallopian tube carcinoma. J Clin Ultrasound 2005;33:372–4.

93. Ludovisi M, DeBlasis I, Virgillio B, et al. Imaging in gynecologic disease (9): clinical and ultrasound characteristic of tubal cancer. Ultrasound Obstet Gynecol 2014;43:328–35.

94. Palmer JR. Advances in the epidemiology of gestational trophoblastic disease. J Reprod Med 1994;39:155–62.

95. Lawler SD, Fisher RA, Dent J. A prospective genetic study of complete and partial hydatidiform moles. Am J Obstet Gynecol 1991;164:1270–7.

96. Fisher RA, Newlands ES. Gestational trophoblastic disease. Molecular and genetic studies. J Reprod Med 1998;43:87–97.

97. Berkowitz RS, Goldstein DP. Clinical practice. Molar pregnancy. N Engl J Med 2009;360:1639–45.

98. Green CL, Angtuaco TL, Shah HR, et al. Gestational trophoblastic disease: a spectrum of radiologic diagnosis. Radiographics 1996;16:1371–84.

99. Shaaban AM, Rezvani M, Haroun RR, et al. Gestational trophoblastic disease: clinical and imaging features. Radiographics 2017;37:681–700.

100. Fowler DJ, Lindsay I, Seckl MJ, et al. Routine pre-evacuation ultrasound diagnosis of hydatidiform mole: experience of more than 1000 cases from a regional referral center. Ultrasound Obstet Gynecol 2006;27:56–60.

101. Lurain JR. Gestational trophoblastic disease. Epidemiology, pathology, clinical presentation and diagnosis of gestational trophoblastic disease, and management of hydatidiform mole. Am J Obstet Gynecol 2010;203:531–9.

102. Allen SD, Lim AK, Seckl MJ, et al. Radiology of gestational trophoblastic neoplasia. Clin Radiol 2006;61:301–13.

103. FIGO Committee on Gynecology Oncology. Current FIGO staging for cancer of the vagina, fallopian tube, ovary, and gestational trophoblastic neoplasia. Int J Gynaecol Obstet 2009;105:3–4.

104. Semer DA, Macfee MS. Gestational trophoblastic disease: epidemiology. Semin Oncol 1995;22:109–12.

105. Baergen RN, Rutgers JL, Young RH, et al. Placental site trophoblastic tumor: a study of 55 cases and review of the literature emphasizing factors of prognostic significance. Gynecol Oncol 2006;100:511–20.

106. Zhou Y, Lu H, Yu C, et al. Sonographic characteristics of placental site trophoblastic tumor. Ultrasound Obstet Gynecol 2013;41:679–84.

[18F]-2-Fluoro-2-Deoxy-D-glucose–PET Assessment of Cervical Cancer

Chitra Viswanathan, MD*, Silvana Faria, MD, PhD,
Catherine Devine, MD, Madhavi Patnana, MD,
Tara Sagebiel, MD, Revathy B. Iyer, MD, Priya R. Bhosale, MD

KEYWORDS

- Cervical cancer • PET/CT • PET/MR imaging • Cancer staging • Treatment planning

KEY POINTS

- PET/computed tomography is a highly valuable imaging modality in the assessment of patients with cervical cancer, providing prognostic and staging information.
- The metabolic parameters of the primary tumor (maximum standardized uptake value [SUVmax], metabolic tumor volume, and total lesion glycolysis) have been shown to correlate with patient outcome and survival.
- The presence of lymph node involvement and the SUVmax of the lymph nodes are significant prognostic factors.
- By combining metabolic imaging with the anatomic detail of the primary tumor, PET/MR imaging enhances treatment and care for patients with cervical cancer with a decreased radiation dose.

INTRODUCTION

According to the American Cancer Society, there will be 12,280 new diagnoses and 4210 deaths attributable to cervical cancer in 2017.[1] Worldwide, cervical cancer is the fourth most common cause of cancer, with a disease incidence of approximately 520,000 cases per year with 265,000 deaths.[2] In the Western world, most cancers are now diagnosed in the preclinical stage as a result of active screening with the Papanicolaou test. This screening has reduced the incidence of cervical cancer significantly by more than 50%. Additionally, human papilloma virus (HPV) has been found to be a causal factor, with HPV subtypes 16 and 18 a cause in 99% of cervical tumors.[3] The implementation of the HPV vaccine has decreased the disease incidence as well. Despite these measures, cervical cancer continues to be a major health issue worldwide.

The clinical staging system used worldwide is the International Federation of Gynecology and Obstetrics (FIGO). Where available, modalities such as computed tomography (CT), MR imaging, PET/CT, that provide anatomic and metabolic information are highly useful and impact patient therapy and treatment. The treatment of most stages of cervical cancer is chemoradiation, and imaging helps guide the treatment planning. The goal of this review is to provide evidence of the utility of PET imaging, primarily PET/CT, in the diagnosis, staging, treatment planning, and evaluation of tumor recurrence in patients with cervical cancer.

DETECTION

In the Western world, the use of active screening Papanicolaou testing in women aged 21 to 70 years allows early detection of preinvasive and early

Department of Diagnostic Radiology, Division of Diagnostic Imaging, The University of Texas MD Anderson Cancer Center, 1400 Pressler Street, Unit 1473, Houston, TX 77030-4008, USA
* Corresponding author.
E-mail address: Chitra.Viswanathan@mdanderson.org

PET Clin 13 (2018) 165–177
https://doi.org/10.1016/j.cpet.2017.11.004
1556-8598/18/© 2017 Elsevier Inc. All rights reserved.

stage cancers (stage 1) before patients present with symptoms and findings on clinical examination. Symptomatic patients with more advanced tumors may present with postcoital bleeding, intermenstrual and postmenstrual bleeding, foul-smelling discharge, chronic anemia, and mass.[4]

Risk factors for cervical cancer include early age of sexual activity, genital warts, cigarette smoking, greater number of sexual partners, immunosuppression, human immunodeficiency virus positive status, and HPV infection serotypes 16 and 18. With the strong causal relationship between HPV and cervical cancer, patients older than 30 years have HPV testing at the time of a Papanicolaou test.[3]

PATHOLOGY

The World Health Organization histological classification includes squamous (epithelial), glandular (adenocarcinoma), and other epithelial tumors, such as adenosquamous, neuroendocrine, and undifferentiated carcinoma. Most cervical cancer cases are of squamous cell histology, accounting for 70% to 80% of cases. Adenocarcinoma histologies account for 20% to 25%.[5] The nonsquamous pathologies are associated with worse prognoses.[3]

STAGING

Cervical cancer first spreads locally to adjacent structures, such as the vagina, bladder, ureters, and rectum. Then, spread occurs via the pelvic, para-aortic, and supraclavicular lymph nodes in a cephalad fashion. Hematogenous spread occurs to the non-nodal distal sites.[6]

Cervical cancer is most commonly staged using the FIGO and the American Joint Committee on Cancer TNM systems (Table 1). FIGO is a clinical staging system that uses a physical examination, including examination under anesthesia, cystoscopy, colposcopy, proctoscopy, hysteroscopy, barium enema examination, intravenous urography (IVU), radiography of the chest and skeleton, and endocervical curettage and biopsy[7] The use of the FIGO system allows for uniform worldwide staging of patients; but the system is limited in that it does not account for information and factors that affect the prognosis and management, such as lymph node status[3]

ANATOMIC IMAGING

CT and MR imaging historically have been performed for anatomic assessment and locoregional involvement before the development of metabolic imaging. CT can assess for regional lymph nodes, distal metastases, and hydronephrosis; it has eliminated the need for lymphoscintigraphy and IVU in areas with access to CT. However, CT is limited in its soft-tissue resolution and assessment of cervical tumor invasion, parametrial invasion, and pelvic sidewall involvement. In this regard, MR imaging is highly valuable in the evaluation of the primary tumor. MR imaging has close to 90% accuracy in the local staging of cervical cancer tumors greater than 1 cm. MR imaging is superior in the evaluation of tumor size, extension, and location. This superiority is very helpful in treatment planning, in separating patients who can undergo surgical resection versus those who receive chemoradiation.[8]

However, the limitation of CT and MR imaging arises in the evaluation of metastatic nodal disease in the preoperative setting. CT and MR imaging are limited in the evaluation of micrometastatic disease in lymph nodes smaller than 1 cm. They also cannot reliably detect reactive nodes versus metastatic nodes greater than 1 cm.

[18F]-2-FLUORO-2-DEOXY-D-GLUCOSE–PET/COMPUTED TOMOGRAPHY

PET is most commonly performed with the radiotracer [18F]-2-fluoro-2-Deoxy-D-glucose (FDG). FDG PET/CT depends on physiologic changes and is based on the degree of uptake and metabolism of glucose, which is abnormal in tumors as compared with surrounding tissues. Historically, PET used to be performed as a standalone procedure. The use of FDG PET alone is an older technique recently replaced with FDG PET/CT given the value of hybrid metabolic and anatomic imaging.

PROTOCOLS

FDG PET/CT can be performed in 2 ways. CT can be performed with a low-dose radiation technique for coregistration and attenuation-correction, or contrast-enhanced (CE) CT can be performed with oral and intravenous contrast administration for diagnosis, attenuation correction, and coregistration.

Patients are asked to fast for 6 hours before the procedure. If diabetic, they are asked to hold their medication or insulin for 6 hours before the study.[8] The intravenous injection of a weight-based amount of FDG (0.22 mCi/kg) is then given. If patients are receiving a CE examination, oral contrast material is given at this time as well. After approximately 60 to 90 minutes to allow for the uptake of radiotracer, the combined PET/CT is obtained. PET acquisition from the proximal thighs to the skull base occurs after patients empty their

Table 1
International Federation of Gynecology and Obstetrics and TNM staging classifications of cervical cancer

FIGO	TNM	Tumor Characteristics	Therapy
	TX	Primary tumor not detectable	—
	T0	No evidence of primary tumor	
	Tis	Carcinoma in situ (preinvasive carcinoma)	Surgery
I	T1	Carcinoma confined to the cervix (disregard extension to uterine corpus)	Surgery
IA	T1a	Invasive carcinoma diagnosed by microscopy; stromal invasion with maximum depth of 5 mm from base of epithelium and horizontal spread ≤7.0 mm	Surgery
IA1	T1a1	Stromal invasion ≤3.0 mm in depth and ≤7.0 mm in horizontal spread	Surgery
IA2	T1a2	Stromal invasion >3.0 mm and ≤5.0 mm with horizontal spread ≤7.0 mm	Surgery
IB	T1b	Clinical lesion confined to cervix or microscopic lesion >T1a/IA2	Surgery
IB1	T1b1	Clinical visible lesion ≤4.0 cm in greatest dimension	Surgery
IB2	T1b2	Clinical visible lesion >4.0 cm in greatest dimension	Surgery
II	T2	Extension beyond uterus but not to pelvic wall or lower one-third of vagina	Surgery
IIA	T2a	Tumor without parametrial invasion	Surgery
IIA1	T2a1	Clinical visible lesion ≤4.0 cm in greatest dimension	CRT ± surgery
IIA2	T2a2	Clinical visible lesion >4.0 cm in greatest dimension	CRT ± surgery
IIB	T2b	Tumor with parametrial invasion	CRT
III	T3	Tumor extends to pelvic wall and/or involves lower one-third of vagina and/or causes hydronephrosis or nonfunctional kidney	CRT
IIIA	T3a	Tumor involves lower one-third of vagina, no extension to pelvic wall	CRT
IIIB	T3b	Tumor extends to pelvic wall and/or causes hydronephrosis or nonfunctional kidney	CRT
IV	T4	Tumor invades bladder or rectum and/or extends below true pelvis	CRT
IVA	T4a	Tumor invades bladder or rectum	CRT
IVB	T4b	Tumor extends beyond true pelvis	CRT/chemotherapy

Abbreviation: CRT, chemoradiation.

bladder to avoid intense bladder activity. CT acquisition occurs after the administration of intravenous contrast material. PET imaging information is reconstructed and available with CT attenuation correction (AC) or without CT AC. The images are sent to a dedicated software platform and fused for image analysis.[9]

STAGING
Primary Tumor

FDG PET/CT has been shown to be useful in the detection of the primary tumor and in the assessment of tumor volume. The normal cervix does not accumulate FDG much over the background tissue. The metabolic activity of the primary tumor,

as measured by maximum standardized uptake value (SUVmax), has been shown in many studies to be a prognostic indicator in patients with cervical cancer (**Fig. 1**). In their study of 59 patients with stage IA2 to IIB cervical cancer who underwent PET/CT followed by surgery, Yagi and colleagues[10] found patients with a higher SUVmax tumors have lower overall survival (OS) and progression-free survival (PFS). These higher SUVmax tumors are also associated with lymph node metastases, advanced stage, lymphovascular invasion, and larger tumors. Kidd and colleagues[11] found that SUVmax of the primary tumor also has other prognostic value, having a correlation with histology and differentiation. Other quantitative data obtained from PET/CT have been

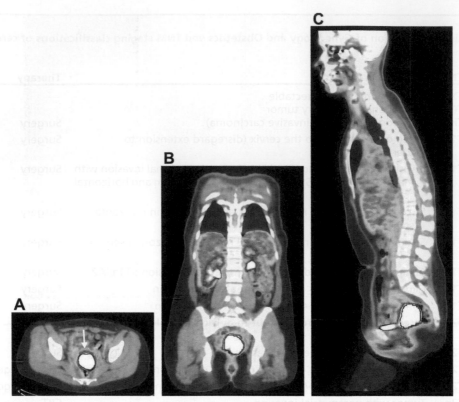

Fig. 1. PET/CT in initial evaluation of cervical cancer primary tumor. A 46-year-old woman with stage IIB squamous cell carcinoma of cervix. (*A–C*) Axial (*A*), coronal (*B*), and sagittal (*C*) fused PET/CT images show an intensely FDG-avid cervical mass (*arrow*) with SUVmax 15.5, metabolic tumor volume 70.64 mL, and total lesion glycolysis 623.0 mL.

shown to be helpful, such as metabolic tumor volume (MTV) and total lesion glycolysis (TLG).[12,13] Zhang and colleagues[14] compared the gross tumor volume (GTV) as assessed by CT, MR imaging, and PET/CT with pathologic volume in 10 patients with stages I to II cervical cancer and found that PET/CT GTV determined to be less than 40% SUVmax had the best correlation with pathology volume. Yang and colleagues[15] found that PET/CT better evaluates the depth of cervical stromal invasion than conventional methods using SUVmax of 7.83 or MTV of 8.76 mL and may allow for better treatment planning.

Lymph Node Metastases

The lymph node status has been shown to be a significant prognostic indicator for survival. In cervical cancer, metastases can involve the pelvic and para-aortic lymph node chains (**Fig. 2**). FDG PET/CT is valuable in detecting metastases in the typical distribution but also in identifying any other lymph nodes.[16] In their 2001 study, Grigsby and colleagues[17] showed in their retrospective study that FDG PET was superior to CT in the detection of abnormal nodes and prediction of treatment outcomes. Kidd and colleagues[18] showed in their larger patient prospective study that the frequency of FDG-avid lymph nodes correlates with the stage. Patients with FDG-avid lymph nodes have poorer outcomes as compared with patients without FDG-avid lymph nodes within the same stage. In their additional study of 83 patients, Kidd and colleagues[19] showed the SUVmax of the pelvic lymph node (PLN) is a prognostic biomarker for cervical cancer response, recurrence, and survival.

Onal and colleagues[20] recently studied 93 patients with pelvic and para-aortic lymph node metastases and found patients with PLN metastases SUVmax of 7.5 or greater had larger lymph node metastases, higher SUVmax primary tumor, higher rate of para-aortic lymph node involvement, and lower post-therapy complete response rates. Rose and colleagues[21] showed that PET has high specificity and sensitivity for predicting pelvic and para-aortic lymphadenopathy and for showing the presence and absence of disease.

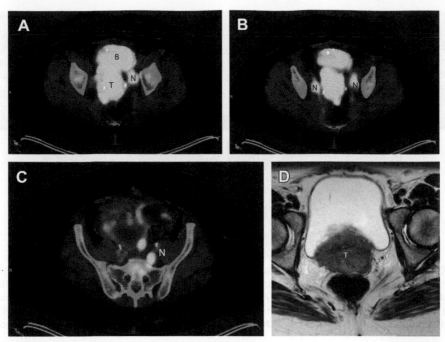

Fig. 2. PET/CT in initial evaluation of cervical cancer primary tumor and lymph nodes. A 57-year-old woman with stage IV squamous cell carcinoma of the cervix. (*A*) Axial fused FDG PET/CT shows cervical tumor (T) with posterior bladder (B) involvement along with anterior rectal invasion and extension to bilateral uterosacral ligaments and upper one-third of vagina. Also note left pelvic sidewall lymphadenopathy (N). (*B*) Axial fused PET/CT shows bilateral pelvic sidewall lymphadenopathy (N), consisting of 2.7-cm left external iliac node and 2.8-cm right external iliac node. (*C*) Axial fused PET/CT shows 1.0-cm left common iliac node (N). As a result of the PET/CT findings, the patient will be treated with definitive chemoradiation to include the pelvis and retroperitoneum. (*D*) Axial T2-weighted MR imaging better shows the rectal and bladder involvement by cervical tumor (T).

PET/CT may be of limited usefulness in early stage cervical tumors. Driscoll and colleagues[22] found PET/CT to be of limited value in their cohort of patients with early stage (stages IA–IB1) MR imaging lymph node–negative cervical cancer. Signorelli and colleagues[23] evaluated 159 women with stages IB1 and IIA cervical cancer and found that PET/CT had low sensitivity for lymph node involvement and did not change management in treatment planning.

Distal Metastatic Disease

FDG PET/CT is valuable in the assessment of distal metastatic disease. Tumors can spread hematogenously to the lungs, liver, and bone marrow (**Fig. 3**). Liu and colleagues[24] studied patients with advanced-stage disease, lymph node metastases, and suspected recurrent disease and found PET/CT to be superior to MR imaging and CT for evaluation of osseous disease (**Fig. 4**). They also found an association between lymph node metastases and osseous metastatic disease. Loft and colleagues[25] found metastatic disease in 10 of 119 patients and concluded

PET/CT has a sensitivity of 100%, specificity of 94%, positive predictive value of 63%, and negative predictive value (NPV) of 100%.

TREATMENT PLANNING

Treatment of cervical cancer includes surgery, radiation, chemotherapy, and/or a combination of these modalities. For most of the stages, chemoradiation is the primary mode of treatment. Aside from its diagnostic and prognostic factors, PET/CT is used for radiation treatment plan modeling and dose allocation.

External Beam Radiation Therapy

Studies have found that PET/CT is useful in radiation treatment planning to assess the treatment volume, treatment dose, and to direct therapy to the lymph nodes. External beam radiation may be given to the pelvis only if patients have a tumor in the pelvis and lymph nodes confined to the pelvis. If there is para-aortic nodal involvement, then radiation will be given to the pelvis and para-aortic region. Radiation treatment planning

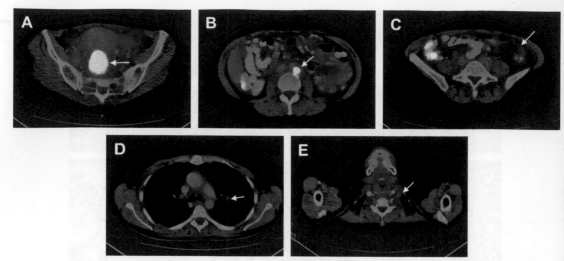

Fig. 3. PET/CT in evaluation of metastatic disease. A 46-year-old woman with stage IVB poorly differentiated cervical carcinoma. (*A*) Axial fused FDG PET/CT shows primary cervical tumor (*arrow*). (*B*) Axial fused PET/CT shows FDG-avid left common iliac node (*arrow*). (*C*) Axial fused PET/CT through upper pelvis shows stranding in left omental fat with mild FDG uptake (*arrow*), in keeping with peritoneal disease. (*D*) Axial fused PET/CT shows an FDG-avid left lung nodule (*arrow*). (*E*) Axial fused PET/CT shows an FDG-avid left supraclavicular node (*arrow*).

contours can be made from the PET/CT images to specifically target the FDG-avid tumor regions and to decrease the dose to adjacent organs not involved with the tumor.[26] The field may be extended to include nodal involvement.[27]

Brachytherapy

Intracavitary brachytherapy can be performed using 2-dimensional techniques, such as radiography, and 3-dimensional (3D) techniques, such as CT, MR imaging, and FDG PET/CT.[28] PET/CT has the advantage of not depending on anatomic details like CT and MR imaging, but rather depending on changes in metabolic activity. The metabolic activity of the tumor on PET/CT can be directly overlaid on the CT image of the intracavitary applicators, and dose calculations can be obtained

accordingly. Changes in metabolic activity can be monitored using PET/CT during the course of radiation therapy.[27]

Evidence

Chung and colleagues[29] found a higher disease-free survival and overall better survival when PET/CT intensity-modulated radiation therapy, image-guided radiation therapy, and 3D brachytherapy treatment planning were used in their study set of 72 patients with advanced cervical cancer with pelvic, para-aortic, and supraclavicular nodes. The main causes of treatment failure were out-of-field disease at the junction of the treatment plan and distal metastatic disease. The use of PET/CT in this regard can be very helpful in targeting the tumor and sparing normal adjacent

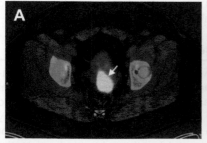
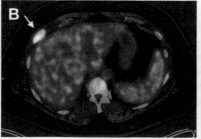
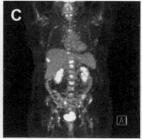

Fig. 4. PET/CT in evaluation of osseous metastatic disease. A 40-year-old woman with stage IIA poorly differentiated adenocarcinoma of the cervix. (*A*) Axial fused FDG PET/CT shows primary cervical tumor (*arrow*). (*B*) Axial fused PET/CT shows FDG-avid right rib lesion (*arrow*). (*C*) Coronal PET maximum-intensity-projection image shows multiple FDG-avid osseous lesions compatible with widespread bone marrow metastases.

tissues. Lazzari and colleagues[30] reported that FDG PET/CT helps accurately determine tumor volumes, which enables a higher dose to smaller areas and may allow for dose escalation. This ability helps decrease patient morbidity from treatment and possible side effects.

FOLLOW-UP EVALUATION
Response Assessment

PET/CT is usually performed 3 to 7 months after chemoradiation to determine the efficacy of the treatment and to determine the follow-up interval required.[28] The response to therapy is related to the prognosis (**Fig. 5**). Kidd and colleagues[31]

studied the SUVmax, MTV, and tumor heterogeneity in 25 patients with stages IA to IV cervical cancer at different time points after treatment. They found that SUVmax declines with treatment and pretreatment and 4-week SUVmax measurements represent the best time points for the assessment of response. There were 5 patients with persistent or new disease on the 3-month follow-up FDG PET/CT, and these patients showed higher SUVmax and tumor heterogeneity at all time points. Schwarz and colleagues[32] did a retrospective analysis of 92 patients after external radiation, brachytherapy, and concurrent chemotherapy and found that the 3-month post-therapy SUVmax is predictive of survival. Seventy percent of the

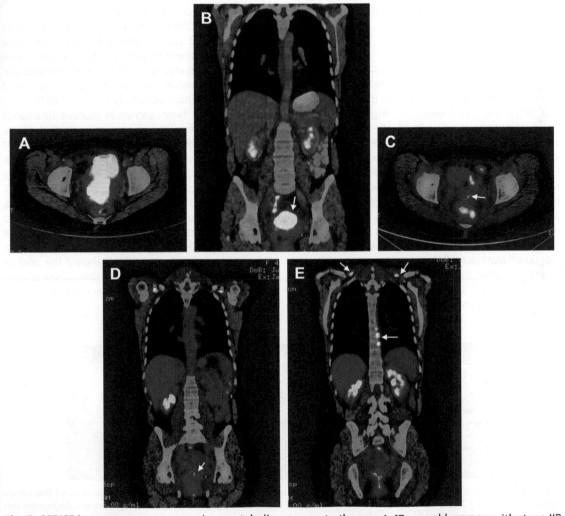

Fig. 5. PET/CT in tumor response: complete metabolic response to therapy. A 47-year-old woman with stage IIB squamous cell carcinoma of the cervix. (*A, B*) Axial (*A*) and coronal (*B*) fused FDG PET/CT images show mass with intense FDG uptake in the cervix with SUVmax 19.6 (*arrow*). (*C–E*) Follow-up axial (*C*) and coronal (*D*) fused PET/CT images after treatment with definitive chemoradiation using external beam radiation therapy and brachytherapy show complete metabolic and anatomic response after therapy (SUVmax 3.4) with radiation fiducial marker in place (*arrow*). Coronal (*E*) fused PET/CT shows FDG uptake in brown fat in the neck and chest (*arrows*).

patients had a complete metabolic response (MR), 15% had a partial MR, and 6% had progressive disease (PD). The 3-year PFS rates were 78% for the complete MR group, 33% for the partial MR group, and 0% for the PD group. Siva and colleagues[33] examined 105 patients who underwent posttreatment PET/CT at 3 to 12 months (average 5 months), based on the discretion of the clinician. In the 73 patients with complete MR, only 1 had tumor recurrence, detected by clinical examination, as the patient was asymptomatic. They concluded that the presence of complete MR is a strong predictor of survival. In the patients with complete MR after treatment, conservative follow-up can be performed[34]. Herrera and colleagues[35] found that the parameters of TLG, pretreatment mean standardized uptake value of 5 or greater, and partial MR to be associated with unfavorable outcome.

Recurrence/Restaging

Tumor recurrence is the development of a tumor at least 6 months after the initially treated disease has responded to therapy[9,36] (**Fig. 6**). As many as one-third of patients with locally advanced cervical cancer develop recurrent disease, usually within 2 years.[35] Wong and colleagues[37] found PET/CT to be an accurate tool in diagnosing local recurrence and distant metastases. The sensitivity, specificity, and accuracy of PET/CT was 82%, 97%, and 92%, respectively, for local tumor recurrence and 100%, 90%, and 94%, respectively, for distant metastatic disease. Ryu and colleagues[38] evaluated 249 patients with no evidence of cancer after treatment with surveillance PET. They found PET to be effective in the detection of tumor recurrence, with a sensitivity of 90.3%

and a specificity of 76.1%. Eighty-two percent of the recurrent cases occurred within 6 to 18 months after therapy, and 89% of recurrent cases occurred in patients with stage IIB and III disease. Lee and colleagues[39] studied 51 patients with treated cervical cancer and found tumor recurrence or metastasis in 37 patients. They found PET/CT to have a sensitivity of 97.3%, a specificity of 71.4%, and an accuracy of 90.2%. PET/CT has been shown to detect metastases in asymptomatic patients and in patients with increasing tumor markers.

Brooks and colleagues[40] performed a prospective study that followed asymptomatic patients who had a complete response on their 3-month evaluation and found that PET/CT detected tumor recurrence in patients who could potentially benefit from salvage therapy.

Chong and colleagues[41] evaluated patients with an unexplained tumor marker elevation following a complete treatment response with PET/CT. These patients had an elevation of carcinoembryonic antigen or squamous cell carcinoma antigen, and PET/CT had a high sensitivity and high NPV.

PET/CT has been shown in studies to impact clinical management and change treatment plans. Chung and colleagues[42] showed posttreatment PET/CT to have significant prognostic impact, showing patients with a negative PET/CT to have a better PFS and OS. In their study, PET/CT changed treatment plans in 24.2% of the patients. Recent meta-analyses performed in the United Kingdom found that PET/CT is not cost-effective for the evaluation of recurrent disease; however, the recommendations could change if the cost of PET/CT decreases and more studies show a therapeutic impact in patients with recurrent or persistent disease.[43,44]

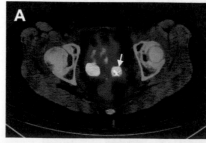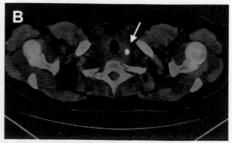

Fig. 6. PET/CT in recurrent cervical cancer. A 39-year-old woman with FIGO stage IB adenocarcinoma of the cervix initially diagnosed 2 years prior and treated with radical hysterectomy and bilateral PLN dissection. Although the lymph nodes were negative, there was deep cervical involvement and radiation therapy was implemented. Follow-up PET/CT was obtained because of symptoms and elevated carcinoembryonic antigen levels. (*A*) Axial fused FDG PET/CT shows an FDG-avid focus in the left pelvis in the region of the radiation marker, representing recurrent disease (*arrow*). (*B*) Axial fused PET/CT also shows an FDG-avid left supraclavicular lymph node (*arrow*) suspicious for metastasis. Biopsy was obtained to exclude metastatic disease, with no evidence of malignancy noted on pathology.

PET/COMPUTED TOMOGRAPHY PITFALLS
Benign Conditions

There are potential imaging pitfalls that can occur with PET/CT. One is FDG uptake in brown fat, which can be distinguished from lymphadenopathy by its characteristic distribution in the neck and thorax and absence of lymph nodes in the areas of uptake. It can be prevented by the use of blankets or with anxiolytics in the case of anxiety as tolerated by patients.[8] Physiologic uptake in the endometrium and ovaries can occur in younger patients because of the menstrual cycle. Physiologic uptake in the ureter can mimic a lymph node. Infection or inflammation can also have FDG uptake and mimic malignancy.

Post-Therapy Changes

The inflammatory response at the primary site caused by radiation therapy can be hypermetabolic. Therefore, follow-up PET/CT is generally performed 8 to 12 weeks after radiation therapy has been completed to allow these changes to abate.[45] However, in some cases, they may persist for months; biopsy may be required for further evaluation.

Gastrointestinal side effects of radiation and chemotherapy, such as enteritis, proctitis, fistulas, and strictures, can also cause findings at PET/CT that should not be confused as progression of disease.[46]

Post-therapeutic changes in the osseous structures can also be hypermetabolic or hypometabolic. Causes of increased metabolic uptake include bone marrow stimulation, inflammatory change due to radiation, or postradiation fractures. Decreased metabolic uptake may be seen in delayed reactions, such as bone marrow suppression.[46]

TUMOR HYPOXIA

Hypoxic tumors have a decreased response to chemotherapy and radiation therapy, and assessing the presence of hypoxia would be helpful to alter therapy. Hypoxia may be a significant prognostic factor, given that patients with hypoxic tumors have worse outcomes than patients who do not and may be a factor in resistance to therapy.[47] Hypoxia studies have been performed with the copper-labeled radiotracers ^{60}C-diacetyl-bis (N^4-methylthiosemicarbazone) (^{60}Cu-ATSM) and ^{64}C-diacetyl-bis (N^4-methylthiosemicarbazone) (^{64}Cu-ATSM) along with ^{18}F-fluoromisonidazole PET/CT. Studies by Dehdashti and colleagues[48] with the use of ^{60}Cu-ATSM in pretreatment planning concluded that tumor uptake, specifically tumor-to-muscle uptake of 3.5, was correlated to recurrent disease along with shorter PFS and cause-specific survival. Lewis and colleagues[49] did a comparison of ^{60}Cu-ATSM and ^{64}Cu-ATSM and concluded ^{64}Cu-ATSM is a safe radiotracer for producing high-quality PET images in the evaluation of hypoxia. There is currently an ongoing American College of Radiology Imaging Network clinical trial to study how well ^{64}Cu-ATSM PET performs in predicting disease progression in patients with cervical cancer.[47,50]

[18F]-2-FLUORO-2-DEOXY-D-GLUCOSE PET/MR IMAGING

PET/MR imaging is now coming to the forefront as a new diagnostic tool in the treatment of cervical cancer, after some initial technical challenges. PET/MR imaging systems can either operate simultaneously or sequentially. In the simultaneous model, PET and MR imaging elements are housed in the same gantry, with simultaneous acquisition of data from the same body section. In the sequential model, the MR imaging and PET elements are connected via moving tables.[51–54]

Study results are very promising. Kitajima and colleagues[55] evaluated 30 patients with PET/CT, MR imaging, nonfused PET and MR imaging, and fused PET/MR imaging. In the evaluation of the primary tumor, PET/MR imaging detected a tumor in 100% of the cases versus 93.3% with PET/CT. CE-fused PET/MR imaging has the advantage of a more detailed assessment of the extension of the primary tumor and spread into the parametrium, vagina, pelvic sidewall, and bladder because of a small field of view (**Fig. 7**). However, the difference between the two modalities was not statistically significant. In the evaluation of the primary tumor, PET/MR imaging is significantly more accurate, with accuracy of 83.3% versus PET/CT's accuracy of 53.3%. For assessment of the lymph nodal stage, PET/MR imaging and PET/CT showed similar sensitivity, specificity, and accuracy of 92.3%, 88.2%, and 90.0%, respectively. Grueneisen and colleagues[56] showed PET/MR imaging to have excellent performance in the evaluation of T stage, regional nodal involvement, and metastatic disease.

Functional and multi-parametric techniques used in MR imaging may also allow greater quantitative assessment between biomarkers in PET and MRI.[57] Grueneisen and colleagues[56] found that pathologic grade and tumor size were significantly correlated with SUVmax and apparent diffusion coefficient (ADC). Surov and colleagues[58] performed

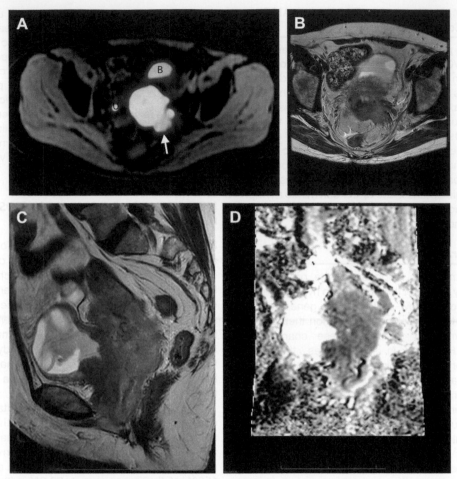

Fig. 7. PET/MR imaging in primary evaluation. A 53-year-old woman with stage IVA squamous cell carcinoma of the cervix. (*A*) Axial fused FDG PET/MR imaging shows FDG-avid large circumferential cervical tumor involving the left parametrium (*arrow*), lower one-third of vagina, uterus, and urinary bladder (B). Significant thickening is seen in the distal portions of bilateral ureters (right ureter [U]), likely representing tumor extension. The patient had bilateral ureteral stents in place. (*B*) Axial T2-weighted MR imaging at the same level of fused PET/MR imaging shows the primary cervical tumor and local extension into the surrounding tissues as described in (*A*) with improved conspicuity, demonstrating the value of MR imaging in local tumor evaluation. (*C*) Sagittal T2-weighted MR imaging shows the full extent of cervical tumor, along with extension into the posterior urinary bladder and into the vagina. (*D*) Sagittal ADC map MR imaging reveals low signal intensity of the primary cervical tumor, in keeping with restricted diffusion.

PET/MR imaging on 21 patients and found a statistically significant correlation between the proliferation index KI67 and SUVmax, SUVmean, minimum ADC (ADCmin), and SUVmax/ADCmin.

PET/MR imaging has advantages in follow-up after radiation treatment planning. In the posttreatment evaluation, PET/MR imaging may be better able to detect radiation changes from a recurrent tumor, such as post-therapeutic scarring.[59] Furthermore, the reduced radiation exposure in PET/MR imaging is an advantage in patients with cancer who undergo multiple serial examinations. As the current recommendation by most governing bodies, such as the National Comprehensive Cancer Network (NCCN), American College of Radiology, and European Society of Gynecologic Oncology, is to obtain PET/CT and MR imaging, this obviates 2 examinations as well.[34,47,57,60]

SUMMARY

Cervical cancer continues to be a significant worldwide health issue. The use of PET/CT has continued to evolve, and the modality has significant use in the detection of disease, prognosis and treatment planning. The NCCN, the American College of Radiology, and the US Center for Medicare and Medicaid Services all acknowledge the utility of PET/CT in the initial evaluation of cervical cancer.[61,62] Radiation treatment planning can be better performed with a more targeted therapy and less effect on adjacent structures with the use of PET/CT. The use of tumor values from PET, such as SUVmax, MTV, and TLG, in combination with the parameter ADC from PET/MR imaging, continues to enhance the impact of these imaging modalities on disease prognostication and treatment planning.

REFERENCES

1. Siegel RL, Miller KD, Jemal A. Cancer statistics, 2017. CA Cancer J Clinicians 2017;67(1):7–30.
2. Bruni L, B.-R.L., Albero G, Serrano B, Mena M, Gómez D, Muñoz J, Bosch FX, de Sanjosé and S., ICO Information Centre on HPV and Cancer (HPV Information Centre). Human Papillomavirus and Related Diseases in the World. Summary report.
3. Marth C, Landoni F, Mahner S, et al. Cervical cancer: ESMO clinical practice guidelines for diagnosis, treatment and follow-up†. Ann Oncol 2017; 28(suppl_4):iv72–83.
4. Comprehensive cervical cancer control: a guide to essential practice. 2nd edition. Annex 10, cervical cancer treatment by FIGO stage. Geneva, Switzerland: World Health Organization; 2014. Available at: https://www.ncbi.nlm.nih.gov/books/NBK269617/.
5. Howlader N, Noone AM, Krapcho M, et al (editors). SEER cancer satistics review, 1975-2014. Bethesda (MD): National Cancer Institute. Available at: https://seer.cancer.gov/csr/1975_2014/. based on November 2016 SEER data submission, posted to the SEER web site, April 2017.
6. Benedetti-Panici P, Maneschi F, Scambia G, et al. Lymphatic spread of cervical cancer: an anatomical and pathological study based on 225 radical hysterectomies with systematic pelvic and aortic lymphadenectomy. Gynecol Oncol 1996;62(1):19–24.
7. Pecorelli S. Revised FIGO staging for carcinoma of the vulva, cervix, and endometrium. Int J Gynaecol Obstet 2009;105:103.
8. Kusmirek J, Robbins J, Allen H, et al. PET/CT and MRI in the imaging assessment of cervical cancer. Abdom Imaging 2015;40(7):2486–511.
9. Mirpour S, Mhlanga JC, Logeswaran P, et al. The role of PET/CT in the management of cervical cancer. Am J Roentgenology 2013;201(2):W192–205.
10. Yagi S, Yahata T, Mabuchi Y, et al. Primary tumor SUVmax on preoperative FDG-PET/CT is a prognostic indicator in stage IA2-IIB cervical cancer patients treated with radical hysterectomy. Mol Clin Oncol 2016;5(3):216–22.
11. Kidd EA, Siegel BA, Dehdashti F, et al. The standardized uptake value for F-18 fluorodeoxyglucose is a sensitive predictive biomarker for cervical cancer treatment response and survival. Cancer 2007; 110(8):1738–44.
12. Hong JH, Jung US, Min KJ, et al. Prognostic value of total lesion glycolysis measured by 18F-FDG PET/CT in patients with locally advanced cervical cancer. Nucl Med Commun 2016;37(8): 843–8.
13. Hong JH, Min KJ, Lee JK, et al. Prognostic value of the sum of metabolic tumor volume of primary tumor and lymph nodes using 18F-FDG PET/CT in patients with cervical cancer. Medicine (Baltimore) 2016; 95(9):e2992.
14. Zhang Y, Hu J, Li J, et al. Comparison of imaging-based gross tumor volume and pathological volume determined by whole-mount serial sections in primary cervical cancer. Onco Targets Ther 2013;6: 917–23.
15. Yang Z, Xu W, Ma Y, et al. 18F-FDG PET/CT can correct the clinical stages and predict pathological parameters before operation in cervical cancer. Eur J Radiol 2016;85(5):877–84.
16. Fontanilla HP, Klopp AH, Lindberg ME, et al. Anatomic distribution of [18F] fluorodeoxyglucose-avid lymph nodes in patients with cervical cancer. Pract Radiat Oncol 2013;3(1):45–53.
17. Grigsby PW, Siegel BA, Dehdashti F. Lymph node staging by positron emission tomography in patients with carcinoma of the cervix. J Clin Oncol 2001; 19(17):3745–9.
18. Kidd EA, Siegel BA, Dehdashti F, et al. Lymph node staging by positron emission tomography in cervical cancer: relationship to prognosis. J Clin Oncol 2010; 28(12):2108–13.
19. Kidd EA, Siegel BA, Dehdashti F, et al. Pelvic lymph node F-18 fluorodeoxyglucose uptake as a prognostic biomarker in newly diagnosed patients with locally advanced cervical cancer. Cancer 2010; 116(6):1469–75.
20. Onal C, Guler OC, Reyhan M, et al. Prognostic value of 18F-fluorodeoxyglucose uptake in pelvic lymph nodes in patients with cervical cancer treated with definitive chemoradiotherapy. Gynecol Oncol 2015; 137(1):40–6.
21. Rose PG, Adler LP, Rodriguez M, et al. Positron emission tomography for evaluating para-aortic nodal metastasis in locally advanced cervical cancer before surgical staging: a surgicopathologic study. J Clin Oncol 1999;17(1):41–5.
22. Driscoll DO, Halpenny D, Johnston C, et al. 18F-FDG-PET/CT is of limited value in primary staging of early stage cervical cancer. Abdom Imaging 2015;40(1):127–33.
23. Signorelli M, Guerra L, Montanelli L, et al. Preoperative staging of cervical cancer: is 18-FDG-PET/CT really effective in patients with early stage disease? Gynecol Oncol 2011;123(2):236–40.

24. Liu FY, Yen TC, Chen MY, et al. Detection of hematogenous bone metastasis in cervical cancer: 18F-fluorodeoxyglucose-positron emission tomography versus computed tomography and magnetic resonance imaging. Cancer 2009;115(23):5470–80.

25. Loft A, Berthelsen AK, Roed H, et al. The diagnostic value of PET/CT scanning in patients with cervical cancer: a prospective study. Gynecol Oncol 2007; 106(1):29–34.

26. Haynes-Outlaw ED, Grigsby PW. The role of FDG-PET/CT in cervical cancer: diagnosis, staging, radiation treatment planning and follow-up. PET Clin 2010;5(4):435–46.

27. Grigsby PW. PET/CT imaging to guide cervical cancer therapy. Future Oncol 2009;5(7):953–8.

28. Mackay HJ, Wenzel L, Mileshkin L. Nonsurgical management of cervical cancer: locally advanced, recurrent, and metastatic disease, survivorship, and beyond. Am Soc Clin Oncol Educ Book 2015; e299–309.

29. Chung YL, Horng CF, Lee PI, et al. Patterns of failure after use of 18F-FDG PET/CT in integration of extended-field chemo-IMRT and 3D-brachytherapy plannings for advanced cervical cancers with extensive lymph node metastases. BMC Cancer 2016;16(1):179.

30. Lazzari R, Cecconi A, Jereczek-Fossa BA, et al. The role of [(18)F]FDG-PET/CT in staging and treatment planning for volumetric modulated Rapidarc radiotherapy in cervical cancer: experience of the European Institute of Oncology, Milan, Italy. Ecancermedicalscience 2014;8:409.

31. Kidd EA, Thomas M, Siegel BA, et al. Changes in cervical cancer FDG uptake during chemoradiation and association with response. Int J Radiat Oncol Biol Phys 2013;85(1):116–22.

32. Schwarz JK, Siegel BA, Dehdashti F, et al. Association of post-therapy positron emission tomography with tumor response and survival in cervical carcinoma. JAMA 2007;298(19):2289–95.

33. Siva S, Herschtal A, Thomas JM, et al. Impact of post-therapy positron emission tomography on prognostic stratification and surveillance after chemoradiotherapy for cervical cancer. Cancer 2011; 117(17):3981–8.

34. Zola P, Macchi C, Cibula D, et al. Follow-up in gynecological malignancies: a state of art. Int J Gynecol Cancer 2015;25(7):1151–64.

35. Herrera FG, Breuneval T, Prior JO, et al. [18F]FDG-PET/CT metabolic parameters as useful prognostic factors in cervical cancer patients treated with chemo-radiotherapy. Radiat Oncol 2016;11(1):43.

36. Heron CW, Husband JE, Williams MP, et al. The value of CT in the diagnosis of recurrent carcinoma of the cervix. Clin Radiol 1988;39(5):496–501.

37. Wong TZ, Jones EL, Coleman RE. Positron emission tomography with 2-deoxy-2-[(18)F]fluoro-D-glucose for evaluating local and distant disease in patients with cervical cancer. Mol Imaging Biol 2004;6:55.

38. Ryu SY, Kim MH, Choi SC, et al. Detection of early recurrence with 18F-FDG PET in patients with cervical cancer. J Nucl Med 2003;44(3): 347–52.

39. Lee M, Lee Y, Hwang KH, et al. Usefulness of F-18 FDG PET/CT in assessment of recurrence of cervical cancer after treatment. Nucl Med Mol Imaging 2011; 45(2):111–6.

40. Brooks RA, Rader JS, Dehdashti F, et al. Surveillance FDG-PET detection of asymptomatic recurrences in patients with cervical cancer. Gynecol Oncol 2009;112(1):104–9.

41. Chong A, Ha JM, Jeong SY, et al. Clinical usefulness of 18F-FDG PET/CT in the detection of early recurrence in treated cervical cancer patients with unexplained elevation of serum tumor markers. Chonnam Med J 2013;49(1):20–6.

42. Chung HH, Kim JW, Kang KW, et al. Predictive role of post-treatment [18F]FDG PET/CT in patients with uterine cervical cancer. Eur J Radiol 2012;81(8): e817–22.

43. Meads C, Davenport C, Małysiak S, et al. Evaluating PET-CT detection management recurrent cervical cancer: systematic reviews diagnostic accuracy subjective elicitation. BJOG 2014;121(4): 398–407.

44. Auguste P, Barton P, Meads C, et al. Evaluating PET–CT in routine surveillance and follow-up after treatment for cervical cancer: a cost-effectiveness analysis. BJOG 2014;121(4):464–76.

45. Ulaner GA, Lyall A. Identifying and distinguishing treatment effects and complications from malignancy at FDG PET/CT. Radiographics 2013;33(6): 1817–34.

46. Viswanathan AN, Lee LJ, Eswara JR, et al. Complications of pelvic radiation in patients treated for gynecologic malignancies. Cancer 2014;120(24): 3870–83.

47. Khiewvan B, Torigian DA, Emamzadehfard S, et al. Update of the role of PET/CT and PET/MRI in the management of patients with cervical cancer. Hell J Nucl Med 2016;19(3):254–68.

48. Dehdashti F, Grigsby PW, Lewis JS, et al. Assessing tumor hypoxia in cervical cancer by PET with 60Cu-labeled diacetyl-bis(N4-methylthiosemicarbazone). J Nucl Med 2008;49:201.

49. Lewis JS, Laforest R, Dehdashti F, et al. An imaging comparison of 64Cu-ATSM and 60Cu-ATSM in cancer of the uterine cervix. J Nucl Med 2008;49:1177.

50. ACRIN; Available at: https://www.acrin.org/6682_protocol.aspx. Accessed August 13, 2017.

51. Lee SI, Catalano OA, Dehdashti F. Evaluation of gynecologic cancer with MR imaging, 18F-FDG PET/CT, and PET/MR imaging. J Nucl Med 2015;56(3): 436–43.

52. Zaidi H, Ojha N, Morich M, et al. Design and performance evaluation of a whole-body Ingenuity TF PET-MRI system. Phys Med Biol 2011;56(10):3091–106.

53. Delso G, Fürst S, Jakoby B, et al. Performance measurements of the Siemens mMR integrated whole-body PET/MR scanner. J Nucl Med 2011;52(12): 1914–22.

54. Torigian DA, Zaidi H, Kwee TC, et al. PET/MR imaging: technical aspects and potential clinical applications. Radiology 2013;267(1):26–44.

55. Kitajima K, Suenaga Y, Ueno Y, et al. Fusion of PET and MRI for staging of uterine cervical cancer: comparison with contrast-enhanced (18)F-FDG PET/CT and pelvic MRI. Clin Imaging 2014;38(4):464–9.

56. Grueneisen J, Schaarschmidt BM, Heubner M, et al. Integrated PET/MRI for whole-body staging of patients with primary cervical cancer: preliminary results. Eur J Nucl Med Mol Imaging 2015;42(12): 1814–24.

57. Ponisio MR, Fowler KJ, Dehdashti F. The emerging role of PET/MR imaging in gynecologic cancers. PET Clin 2016;11(4):425–40.

58. Surov A, Meyer HJ, Schob S, et al. Parameters of simultaneous (18)F-FDG-PET/MRI predict tumor stage and several histopathological features in uterine cervical cancer. Oncotarget 2017;8(17): 28285–96.

59. Nie J, Zhang J, Gao J, et al. Diagnostic role of 18F-FDG PET/MRI in patients with gynecological malignancies of the pelvis: a systematic review and meta-analysis. PLoS One 2017;12(5): e0175401.

60. Gaffney DK, Erickson-Wittmann BA, Jhingran A, et al. ACR appropriateness criteria on advanced cervical cancer expert panel on radiation oncology & gynecology. Int J Radiat Oncol Biol Phys 2011; 81(3):609–14.

61. Siegel CL, Andreotti RF, Cardenes HR, et al. ACR appropriateness criteria pretreatment planning of invasive cancer of the cervix. J Am Coll Radiol 2012;9(6):395–402.

62. 2013 NCCN clinical practice guidelines in oncology™ cervical cancer v.2.2013. Available at: http://www.nccn.org/professionals/physician_gls/PDF/cervical.pdf. Accessed September 5, 2017.

Fludeoxyglucose F 18 PET/CT Assessment of Ovarian Cancer

Maria Cristina Marzola, MD*, Sotirios Chondrogiannis, MD,
Domenico Rubello, MD

KEYWORDS

• Ovarian cancer • FDG PET/CT • Staging • Biomarkers • Prognosis • Response to treatment

KEY POINTS

- Fludeoxyglucose F 18 (FDG) PET/MR imaging is an emerging hybrid modality that may be useful in the assessment of many malignant disease conditions, including ovarian and others pelvic tumors.
- Thanks to its morphologic high soft tissue contrast and the use of diffusion-weighted imaging–MR imaging with intravenous contrast administration, PET/MR imaging is able to overcome some limitations of FDG PET/CT in the detection of the primary tumor in patients with a high suspicion of disease and also in the delineation of the tumor mass for pretreatment planning, which may have an impact on the therapeutic approach.
- The reason for the high death rate is the late presentation in most cases, due to its silent nature earlier in the course of disease.

INTRODUCTION

Ovarian cancer is one of the most common gynecologic malignancies, is the most fatal gynecologic malignancy, and is the fifth most common cause of female cancer–related death.[1] The reason for the high death rate is the late presentation in most cases, due to its silent nature earlier in the course of disease. Thus, patients often present with advanced disease, widely spread within the abdomen (75% of cases), in the absence of specific signs or symptoms. One of the most important factors influencing survival is represented by the disease stage at diagnosis.[2] Despite advances in medicine over the past decades, only minor improvement in 5-year survival has been achieved in patients diagnosed with advanced epithelial ovarian cancer.[3]

EPIDEMIOLOGY OF OVARIAN CANCER

Ovarian cancer is one of the most commonly diagnosed cancers and one of the leading causes of cancer death in women worldwide, accounting for approximately 3.6% (238,719) of total new cancer cases and 4.3% (151,917) of total cancer deaths among women in 2012.[4] Published epidemiologic data estimate approximately 22,440 new cases in the United States in 2017, accounting for approximately 2.6% of all new malignancies in women. According to the same data, ovarian cancer is the leading cause of gynecologic cancer–related deaths (14,080 deaths estimated for 2017) and the fifth most frequent cause of cancer mortality in women (5% of all cancer deaths) after lung and bronchus (25%), colon-rectum (14%), breast (8%), and pancreas (7%) cancers.[5]

The authors declare they have neither commercial or financial conflicts of interest nor funding sources.
Department of Nuclear Medicine PET/CT Centre, S. Maria della Misericordia Hospital, Viale 3 Martiri, 140, Rovigo 45100, Italy
* Corresponding author.
E-mail address: crinuk@iol.it

PET Clin 13 (2018) 179–202
https://doi.org/10.1016/j.cpet.2017.11.005

According to the 2017 Surveillance, Epidemiology, and End Results program statistics of the National Cancer Institute, the number of new cases of ovarian cancer was 11.7 per 100,000 women per year, and the number of deaths was 7.4 per 100,000 women per year (rates age adjusted and based on the 2010–2014 period). According to the same data for patients with disease limited to the ovaries, the 5-year survival rate is approximately 92.5%, whereas for patients presenting with advanced disease, the 5-year survival rate is approximately 30%.[5] Unfortunately, approximately 70% of patients are diagnosed with advanced ovarian cancer.

SPREAD

Ovarian cancer spreads via 3 different routes: (1) the peritoneum, (2) the lymphatic system, and (3) the bloodstream.

1. The peritoneum is the most frequent target, due to the distribution of cells within the normal peritoneal fluid circulation. Tumor cells from the primary tumor spread into the peritoneal cavity and then are transported by peritoneal fluid toward the upper abdominal quadrants. During breathing movements, the negative pressure at the subphrenic level increases to a positive one, so fluid moves from the paracolic gutters up to the right subhepatic space and the right subdiaphragmatic space.[6] The more common sites of tumor disseminations include greater omentum, paracolic gutters, pouch of Douglas, liver (especially glissonian capsule), diaphragmatic and bowel surface, and, less frequently, mesentery, splenic surface, porta hepatis, and gastrosplenic ligament. Peritoneal involvement may appear as nodular soft tissue lesions, linear or plaque-like thickening of the parietal or visceral peritoneum, or, in histologically serous tumors, tiny calcifications,[3]
2. Lymph node dissemination can follow 3 different routes: (a) along the ovarian vessels (more frequently), reaching the upper common iliac and para-aortic lymph nodes; (b) along the broad ligament and parametrium, reaching the external iliac and obturator lymph nodes; (c) rarely, along the round ligaments, toward the external iliac and inguinal lymph nodes.[7–9]
3. Through the bloodstream, tumor dissemination usually occurs to the liver, lung, spleen, and skeleton.[7]

STAGING: INTERNATIONAL FEDERATION OF GYNECOLOGY AND OBSTETRICS, TNM, AND WORLD HEALTH ORGANIZATION CLASSIFICATIONS
International Federation of Gynecology and Obstetrics Classification

After the diagnosis of cancer, staging is an essential step in disease management, with the aim to define, with standard terminology, tumor characteristics and extension and to assign patients to prognostic groups to optimize/personalize treatment options to achieve a more favorable outcome.

At present, the staging system worldwide used for ovarian cancer is represented by the International Federation of Gynecology and Obstetrics (FIGO) staging classification,[7] which was first published in 1973, then revised in 1988 and, more recently, in 2014. Numerous publications in recent years have enlightened various controversial aspects of the disease. It is recognized that "ovarian cancer" is not a homogeneous disease but is instead a group of diseases, each with different etiology, pathogenesis, morphology, and prognosis, which can present in the ovaries, fallopian tubes, and peritoneum.[10] In the new FIGO staging classification of 2014, ovarian, fallopian tube, and primary peritoneal cancers are considered collectively as 1 entity. Ovarian cancers differ primarily based on histologic type. Approximately 90% of ovarian, fallopian tubes, and primary peritoneum tumors are carcinomas, with at least 5 main types accounting for 98% of them (based on histopathology, immunohistochemistry, and molecular genetic analysis):

1. High-grade serous carcinoma (HGSC [70%])
2. Endometrioid carcinoma (EC [10%])
3. Clear cell carcinoma (10%)
4. Mucinous carcinoma (3%)
5. Low-grade serous carcinoma (<5%)[11]

Much less common types are malignant germ cell tumors (dysgerminomas, yolk sac tumors, and immature teratomas [3% of ovarian cancers]) and potentially malignant sex cord–stromal tumors [1%–2%, mainly granulosa cell tumors].[10] Despite differences in tumor biology, dissemination pattern, response to chemotherapy, and outcome, the FIGO staging classification is the same for each type of ovarian carcinoma for the sake of simplicity, considering the most relevant prognostic parameters shared by all tumor types.[11]

Stage I
Stage I includes tumors limited to the ovaries or fallopian tubes, although tumor cells may be

present in peritoneal fluid. Stage I ovarian cancer is rare (less than 5% of HGSCs are stage I tumors) because most patients are diagnosed in advanced stages (III and IV) and is associated with excellent survival rates.[11,12]

Stage II

Stage II includes tumors that involve 1 or both ovaries or fallopian tubes with pelvic extension below the pelvic brim or primary peritoneal cancer. It comprises a small and heterogeneous group making up less than 10% of HGSCs.[10,11] All malignant peritoneal metastases of the inferior pelvis are classified as stage II. Therefore, there are no stage I peritoneal carcinomas.

Stage III

Stage III includes advanced cancers that involve 1 or both ovaries or fallopian tubes, or primary peritoneal cancer, with cytologically or histologically confirmed spread to the peritoneum outside the pelvis and/or metastasis to the retroperitoneal lymph nodes. Most ovarian cancers are HGSCs that usually present in stage III, with the vast majority (84%) stage IIIC.

Stage IV

Stage IV includes all tumors with distant metastases excluding peritoneal metastasis, which are included in stages II (if located below the pelvic brim) or III; 12%-21% of patients present with stage IV disease.[13]

The 2014 FIGO staging classification is reported in detail in **Table 1** and compared with the equivalent TNM classification of the American Joint Committee on Cancer (AJCC) staging system published in 2017.[11]

TNM Classification According to the American Joint Committee on Cancer

Primary tumor

Primary tumor (T) categories correspond to the stages proposed by the FIGO 2014 classification. In clinical category T1, disease is limited to the ovaries (1 or both) or fallopian tube(s). In T2 disease, tumor involves 1 or both ovaries or fallopian tubes with pelvic extension (below pelvic brim) or primary peritoneal cancer. T3a/b includes cytologically or histologically confirmed spread to the peritoneum outside the pelvis and/or metastasis to the retroperitoneal (pelvic or para-aortic) lymph nodes. T3c includes surface involvement of the liver and spleen without any parenchymal metastases (see **Table 1**).

Regional lymph node

The lymphatic spread of the disease involves the external iliac, internal iliac, obturator, common iliac, para-aortic, pelvic, and retroperitoneal lymph nodes. Regional lymph node (N) categories define N1 disease when histologically confirmed regional lymph node involvement is present (N1a: metastasis up to 10 mm in greatest dimension, N1b: more than 10 mm in greatest dimension), NX disease when regional lymph nodes cannot be assessed, N0 disease when no regional lymph node metastases are present, and N0(i+) disease when isolated tumor cells in regional lymph node(s) are no greater than 0.2 mm[11] (**Table 2**).

Distant metastasis

Spread in the peritoneum (including the omentum) and diaphragmatic and liver surface involvement are common but are not considered distant metastases. Metastatic sites include liver, lung, spleen, transmural involvement of intestine, and skeletal metastases as well as involvement of the inguinal, supraclavicular, and axillary nodes.

Consistently with the FIGO classification, AJCC TNM categories of distant metastasis (M) include M0 when there are no distant metastasis; M1, distant metastasis, including pleural effusion with positive cytology (M1a), liver or splenic parenchymal metastases or metastases to extra-abdominal organs (including inguinal lymph nodes and lymph nodes outside the abdominal cavity), or transmural involvement of intestine (M1b)[11] (**Table 3**).

Histopathologic Classification (World Health Organization and American Joint Committee on Cancer)

In parallel with the FIGO classification for the staging of ovarian cancer, the World Health Organization (WHO) classification was also revised in 2014. Whereas the FIGO classification focuses on the separation into tumor stages, the WHO classification indicates the histopathologic and molecular tumor type.

Tumor stage (FIGO classification) and tumor type (WHO classification) are both essential for the treatment decision-making process and represent the most important prognostic factors.

AJCC endorses the FIGO staging classification and recommends a simplified version of the WHO histologic typing of epithelial ovarian tumors revised in 2014[14,15] (**Box 1**).

Surgical pathologic evaluation of the abdomen and pelvis is necessary to establish a definitive diagnosis of ovarian/fallopian tube/peritoneal cancer and should include resection of the primary mass, hysterectomy, selective pelvic and para-aortic lymphadenectomy, and biopsy or resection of any suspicious lesion as well as random biopsies of all frequently involved sites (omentum,

Table 1
The revised 2014 International Federation of Gynecology and Obstetrics classification of ovarian cancer with the equivalent TNM prognostic stage group classification of the American Joint Committee on Cancer

Prognostic Stage Group (International Federation of Gynecology and Obstetrics)	TNM (American Joint Committee on Cancer)	Criteria
	TX	Primary tumor cannot be assessed
	T0	No evidence of primary tumor
I	T1-N0-M0	Tumor confined to ovaries (1 or both) or fallopian tube(s)
IA	T1a-N0-M0	Tumor limited to 1 ovary (capsule intact) or fallopian tube; no tumor on ovarian or fallopian tube surface; no malignant cells in ascites or peritoneal washings
IB	T1b-N0-M0	Tumor limited to both ovaries (capsules intact) or fallopian tubes; no tumor on ovarian or fallopian tube surface; no malignant cells in ascites or peritoneal washings
IC	T1c-N0-M0	Tumor limited to 1 or both ovaries or fallopian tubes, with any of the following
IC1	T1c1-N0-M0	Surgical spill
IC2	T1c2-N0-M0	Capsule ruptured before surgery or tumor on ovarian or fallopian tube surface
IC3	T1c3-N0-M0	Malignant cells in ascites or peritoneal washings
II	T2-N0-M0	Tumor involves 1 or both ovaries or fallopian tubes with pelvic extension below pelvic brim or primary peritoneal cancer
IIA	T2a-N0-M0	Extension and/or implants on the uterus and/or fallopian tube(s) and/or ovaries
IIB	T2b-N0-M0	Extension to and/or implants on other pelvic tissues
III	T1/T2/T3-NX/N0/N1-M0	Tumor involves 1 or both ovaries or fallopian tubes, or primary peritoneal cancer, with microscopically confirmed peritoneal metastasis outside the pelvis and/or metastasis to the retroperitoneal (pelvic and/or para-aortic) lymph nodes
IIIA1	T1/T2-N1-M0	Positive retroperitoneal lymph nodes only (histologically confirmed)
i		Metastasis up to and including 10 mm in greatest dimension
ii		Metastasis more than 10 mm in greatest dimension
IIIA2	T3a-NX/N0/N1-M0	Microscopic extrapelvic (above the pelvic brim) peritoneal involvement with or without positive retroperitoneal lymph nodes
IIIB	T3b-NX/N0/N1-M0	Macroscopic peritoneal metastasis beyond the pelvis 2 cm or less in greatest dimension with or without metastasis to the retroperitoneal lymph nodes
IIIC	T3c-NX/N0/N1-M0	Macroscopic peritoneal metastasis beyond the pelvis more than 2 cm in greatest dimension with or without metastasis to the retroperitoneal lymph nodes (includes extension of tumor to capsule of liver and spleen without parenchymal involvement of either organ)
IV	Any T, any N, M1	Distant metastasis, including pleural effusion with positive cytology; liver or splenic parenchymal metastasis; metastasis to extra-abdominal organs (including inguinal lymph nodes and lymph nodes outside the abdominal cavity); and transmural involvement of intestine

(continued on next page)

Table 1 (continued)		
Prognostic Stage Group (International Federation of Gynecology and Obstetrics)	**TNM (American Joint Committee on Cancer)**	**Criteria**
IVA	Any T, any N, M1a	Pleural effusion with positive cytology
IVB	Any T, any N, M1b	Liver or splenic parenchymal metastases; metastases to extra-abdominal organs (including inguinal lymph nodes and lymph nodes outside the abdominal cavity); transmural involvement of intestine

Data from Prat J. FIGO Committee on Gynecologic Oncology Staging classification for cancer of the ovary, fallopian tube, and peritoneum. Int J Gynaecol Obstet 2014;124(1):1–5; and Prat J, Olawaiye AB, Bermudez A, et al. Ovary fallopian tube and primary peritoneal carcinoma. AJCC Cancer Staging Manual. 8th edition. Chapter 55. Springer International Publishing; 2017. p. 681–90.

Table 2
Definition of regional lymph node involvement according to the American Joint Committee on Cancer and corresponding International Federation of Gynecology and Obstetrics stage

N Category	International Federation of Gynecology and Obstetrics Stage	Criteria
NX		Regional lymph nodes cannot be assessed
N0		No regional lymph nodes metastasis
N0(i+)		Isolated tumor cells in regional lymph node(s) no >0.2 mm
N1	IIIA1	Positive retroperitoneal lymph nodes only (histologically confirmed)
N1a	IIIA1i	Metastasis up to and including 10 mm in greatest dimension
N1b	IIIA1ii	Metastasis more than 10 mm in greatest dimension

Data from Prat J. FIGO Committee on Gynecologic Oncology Staging classification for cancer of the ovary, fallopian tube, and peritoneum. Int J Gynaecol Obstet 2014;124(1):1–5; and Prat J, Olawaiye AB, Bermudez A, et al. Ovary fallopian tube and primary peritoneal carcinoma. AJCC Cancer Staging Manual. 8th edition. Chapter 55. Springer International Publishing; 2017. p. 681–90.

mesentery, diaphragm, peritoneal surfaces, pelvic nodes, and para-aortic nodes).[11,14] In addition to the postsurgical histologic findings, clinical and imaging evaluation is considered for final staging. Moreover, complete macroscopic tumor resection and postoperative residual tumor are the strongest independent prognostic factors, together with tumor stage.[16,17]

IMAGING PROCEDURES

An early identification of malignant lesions and a precise and complete staging at diagnosis are crucial for deciding the subsequent therapeutic approach. A tailored approach is based on the overall extent of the disease, and several imaging modalities can contribute to the subsequent steps: diagnosis (in terms of characterization of an adnexal mass), staging and pretreatment evaluation, assessment of treatment response and prognosis, and restaging.

Ultrasonography (US) is particularly useful for the assessment of an ovarian mass and for defining the limits of the local disease. CT can be used for staging, evaluation of treatment response, and restaging given its ability to evaluate lymphatic, hematogenous, and peritoneal spread.[18] MR imaging can be especially useful as a complementary tool for a better characterization of adnexal masses discovered but indeterminate at US.

The major limitation of radiological evaluation of an early ovarian cancer lies in its inability to consistently detect small lesions.[18,19]

Fludeoxyglucose F 18 (FDG) PET/CT is a hybrid technique combining metabolic and morphologic tomographic images. Its usefulness has been well demonstrated in many malignant tumors, given their glucose avidity, which is an expression of the tumor glycolytic metabolism. Typically,

Table 3
Definition of distant metastases according to the American Joint Committee on Cancer and corresponding International Federation of Gynecology and Obstetrics stage

M Category	International Federation of Gynecology and Obstetrics Stage	Criteria
M0		No distant metastasis
M1	IV	Distant metastasis, including pleural effusion with positive cytology; liver or splenic parenchymal metastasis; metastasis to extra-abdominal organs (including inguinal lymph nodes and lymph nodes outside the abdominal cavity); and transmural involvement of intestine
M1a	IVA	Pleural effusion with positive cytology
M1b	IVB	Liver or splenic parenchymal metastasis; metastasis to extra-abdominal organs (including inguinal lymph nodes and lymph nodes outside the abdominal cavity); and transmural involvement of intestine

Data from Prat J. FIGO Committee on Gynecologic Oncology Staging classification for cancer of the ovary, fallopian tube, and peritoneum. Int J Gynaecol Obstet 2014;124(1):1–5; and Prat J, Olawaiye AB, Bermudez A, et al. Ovary fallopian tube and primary peritoneal carcinoma. AJCC Cancer Staging Manual. 8th edition. Chapter 55. Springer International Publishing; 2017. p. 681–90.

malignant cells have a higher FDG uptake than normal tissues due to a higher glycolytic turnover. Most ovarian cancers demonstrate a high affinity for FDG, so detection of significant FDG uptake within the ovary in a postmenopausal woman, especially if associated with an adnexal mass, raises suspicious for ovarian cancer. Moreover, the associated CT images allow for a better visualization and anatomic characterization of the mass itself, with high resolution and suitable localization of FDG-avid components.

The role of FDG PET/CT in diagnosis, staging, restaging, and providing prognostic information is explained.

THE ROLE OF CANCER ANTIGEN 125 IN DIAGNOSIS OF OVARIAN CANCER

Serum measurement of cancer antigen (CA)-125 as tumor marker can also play a role in ovarian cancer diagnosis. In the presence of an increased CA-125 level (especially when >400 U/mL), an adnexal mass in a postmenopausal woman is considered probably malignant with a sensitivity of 94% and a specificity of 82%, and US has been validated as a part of the risk of malignancy index in combination with menopausal status and serum CA-125 measurement in the initial investigation of an adnexal mass.[20] Unfortunately, CA-125 is elevated in fewer than half of patients with early stage disease.[21] Moreover, the marker specificity is too low in premenopausal women (60%), because CA-125 can increase in conditions

other than malignancies, such as endometriosis, cystadenomas, pelvic inflammatory disease, and also in nonovarian cancer with peritoneal involvement.[22] Yet, it is considered a good marker of tumor recurrence.

THE ROLE OF IMAGING IN DIAGNOSIS OF OVARIAN CANCER: CONVENTIONAL IMAGING AND FLUDEOXYGLUCOSE F 18 PET/CT
Conventional Imaging

Ovarian masses are common in postmenopausal women. They include, however, both benign and malignant lesions, where most are benign,[23] including endometriomas, thecomas, corpus luteum cysts, and serum cystadenomas.[2] Thus, the clinical impact of defining whether an adnexal mass is benign or malignant is of key importance.

Transvaginal US (TVUS) combined with Doppler techniques is the first-line imaging technique (in some cases also performed with complementary transabdominal US [TAUS]) and is the most appropriate imaging investigation in patients suspected of having adnexal pathology, with the aim of determining the site of origin and to characterize it as benign or malignant. US is available worldwide, noninvasive, relatively inexpensive, and also useful for screening of high-risk patients.[24,25] Masses presenting with thick irregular walls or with papillary projections and solid echogenic foci are usually considered malignant,[26] especially if presenting together with ascites or peritoneal

Box 1
The American Joint Committee on Cancer simplified version of the 2014 World Health Organization histopathologic classification of epithelial tumors of the ovary

Epithelial ovarian tumors

Serous tumors

  Benign serous cystadenoma

  Serous borderline tumor: serous cystadenoma with epithelial proliferation and nuclear atypia but with no destructive stromal invasion

  Serous low-grade carcinoma

  HGSC

    Transitional cell variant

Mucinous tumors

  Benign mucinous cystadenoma

  Mucinous borderline tumor: mucinous cystadenoma with epithelial proliferation and nuclear atypia, but with no destructive stromal invasion

  Mucinous carcinoma

Endometrioid tumors

  Benign endometrioid cystadenoma

  Endometrioid borderline tumor with epithelial proliferation and nuclear atypia, but with no destructive stromal invasion

  EC

Clear cell tumors

  Benign clear cell tumors

  Borderline clear cell tumors with epithelial proliferation and nuclear atypia, but with no destructive stromal invasion

  Clear cell carcinoma

Brenner tumors

  Borderline Brenner tumor

  Malignant Brenner tumor

Seromucinous tumors

  Borderline seromucinous tumor

  Seromucinous carcinoma

Undifferentiated carcinoma

  A malignant tumor that is too poorly differentiated to be placed in any other group

Mixed epithelial tumor

  Tumors composed ($\geq$10%) of 2 or more of the 5 major cell types of common epithelial tumors

Data from Prat J, Olawaiye AB, Bermudez A, et al. Ovary fallopian tube and primary peritoneal carcinoma. AJCC Cancer Staging Manual. 8th edition. Chapter 55. Springer International Publishing; 2017. p. 681–90; and Kurman R, Carcangiu ML, Herrington CS, et al. WHO classification of tumors of female reproductive organs. 4th edition. Lyon (France): The International Agency for research on Cancer; 2014.

nodules. Moreover, power Doppler examination can help identify tumor neovascularity within solid masses.[27]

Body habitus and bowel gas account, however, for variability and diagnostic accuracy of US,[12,28] and US is an operator-dependent technique. Therefore, 5% to 20% of ovarian masses remain indeterminate or difficult to classify.[29] In these cases, MR imaging can be used as a complementary tool, providing tissue differentiation with a greater accuracy in distinguishing benign from malignant masses.[30] On MR imaging, a malignant lesion may have mural thickening or irregularity, intramural nodules, papillary projections, and solid enhancing components.

Contrast-enhanced CT (ceCT) may be useful in detecting solid enhancing components within adnexal masses as well as peritoneal spread of tumor.[31] In particular, the advent of multislice CT has improved spatial resolution and allows for multiplanar reconstruction. Yet, it has not been used traditionally for the initial evaluation of adnexal masses presenting as indeterminate at US due to the poor soft tissue contrast compared with MR imaging.

Fludeoxyglucose F 18 PET/CT

Several studies have evaluated the diagnostic value of FDG PET/CT for ovarian cancer in patients presenting with a pelvic mass, with the aim of improving identification of patients who warrant surgical intervention while avoiding unnecessary laparotomies in women with benign tumor. In many cases, additional value in comparison to conventional imaging has been demonstrated.[32,33] For diagnosing malignancies in 50 consecutive patients with a pelvic lesion who were already scheduled for surgery, Castellucci and colleagues[34] obtained similar sensitivity rates (87% for PET/CT vs 90% for TVUS), whereas PET/CT demonstrated a higher specificity (100% for PET/CT vs 61% for TVUS) and accuracy (92% for PET/CT vs 80% for TVUS). In a prospective study of 30 women with pelvic masses, Risum and colleagues[35] confirmed the high specificity of PET/CT for diagnosing malignancy of pelvic masses and observed a very high sensitivity rate in their population (with sensitivity and specificity of 100% and 92.5%, respectively). Nam and colleagues[36] obtained PET/CT accuracy (92%) superior to that of pelvic Doppler US (83%) and of CT/MR imaging (74%) in discriminating benign versus borderline/malignant ovarian lesions. Glucose transporter 1 (GLUT-1) overexpression in ovarian cancer and microvessel density/tumor proliferation, which are markers of more aggressive malignancy and poorer prognosis, represent the pathophysiologic bases of these observations. Thus, the investigators suggest that PET/CT is a useful tool to improve patient selection for surgical intervention and guiding cytoreductive surgery.[37,38] Furthermore, staging by PET/CT was concordant with surgical staging in 78% of patients, suggesting that PET/CT could be used in the preoperative evaluation of patients suspected to have ovarian cancer.[36] Yet, although Yamamoto

and colleagues[39] and Kitajima and colleagues[33] confirmed high PET/CT sensitivity and specificity in discriminating malignant from benign ovarian lesions (where the likelihood of malignancy increased with increasing glucose uptake measured by maximum standardized uptake value [SUVmax]), they observed a low diagnostic value in differentiating between borderline-malignant and benign tumors (with no significant difference in terms of SUVmax).[33,39] Moreover, despite the satisfactory results obtained in diagnosing ovarian cancer with PET/CT, Fenchel and colleagues[32] and Tanizaki and colleagues[40] reported both false-negative and false-positive results with this technique. The false-negative cases were due to lack of FDG accumulation in early tumors and low FDG uptake in clear cell, mucinous, and cystic carcinomas (compared with serous carcinoma and EC),[41] related to low GLUT-1 concentrations inside of the cells and, consequently, of the cytoplasmic hexokinase activity, blood supply, cellular proliferation, extent of hypoxia, and so forth.[42,43] The false-positive results were usually due to a moderately intense FDG accumulation in benign conditions, such as cystadenomas, endometriomas, and acute inflammatory processes, or in premenopausal ovaries due to the cyclic functional activity changes. Moreover, it has been widely demonstrated that the likelihood of malignancy increases with the FDG uptake, as measured by SUVmax,[33,39] although there is unfortunately overlap between the degree of FDG uptake in malignant, borderline-malignant, and benign conditions.

In summary, PET/CT has a high accuracy in differentiating ovarian cancer from benign tumors but suboptimal accuracy in discriminating borderline-malignant tumors from benign tumors. A single threshold SUVmax value does not exist for defining presence of malignancy or for differentiating histologic types, in particular borderline and benign tumors of serous and mucinous subtypes.[40]

Thus, many investigators have suggested combining FDG PET/CT with US and MR imaging in diagnosing ovarian malignancies, although the use of PET/CT alone does not seem to provide enough information. Moreover, Karantanis and colleagues[44] did not find any significant correlation between SUVmax and tumor grade and histologic subtype tumor grade in 1171 patients with histopathologically confirmed epithelial ovarian cancer patients, implying that FDG PET/CT cannot be used to predict tumor aggressiveness or histology.

For these reasons, despite the high sensitivity and specificity in diagnosing ovarian cancer, the significant variability in results cannot support the routine use of FDG PET/CT in the diagnosis of the disease. Using CA-125 together with US, a second-stage examination seems to be required in only fewer than 10% of cases.[45,46]

THE ROLE OF FLUDEOXYGLUCOSE F 18 PET/CT IN STAGING OVARIAN CANCER

The best treatment of ovarian cancer is debulking surgery followed by systemic therapy. The complete resection of tumor implants is related to the best survival rates, and postsurgical residual tumor is one of the most important negative prognostic factors.[47,48] For these reasons, early detection of sites of tumor spread sites is important,[49] but unfortunately in most cases of ovarian cancer, they are usually discovered when ascites or others signs of metastatic spread are clinically evident. Furthermore, there are some particularly important key features to keep in mind in staging ovarian cancer[50]:

- In suspected ovarian cancer, the presence of ascites in the upper abdomen is indicative of peritoneal spread of tumor, even without visible implants.[51]
- The presence of extensive lymph node involvement at diagnosis predicts an undifferentiated cancer (or a dysgerminoma).
- Liver metastases are rare at diagnosis, but glissonian capsule involvement is frequent, strongly influencing surgical management.[52]
- The presence of pleural effusion and/or cardiophrenic lymph nodes larger than 5 mm at diagnosis shifts the stage toward stage IV disease.

Primary cytoreductive surgery followed by platinum-based chemotherapy has been considered standard of care for ovarian cancer.[53,54] Neoadjuvant chemotherapy followed by interval debulking surgery can be a potential alternative in stages IIIC/IV with similar survival and lower morbidity.[55,56] The precise assessment of tumor extent (primary tumor and peritoneal sites, regional lymph nodes, and distant sites) is the basis for the evaluating whether primary surgery may be feasible or whether the patient should receive neoadjuvant treatment.

Thus, surgery (in particular, exploratory laparotomy) is the cornerstone for staging (using FIGO and TNM classification), prognosis assessment, and subsequent treatment planning, even if several anatomic locations (retrohepatic areas, retroperitoneal spaces, porta hepatis, and so forth)[57,58] are difficult to explore. Unfortunately, in up to 30% of patients, the tumor is understaged at laparotomy, especially due to unexpected peritoneal or extra-abdominal (nodal or extranodal)

spread. Thus, it is still reserved for limited indications.

Even though surgical staging remains, at present, the reference standard, a reliable presurgical staging technique is essential for assessing the overall tumor extent and the feasibility of surgery, the diagnosis of potential complications (such as bowel obstruction, hydronephrosis, and so forth), and the exclusion of other potential primary tumor sites (such as the gastrointestinal tract, pancreas, and so forth). Therefore, in the past few years, a comprehensive pretherapeutic imaging approach has been adopted as an integral part of the initial patient management, where cross-sectional (multiplanar) imaging techniques have been widely applied in clinical routine.

CT can provide information regarding not only the primary tumor but also the metastatic lesions. Its accuracy in staging ovarian cancer ranges from 53% to 92%, and CT is currently considered the imaging modality of choice for staging ovarian cancer.[7] CT has the advantage of speed and coverage, delivering imaging within less than a minute. CT imaging is limited, however, in its ability to reliably detect small cancer implants on bowel surfaces (visceral) and in the mesentery and parietal peritoneum, especially if no ascites is present (with the CT sensitivity in detecting implants of <1 cm in diameter of only 25%–50%).[16] CT also lacks accuracy in characterizing malignant lymph nodes based on nodal size criteria, where abdominopelvic lymph nodes with a short axis greater than 10 mm or cardiophrenic lymph nodes greater than 5 mm are usually classified as metastatic, because CT could miss normal-size metastatic lymph nodes or could erroneously lead to mischaracterization of enlarged inflammatory lymph nodes (>1 cm) as due to metastatic disease. Therefore, additional morphologic criteria may be useful to improve the specificity for tumor infiltration, such as more rounded lymph node shape and presence of central necrosis.[33] Overall, several studies reported that CT had an accuracy of 70% to 90% for preoperative staging of ovarian cancer with a good specificity (82%–96%), although with a variable sensitivity (63%–92%) for the detection of peritoneal involvement[51,59] and metastatic lymph nodes, and with overall sensitivity, specificity, positive predictive value (PPV), negative predictive value (NPV), and accuracy of 64%, 75%, 85%, 47%, and 58%, respectively.[48]

MR imaging demonstrates some advantages relative to CT in evaluating metastatic spread in ovarian cancer, in particular due to its higher soft tissue contrast and lack of radiation exposure. Moreover, the addition of diffusion-weighted imaging (DWI) allows for a higher interobserver agreement. Michielsen and colleagues[60] demonstrated a high MR imaging accuracy of DWI–MR imaging versus CT not only for primary lesions but also for peritoneal and distant metastases, reducing misinterpretation especially for mesenteric and serosal deposits and for lesions obscured by the spleen or by distortion artifacts. MR imaging does not, however, overcome the problem of diagnosing lymph nodal and peritoneal sites of malignancy by size criteria. MR imaging can accurately identify the invasion of pelvic organs given its superior soft tissue contrast resolution, playing an important role in detecting the extent of peritoneal disease in patients who are considered for cytoreductive surgery.[12]

Although several studies concluded that MR imaging was superior to CT for staging ovarian cancer, this advantage has been largely superseded by the advent of multislice CT. Currently, MR imaging could be considered a second-line technique, in patients with contraindications to CT and/or in patients with inconclusive CT findings.[60,61]

In the recent past, FDG PET/CT has been used not only for better evaluation of the primary tumor but also for staging of the disease. Although the use of this imaging modality as a staging tool has not yet been fully established, it seems that it could overcome some major limitations of conventional imaging. In the preoperative staging of 50 ovarian cancer patients, Castellucci and colleagues[34] observed that PET/CT correctly identified metastatic lesions in 69% of patients compared with 53% of patients using CT only. In a group of 133 women evaluated before surgery, FDG PET/CT was concordant with surgery in staging ovarian cancer in 78% of patients.[36] Moreover, Kitajima and colleagues[62] observed an improvement, compared with ceCT, in the overall lesion-based sensitivity (from 37% to 69.8%), specificity (from 97.1% to 97.5%), and accuracy (from 89.7% to 94%), with a minimum size of lesions detectable by PET/CT of 4 mm and a maximum size of lesions not detected by PET/CT of 6 mm.

PET/CT seems to improve diagnostic performance compared with conventional imaging for the evaluation of the lymph node involvement, extra-abdominal spread, and detection of unsuspected malignant tumors (given that it is a whole-body technique).

Lymphatic spread is not uncommon in ovarian cancer, even when the tumor is apparently limited to the ovaries or pelvis. Systematic pelvic and aortic lymphadenectomy (SAPL) is a part of optimal debulking in advanced disease stages, although in early stages it can be considered as a primary staging procedure. Moreover, SAPL is a major surgical procedure that is associated with increased morbidity and costs, and in ovarian cancers macroscopically confined to the pelvis, the removed lymph nodes are often not involved by tumor. For these reasons, a presurgical imaging procedure to allow for accurate nodal staging is desirable to improve the selection of women who will benefit from SAPL.[63] Kitajima and colleagues[62] observed a better sensitivity and accuracy for FDG PET/CT in detecting metastatic lymph nodes compared with CT only (89% and 94% for PET/CT vs 37% and 87% for CT, respectively), and Nam and colleagues[36] confirmed these results, obtaining sensitivity, specificity, PPV, and NPV of 83.8%, 92.6%, 81.6%, 93.6%, respectively, for PET/ceCT, and 62.5%, 83.6%, 60%, and 85%, respectively, for ceCT. A meta-analysis by Yuan and colleagues[64] (including 882 patients from 18 studies) demonstrated that FDG PET/CT was more accurate than both CT and MR imaging in detecting metastatic lymph nodes (sensitivity of 73% and specificity of 96%, vs 42% and 95%, respectively, for CT and 54% and 88%, respectively, for MR imaging) and that 70% of metastatic lymph nodes and 97% of negative lymph nodes could be correctly diagnosed by PET or PET/CT. Moreover, preoperatively evaluating nodal metastases in patients with ovarian cancer grossly confined to the pelvis and addressed to surgical intervention inclusive of SAPL, Signorelli and colleagues[63] confirmed the previous result: a preoperative FDG PET/CT correctly identified metastatic lymph nodes with good sensitivity, specificity, PPV, NPV, and accuracy for both per patient (83.3%, 98.2%, 90.9%, 96.5%, and 95.6%, respectively) and per node analysis (75.5%, 99.4%, 87.5%, 98.6%, and 98.1%, respectively). The investigators concluded that FDG PET/CT could be considered an accurate tool in selecting women who could benefit from systematic lymphadenectomy. Moreover, the high NPV could avoid SAPL in many patients, minimizing surgical and postsurgical complications. PET/CT is able, in some cases, to identify metastatic lymph nodes smaller than 8 mm to 10 mm if they have high FDG avidity, The sensitivity of PET/CT, however, is suboptimal for the assessment of small lymph nodes, leading to false-negative results in nodes with size smaller than 5 mm[62] or when the volume of malignant cells is too low to obtain a glucose uptake high enough to be evident in PET images.[65] Also, some non-neoplastic lymph nodes (inflammatory, hyperplastic, and so forth) may have increased FDG uptake, leading to false-positive results.

Given the extended craniocaudal scan coverage of PET/CT, it can improve presurgical staging by also detecting extra-abdominal spread missed at conventional imaging,[35,46,66] including lymph nodes located outside of the abdominopelvic area (ie, supraclavicular or cardiophrenic nodes) as well as unsuspected extraovarian tumors.[34,36] In a study retrospectively involving 95 patients already operated on for advanced ovarian cancer (stages III and IV), Fruscio and colleagues[46] confirmed superiority of PET/CT in discovering distant metastases compared with conventional imaging. Metastatic sites detected by PET/CT were predominantly supradiaphragmatic (pleura and mediastinal-supraclavicular lymph nodes), with a percentage of mediastinal involvement of 37.7%.[46,66,67] Moreover, with use of FDG PET/CT in presurgical staging of patients with advanced ovarian cancers, up-staging from stage III to IV occurs in a remarkably high proportion of patients, associated with an increase of the percentage of stage IV patients from 26% to 40%. The importance of early identification of stage IV patients was restated by Risum and colleagues[68] in a prospective study, involving preoperative staging of 201 patients with PET/CT and then analyzing the overall survival (OS) 2 years later and the prognostic variables in the 66 advanced (stages III and IV) cancer patients. In this cohort, the investigators demonstrated a shift of 41% of the stage III patients toward stage IV, with important outcomes in terms of therapeutic decision making, where a patient who is under-staged might be deprived a potential survival benefit from removal of distant metastases or may receive suboptimal postoperative chemotherapy. PET/CT can also help to better identify stage III/IV patients for whom optimal debulking is not possible to direct them toward different therapies (ie, neoadjuvant chemotherapy).[33]

It has been demonstrated that stage IV patients with different amounts of residual disease may have similar progression; thus, an early diagnosis of stage IV disease can meaningfully change the therapeutic approach (eg, by excluding some patients as candidates for aggressive surgery). Thus, PET/CT can be considered a powerful diagnostic tool for the whole-body detection of metabolically active disease in patients with ovarian cancer, and a preoperative FDG uptake at distant sites might be considered a functional marker of aggressive behavior. The investigators also observed, however, that this might not be clinically crucial (up-staged patients have a similar prognosis to stage III patients), probably because the intra-abdominal disease is more likely to lead patients to death than distant lesions.[35,69]

Although the role of PET in the evaluation of peritoneal carcinomatosis in staging ovarian cancer has not yet clearly been established, several studies have shown promising results. PET/CT seems to have a satisfactory diagnostic accuracy for tumoral implants larger than 5 mm. In patients with diffuse peritoneal carcinomatosis, an apron sign or shield sign may be seen on PET/CT, appearing as FDG uptake along the anterior abdomen (sometimes in association with increased peritoneal thickening or omental fat stranding on CT).[48] Moreover, it is important to consider that the imaging sensitivity is not the same in the different portions of the abdominopelvic cavity. Hynninen and colleagues[66] compared the performance of presurgical PET/CT and diagnostic ceCT with histopathologic assessment, with the aim of predicting the debulking results. On a lesion-based analysis, PET/CT was significantly superior to conventional CT in predicting carcinomatosis along subdiaphragmatic peritoneal surfaces and in the bowel mesentery but not in certain other areas of the peritoneal cavity, such as in the small bowel mesentery and right upper abdomen. Moreover, false-positive results were accounted for by the presence of an inflammatory reaction in the peritoneum next to large or multiple tumor implants. On the other hand, negative results often depended on the presence of nodules smaller than 5 mm; on miliary carcinomatous spread involving the hepatic dome, epigastrium, or left upper abdomen; and also on mass lesions resulting from large amounts of fibrosis in conjunction with tiny tumoral implants.[70]

In summary, for staging patients with ovarian cancer, PET/CT might be useful for the assessment of retroperitoneal lymph nodes, and especially for detecting metastatic lymph nodes ranging from 5 mm to 9 mm in size that are not diagnosed at CI.[63] Also, given its capability to detect distant metastases, it might provide for more accurate evaluation of disease extent, especially in those areas that are difficult to investigate by CT and MR imaging, such as some peritoneal reflections, the mediastinum, and the supraclavicular region.[2,27] Moreover, false-negative results tend to occur with small lesions and with diffuse peritoneal spread, whereas false-positive results may occur in the presence of inflammatory lymph nodes. Currently, there are still conflicting data regarding the routine use of this imaging modality in ovarian cancer staging, so more studies are required. At present, it is considered complementary to conventional imaging and surgical techniques for disease staging.

THE PROGNOSTIC VALUE OF FLUDEOXYGLUCOSE F 18 PET/CT IN PRIMARY OVARIAN CANCER AND IN PREDICTING RESPONSE TO NEOADJUVANT CHEMOTHERAPY

FDG PET/CT can provide not only important information in detecting additional metastatic lesions but also on the tumor biology and behavior and their potential impact on prognosis. Different tumor histologic types are different in molecular biology, clinical presentation, and dissemination pattern and also in terms of glucose metabolism. Nakamura and colleagues[71] demonstrated a statistically significant association between glucose uptake measured by SUVmax of the primary tumor and FIGO stage, histology (serous/nonserous carcinoma), presence of nodal metastasis, and poor prognosis with a significantly different OS rate between patients with high SUVmax (>13.5) and low SUVmax of the primary tumor. Konishi and colleagues[72] confirmed these results, demonstrating a significantly lower SUVmax in mucinous (mean value 2.8) and clear cell (mean value 4.9) ovarian cancers (usually presenting with low aggressiveness) than in adenocarcinomas (mean value 11.4). Recently, González García and colleagues[73] reported similar results, confirming the utility of FDG PET/CT in identifying high-risk histologies. From a pathophysiologic point of view, this may depend on a different glucose-transporter concentration in the different tumor types. Cho and colleagues[38] observed a strong correlation between membrane GLUT-1 overexpression in the primary tumor and disease aggressiveness as well as with poor OS.

Volumetric metabolic PET parameters have also been proposed as prognostic factors in ovarian cancer prior to treatment, including metabolic tumor volume (MTV) and total lesional glycolysis (TLG).[74] Some investigators have demonstrated that a poor outcome is usually associated with high values of these parameters. Chung and colleagues[75] observed that preoperative MTV and TLG measured by FDG PET/CT were statistically significant independent prognostic factors for the progression-free interval in patients with ovarian cancer. Lee and colleagues[74] demonstrated that TLG along with tumor stage was an independent prognostic factor for disease progression after cytoreductive surgery and that these 2 combined parameters could stratify the risk of progression. The previous results were recently confirmed by Gallicchio and colleagues[76] for MTV. Moreover, Risum and colleagues,[77] with the aim of selecting the patients unlikely to benefit from primary surgery, demonstrated that stage IV disease on

FDG PET/CT, pleural exudates, and PET-positive large bowel serosal implants were correlated with a lower OS and suggested these PET criteria for referral of patients to neoadjuvant chemotherapy.

Thus, FDG PET provides information not only in detecting additional metastatic lesions but also on the risk of residual cancer after surgery, which may have a potential impact on planning treatment.

Metabolic parameters can also be used before primary cytoreductive surgery in predicting response to neoadjuvant therapy. Avril and colleagues[78] demonstrated in their cohort of patients, who received 3 cycles of neoadjuvant therapy, that PET metabolic responders had a significantly better OS than nonresponders, and that FDG PET/CT could predict patient outcome as early as the first cycle of neoadjuvant chemotherapy, allowing for selection of patients who could benefit from receiving the other 2 cycles of chemotherapy. Similar results have been obtained by Martoni and colleagues,[79] demonstrating that PET monitoring during neoadjuvant chemotherapy could predict early pathologic response and that patients with SUVmax normalization after the first 3 cycles have a high likelihood of benefiting from 3 additional cycles. Recently, Vallius and colleagues[80] demonstrated that a poor metabolic response to neoadjuvant chemotherapy (ie, based on an SUVmax decrease of <57% at FDG PET/CT) was able to identify those histopathological nonresponders who would, therefore, benefit from second-line chemotherapy instead of interval debulking surgery.

THE ROLE OF FLUDEOXYGLUCOSE F 18 PET/CT IN RECURRENT OVARIAN CANCER

Approximately 75% to 80% of all ovarian cancer patients and 90% to 95% of stage III/IV patients recur within 2 years after primary treatment.[81] Tumor recurrence is one of the main determining factors of prognosis, because potentially available therapeutic options progressively decrease during the course of the disease.[19] For this reason, early identification of tumor recurrence is crucial for defining the subsequent therapeutic approach. There are many surveillance options after primary treatment, but the National Comprehensive Cancer Network guidelines recommend post-treatment surveillance 2 months to 4 months for 2 years, then every 4 months to 6 months for 3 years, and then annually for 5 years.[82]

CA-125 is a sensitive and reliable tumor marker, which is accurate in the detection of disease relapse (with an accuracy of 79%–95% reported in literature), usually increasing 3 months to

6 months prior to clinical manifestations of the recurrence.[83,84] A high CA-125 serum level suggests the presence of disease relapse.[33] CA-125 is elevated, however, regardless the site of the recurrence; that is, it is able to identify the presence of the disease but is not able to localize the relapse sites nor the number or size of lesions. Yet, early localization of recurrent disease is of utmost important to identify patients who will benefit from second-look surgery or who will undergo chemotherapy or radiation therapy. Moreover, CA-125 is a nonspecific marker, because it can increase in several benign conditions, and some patients with tumor recurrence present with normal CA-125 levels. Some investigators have also demonstrated that CA-125 has a low NPV (55%–60%) despite a high PPV (95%).[31,83]

Currently, there is no definitive consensus regarding the specific imaging tool that could better identify the site and extent of disease recurrence,[2] and the combination of CA-125 measurement with ceCT, MR imaging, and FDG PET/CT is commonly applied when disease recurrence is suspected.

Conventional imaging (with CT and MR imaging) has moderate usefulness in determining sites of relapse. CT usually demonstrates limited sensitivity and specificity rates, with a high variability in literature (40%–93% and 50%–98%, respectively), possibly because it is not able to recognize small peritoneal implants or disease inside normal-sized lymph nodes.[31] MR imaging provides a similar sensitivity in lesions larger than 1 cm to 2 cm in comparison to CT but is more useful in the detection of disease along the peritoneal surfaces and bowel serosa. It demonstrates, however, a suboptimal specificity when postsurgical changes are present,[85,86] because it is not always possible to differentiate between postsurgical changes and recurrent tumor.

Besides its high accuracy in detecting residual disease after primary treatment, FDG PET/CT is able to identify recurrent disease in both symptomatic and asymptomatic patients,[87] leading to changes in treatment management in more than 50% of cases.[88]

The improved diagnostic performance provided by PET/CT, which can make a difference in terms of accurate diagnosis of tumor recurrence compared with conventional imaging (CT and MR imaging) is summarized as follows:

- The ability to differentiate, in most of cases, between post-therapy scarring/fibrosis and viable tumor recurrence based on differences in metabolic activity. Conventional imaging can detect space-occupying soft tissue but is not able, in many cases, to distinguish between scar and tumor recurrence.
- The possibility to evaluate the whole body, detecting FDG-avid metastases far from abdomen and pelvis (liver, lung, pleura, and bone marrow as well as supradiaphragmatic metastatic lymph nodes) (**Fig. 1**)
- The ability to identify lesions (especially lymph nodes) of small size that are FDG-avid. Sironi and colleagues[89] observed that all the lesions missed at PET/CT in their cohort were smaller than 5 mm in diameter (**Fig. 2**)

The ranges of sensitivity, specificity, PPV, NPV, and accuracy reported in literature from some meta-analyses are 88% to 98%, 71% to 100%, 85% to 100%, 67% to 100%, and 71% to 97%, respectively.[31,90] Most investigators have found encouraging PPV rates, ranging between 89% and 98%, which is particularly important for detecting recurrent cancer.

In comparison to both CA-125 and conventional imaging (CT and MR imaging), FDG PET/CT has demonstrated a better sensitivity in detecting ovarian cancer recurrence. Several investigators have found a higher pooled sensitivity for PET compared with serum CA-125 (91% vs 63%, respectively, in a meta-analysis published by Gu and colleagues[31] in 2009, and 99% vs 72%, respectively, in an article by Evangelista and colleagues[91]), although with lower specificity (PET specificities of 78% and 88%, respectively, and CA-125 specificities of 91% and 93%, respectively). Pan and colleagues[92] and Bhosale and colleagues,[93] however, reported not only a better sensitivity but also a better specificity of PET/CT in detecting recurrent disease compared with serum CA-125. Finally, Antunovic and colleagues[81] demonstrated a significantly higher PET/CT accuracy in detecting recurrence compared with CA-125, for both high-grade and low-grade tumors. Moreover, a better performance of FDG PET/CT in the setting of rising CA-125 serum levels compared with ceCT and MR imaging has been largely reported. A meta-analysis by Gu and colleagues,[31] including 34 studies and comparing the diagnostic value of CA-125, PET, PET/CT, CT, and MR imaging, reported the best area-under-the-curve value for PET and PET/CT taken together (0.96), versus 0.92, 0.88, and 0.8 for CA-125, ceCT, and MR imaging, respectively. The investigators concluded that PET might be a useful supplement to current surveillance techniques, particularly for those patients with an increasing CA-125 level and negative CT or MR imaging results. These observations have been confirmed by a more recent

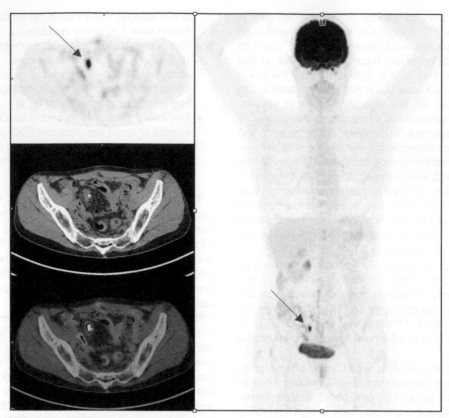

Fig. 1. A 57-year-old woman with ovarian cancer underwent FDG PET/CT imaging for pretreatment purposes (prior to adjuvant chemotherapy) 1 month after surgery. Surgery consisted of hysterectomy, bilateral salpingo-oophorectomy, omentectomy, appendectomy, and lymphadenectomy. The rectosigmoid colon and the terminal part of the ileum were also resected, and multiple biopsies of the peritoneum were also obtained. Histopathologic diagnosis was consistent with mucinous ovarian cancer, moderately differentiated (G3), with a component of signet ring cells, with metastases in 2/26 iliac-obturator lymph nodes and infiltration of the serosa of the ileum and rectosigmoid colon, with presence of mesenteric nodules. Disease was classified as FIGO stage IIIB ovarian cancer, AJCC stage pT3b pN1a cM0. (Upper left) Transverse PET image shows an area of focal abnormal FDG uptake in right iliac fossa (arrow). (Middle left) Transverse CT image shows corresponding mesenteric implant (arrow) adjacent to a metallic clip. (Lower left) Transverse fused PET/CT image again shows 1.7 cm mesenteric implant (arrow) with high pathologic FDG uptake (SUVmax 17) in keeping with residual disease. (Right) Coronal maximum intensity projection PET image. shows residual pelvic disease and confirms absence of distant metastases (cM0).

meta-analysis evaluating 13 studies and involving 661 patients.[90] PET/CT seemed to provide better results in detecting peritoneal implants between 0.5 cm and 2 cm in size and in identifying additional tumor sites, not seen at CT and preceding CT findings by almost 6 months,[94,95] A high overall sensitivity (97%) has been obtained using PET/CT in asymptomatic patients with high serum CA-125 levels and inconclusive results at CT. Thus, the authors strongly recommend use of FDG PET/CT in this context[96,97] (Fig. 3).

PET/CT detected tumor recurrences in patients without any evidence of recurrence on both US and CT.[98] Furthermore, Mangili and colleagues[99] demonstrated that PET/CT was positive in a larger

percentage of patients than CT (93% vs 63%, respectively), and, in particular, PET was positive in 10 of 12 CT-negative patients and was also able to detect more lesions in 8 of the 25 CT positive patients in whom CT demonstrated a single recurrent lesion.

In terms of lesion site, a better FDG PET/CT accuracy was obtained in detecting small peritoneal lesions and metastatic lymph nodes. In a meta-analysis, evaluating 118 studies with 882 patients and comparing FDG PET/CT, CT, and MR imaging results in detecting lymph nodes in recurrent ovarian cancer, Yuan and colleagues[64] observed that PET/CT was the more accurate imaging modality for this goal, with sensitivity

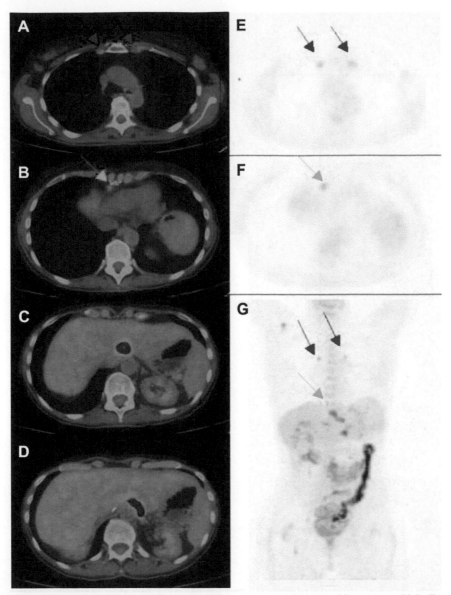

Fig. 2. A 58-year-old woman with serous ovarian carcinoma previously treated by surgery (debulking, hysterectomy, bilateral salpingo-oophorectomy, lymphadenectomy, omentectomy, hemicolectomy) followed by adjuvant chemotherapy. Due to elevation of serum CA-125, the patient underwent FDG PET/CT, which showed diffuse peritoneal involvement, hepatic metastases, para-aortic, anterior diaphragmatic, bilateral internal mammary chain lymphadenopathy. (*Left column*) (*A*) Transverse fused PET/CT image shows small FDG-avid internal mammary chain lymph nodes (*red arrows*); (*B*) transverse fused PET/CT image shows a small FDG-avid right anterior diaphragmatic chain lymph node (*green arrow*); (*C*) transverse fused PET/CT image shows an FDG-avid hepatic lesion; and (*D*) transverse fused PET/CT image shows FDG-avid para-aortic lymph nodes. (*Right column*) (*E*, *F*) Transverse PET images, corresponding to (*A*) and (*B*), and (*G*) coronal maximum intensity projection PET image show many foci of pathologic FDG uptake in liver, lymph nodes, and peritoneum.

and specificity values of 73.2% and 96.7%, respectively, versus 42.6% and 95%, respectively, for CT, and 54.7% and 88.3%, respectively, for MR imaging. In particular, FDG PET or PET/CT was able to correctly diagnose 70% of metastatic lymph nodes and 97.1% of negative lymph nodes. The sensitivity of PET/CT was moderate, even if it was significantly better than that of CT and MR imaging. A possible explanation of this result could be that PET can only detect lesions with sufficient malignant cells to change glucose metabolism and that FDG uptake may not be sufficiently increased in low-grade tumors.[59,65,100]

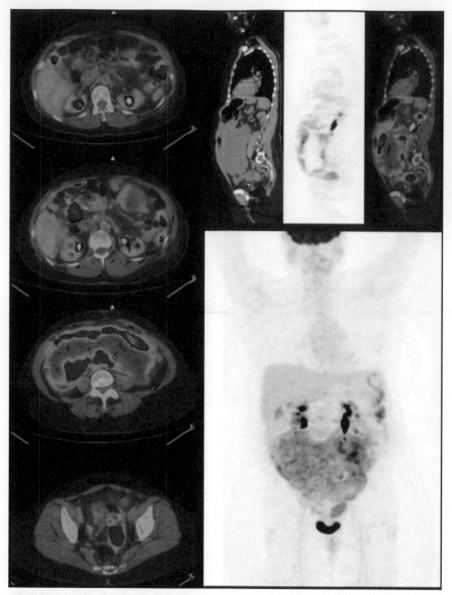

Fig. 3. A 71-year-old woman operated on for low-grade serous ovarian carcinoma infiltrating the appendix, ileum, and peritoneum, followed by chemotherapy. For CA-125 elevation, she underwent FDG PET/CT imaging, which demonstrated diffuse peritoneal uptake of FDG in the anterior abdomen along with several other pathologic foci of FDG uptake in the peritoneum/mesentery and lack of distant metastasis. (*Left images*) Transverse fused PET/CT images reveal FDG-avid foci of uptake in the peritoneum and mesentery. (*Right images, upper*) Sagittal CT, PET, and fused PET/CT images reveal FDG-avid peritoneal carcinomatosis. (*Right image, lower*) Coronal MIP PET image reveals characteristic diffuse abnormal FDG uptake in abdomen indicative of peritoneal spread of tumor.

An elevation of serum CA-125 levels can determine the presence of recurrent disease with a high accuracy (79%–95%), thus preceding a clinically apparent recurrence by 3 months to 6 months; however, a normal CA-125 level cannot exclude a disease relapse and, in particular, it has been demonstrated that, among patients with ovarian cancer in complete clinical remission, a progressive low-level increase in serum CA-125 levels (remaining below the upper limit of normal) is strongly predictive of disease recurrence.[101] Thus, with the aim to achieve very early detection of tumor recurrence, the usefulness of FDG PET/CT in these patients has been evaluated with encouraging results. In a group of patients with a low-level increased serum CA-125 levels, Peng and colleagues[102] demonstrated an FDG PET/CT 90.9% detection rate for recurrent ovarian cancer. In addition, symptomatic patients followed-up due to suspected recurrence despite normal CA-125 and conventional imaging results but with positive PET scan results (initially considered false-positive results) were confirmed to have recurrence 2 years later.[87] In a group of patients who underwent PET/CT for suspicion of disease recurrence or for evaluating response to therapy or follow-up, Evangelista and colleagues[91] observed that at least 35% of PET-positive patients had normal CA-125 serum level, suggesting that PET/CT can detect tumor recurrence at a very early stage; moreover, in all cases, FDG PET/CT affected the clinical management, thanks to an early localization of the relapse site.

After completion of chemotherapy, imaging procedures are usually performed to evaluate if the disease has completely disappeared or if residual tumor persists. Conventional imaging (CT and MR imaging), however, can detect the occupying-space lesions, but are not able, in many cases, to distinguish between scar (tumor necrosis or fibrosis, as a result of previous surgery or chemotherapy) and residual or recurrent viable tumor. For this reason, a second-look laparotomy is often performed to determine patient management and, when disease is not histologically demonstrated, additional chemotherapy can be avoided. Otherwise, reductive surgery followed by further adjuvant chemotherapy could be performed. FDG PET/CT has a better ability to differentiate between viable/nonviable tissue than CT and MR imaging and thus can be used to evaluate for complete versus noncomplete therapeutic response, also potentially reducing the number of second-look laparotomies. Prospectively evaluating the accuracy of FDG PET/CT for detecting tumor persistence after first-line treatment, Sironi and colleagues[89] demonstrated a strong correlation between PET results and second-look histologic findings, with the overall lesion-based sensitivity, specificity, PPV, NPV, and accuracy of 78%, 75%, 89%, 57%, and 77%, respectively. In addition, Kim and colleagues[103] confirmed the previous results and also demonstrated no significant differences in PFI and disease-free interval between the 2 groups of patients who had undergone PET and surgical second look after first-line treatment. Thus, the investigators concluded that both approaches had a high prognostic value. Despite these promising results, however, the size threshold of detected tumor could be set at 0.5 cm (because this was the largest diameter of a lesion missed at PET/CT). Thus, the sensitivity of PET before second-look laparotomy for small-volume persistent disease is relatively low, and additional research should be performed to determine whether FDG PET could be used to replace second-look laparotomy. Moreover, secondary cytoreductive surgery (SCRS) at second-look laparotomy is an important method to treat recurrent ovarian cancer, although its benefits are controversial,[104,105] because the increase in overall postrecurrence survival time is strongly related to an optimal surgical procedure, defined as the achievement of complete resection.[106] At present, however, the best method to identify suitable candidates for SCRS and to offer preoperative guidance has yet to be definitively determined. Peng and colleagues,[107] investigating the potential benefits of FDG PET/CT compared with conventional imaging as a guide for SCRS, demonstrated that patients who undergo PET-guided SCRS have a greater chance of complete tumor resection (fewer residual lesions) and may benefit from SCRS with improved progression-free survival (PFS) and OS.

Moreover, Hebel and colleagues[108] pointed out, in their study, not only the ability of FDG PET/CT to reliably map sites of recurrent tumor in the body but also a relatively high accuracy of a negative FDG PET/CT to predict the absence of disease, because negative scans were associated with 2-year PFS.

Finally, FDG PET/CT can be considered useful not only for the early detection of recurrence but also for the optimization and customization of the treatment plan. It might identify ovarian cancer recurrence long before CT (almost 6 months)[95] and also before the onset of clinical symptoms, especially in patients with rising CA-125 levels. Patients presenting a small amount of residual disease after primary therapy seem to have better outcomes that patients who demonstrate a large volumes disease after surgical treatment. Therefore, if FDG PET is able to enable early detection of small volume tumor recurrence, then patients could undergo surgical resection (second look) with better outcomes, and unnecessary laparotomies could be avoided.[109,110] There is evidence in the literature confirming the ability of PET/CT to change treatment management, by both leading to the use of previously unplanned therapies and avoiding previously planned diagnostic procedures. Mangili and colleagues[99] observed a change in the clinical management in 44% of cases when PET/CT information was added to conventional follow-up and, similarly, Simcock and colleagues[111] reported a major change in the management plan in 57% of patients. A prospective multicenter study demonstrated that FDG PET/CT provided new information that led to major changes in planned management in more than

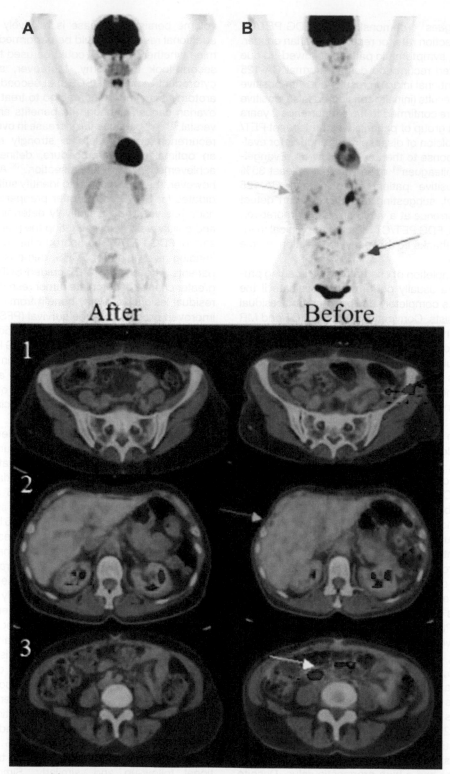

Fig. 4. A 54-year-old woman with serous ovarian carcinoma underwent surgery (bilateral salpingo-oophorectomy, omentectomy, lymphadenectomy, appendectomy, and intestinal resection), which was classified as FIGO stage IIIC (pT3c, G3) ovarian cancer. The patient, after surgery, underwent FDG PET/CT imaging for assessment prior to adjuvant chemotherapy (*right column images*), (*B*) which showed pathologic uptake of FDG in various sites of the peritoneum (right column images 1, 2, 3 with pathologic uptake sites marked with red, yellow, and green arrows), whereas no distant disease was demonstrated. The patient underwent chemotherapy and

30% of patients, where the main clinical impact was the shift from nontreatment to treatment as a result of positive findings on FDG PET/CT.[112] All these studies confirm the results reported from US National Oncology PET Registry, demonstrating that a change in management occurred in 38% to 45% of patients who were restaged using FDG PET/CT.[113,114]

THE PROGNOSTIC VALUE OF FLUDEOXYGLUCOSE F 18 PET/CT IN RECURRENT OVARIAN CANCER AND IN PREDICTING RESPONSE TO ADJUVANT CHEMOTHERAPY

Beyond the stage of the disease at diagnosis, the most independent prognostic factor for OS in ovarian cancer is the absence or residual disease after primary surgery.[55,77,115] Several studies advocate the postsurgical metabolic parameters obtained from PET as predictors of recurrence, especially the volumetric tumor burden measured by MTV and TLG. Vargas and colleagues[116] reported that MTV and TLG, but not SUVmax, measured by PET, were significantly related to both optimal tumor debulking and PFS. Yamamoto and colleagues[39] obtained similar predictive performances in patients who were already operated on and heading toward platinum-based adjuvant chemotherapy. Using PET/CT, they observed that TLG was a statistically significant risk factor for a poor PFS and suggested it as a potential biomarker for recurrence and to identify patients who need more aggressive treatment. Evangelista and colleagues[91] not only confirmed that a positive PET/CT scan in restaging is associated with a poor prognosis but also identified that the peritoneal-disease localization is an independent predictor of poor prognosis. In a multicenter study, lymph nodal and distant involvement detected by PET were independently associated with an increased risk of disease progression. The same investigators observed that not only was a positive PET/CT scan related to a higher risk of progression and reduced OS but also that PET/CT demonstrates an incremental prognostic value in terms of further risk stratification compared with the FIGO staging system, because FIGO stages I–II patients with negative PET had a significantly

better 4-year OS compared with patients with the same FIGO stage but with positive PET scan results.[117]

Two preliminary studies have evaluated the potential role of FDG PET/CT in measuring the response to adjuvant chemotherapy, with the aim of early evaluation of tumor chemosensitivity using PET-based parameters, moving from the hypothesis that changes in FDG uptake early in the course of adjuvant treatment allow for prediction of the effectiveness of chemotherapy and subsequent patient outcome. Kim and colleagues[118] demonstrated that the change in SUVmax (ΔSUVmax) after the third cycle of platinum-based combination chemotherapy was an independent risk factor for recurrence and that PFS significantly differed in the 2 groups categorized by ΔSUVmax after chemotherapy. In a phase Ib study of temsirolimus and pegylated liposomal doxorubicin chemotherapy, Boers-Sonderen and colleagues[119] observed that changes in tumor TLG on PET after 2 weeks of therapy predicted a partial response on CT after 10 weeks and that an increase in SUVmax between 2 weeks and 6 weeks was predictive of future progressive disease and worse PFS. Thus, FDG PET/CT was able to identify early on which patients could benefit from therapy, which may have a positive effect on the quality of life, whereas the early prediction of progressive disease could avoid the continuation of an ultimately ineffective and expensive treatment with associated toxicities, and allow for initiation of an alternative treatment (**Fig. 4**).

FLUDEXOYGLUCOSE F 18 PET/MR IMAGING IN ASSESSMENT OF OVARIAN CANCER

FDG PET/MR imaging is an emerging hybrid modality, which may be useful in the assessment of many malignant disease conditions, including ovarian and other pelvic tumors. It couples the MR imaging features of superior soft tissue contrast compared with CT with the metabolic information provided by PET.[120] Thanks to its morphologic high soft tissue contrast and the use of DWI–MR imaging with intravenous contrast administration, PET/MR imaging is able to overcome some limitations of FDG PET/CT in the

subsequent restaging FDG PET/CT (*left column images* [A]). This new study was completely negative for all sites of peritoneal disease, in keeping with complete metabolic response after systemic treatment. (*Right column images*) Coronal maximum intensity projection PET image and transverse fused PET/CT images show areas of pathologic FDG uptake in the peritoneum after surgery (some of which are labeled with red, yellow, and green arrows). (*Left column images*) Coronal MIP PET image and transverse fused PET/CT images after adjuvant chemotherapy demonstrate resolution of all previously FDG-avid sites of disease, in keeping with complete metabolic response.

detection of the primary tumor in patients with a high suspicion of disease and also in the delineation of the tumor mass for pretreatment planning, which may have an impact on the therapeutic approach. Moreover, the excellent contrast resolution provided by PET might allow better identification of normal-sized pathologic retroperitoneal lymph nodes or small peritoneal or extrapelvic recurrences, with a radiation exposure that is 80% less than that of PET/CT.[90] A study by Queiroz and colleagues[121] comparing the diagnostic performances of PET/CT and PET/MR imaging in different pelvic tumor types has confirmed the superiority of PET/MR imaging in diagnosing the primary tumor (detection and localization) but revealed similar results in identifying regional lymph node involvement and distant metastases. Other investigators, using PET/MR imaging compared with PET/CT for restaging of gynecologic cancers, reported high but comparable diagnostic performances between the 2 imaging modalities, with lesion-based sensitivity, specificity, PPV, NPV, and accuracy for the detection of malignant lesions of 82%, 91%, 97%, 58%, and 84%, respectively, for PET/CT, and 85%, 87%, 96%, 63%, and 86%, respectively, for PET/MR imaging.[122]

PET/MR imaging currently suffers, however, from limited availability and high costs. Therefore, its potential role in clinical arena remains to be explored.

REFERENCES

1. Siegel RL, Miller KD, Jemal A. Cancer statistics, 2017. CA Cancer J Clin 2017;67(1):7–30.
2. Mapelli P, Incerti E, Fallanca F, et al. The role of ^{18}F FDG PET/CT. Q J Nucl Med Mol Imaging 2016;60: 93–102.
3. Forstner R, Meissnitzer M, Cunha TM. Update on imaging of ovarian cancer. Curr Radiol Rep 2016;4:31.
4. Ferlay J, Soerjomataram I, Dikshit R, et al. Cancer incidence and mortality worldwide: sources, methods and major patterns in GLOBOCAN 2012. Int J Cancer 2015;136(5):E359–86.
5. Surveillance, Epidemiology, and End Results (SEER) Program (www.seer.cancer.gov) Research Data (1973-2014), National Cancer Institute, DCCPS, Surveillance Research Program. 2017. Based on the November 2016 submission. Available at: https://seer.cancer.gov/statfacts/html/ovary.html.
6. Meyers MA. Distribution of intra-abdominal malignant seeding: dependency on dynamics of flow of ascitic fluid. Am J Roentgenol Radium Ther Nucl Med 1973;119:198–206.
7. Forstner R. Radiological staging of ovarian cancer: imaging findings and contribution of CT and MRI. Eur Radiol 2007;17:3223–35.
8. Coakley FV. Staging ovarian cancer: role of imaging. Radiol Clin North Am 2002;40:609–36.
9. Mitchell CL, O'Connor JP, Jackson A, et al. Identification of early predictive imaging biomarkers and their relationship to serological angiogenic markers in patients with ovarian cancer with residual disease following cytotoxic therapy. Ann Oncol 2010; 21:1982–9.
10. Prat J. FIGO Committee on Gynecologic Oncology Staging classification for cancer of the ovary, fallopian tube, and peritoneum. Int J Gynaecol Obstet 2014;124(1):1–5.
11. Prat J, Olawaiye AB, Bermudez A, et al. Ovary fallopian tube and primary peritoneal carcinoma. AJCC Cancer Staging Manual. 8th edition. Springer International Publishing; 2017. p. 681–90. Chapter 55.
12. Javadi S, Ganeshan DM, Qayyum A, et al. Ovarian cancer, the revised FIGO staging system and the role of imaging. AJR Am J Roentgenol 2016;206: 1351–60.
13. Prat J. FIGO Committee on Gynecologic Oncology Abridged republication of FIGO's staging classification for cancer of the ovary, fallopian tube, and peritoneum. Cancer 2015;121(19):3452–4.
14. Berek JS, Crum C, Friedlander M. Cancer of the ovary, fallopian tube, and peritoneum. Int J Gynaecol Obstet 2015;131(Suppl 2):S111–22.
15. Kurman R, Carcangiu ML, Herrington CS, et al. WHO classification of tumors of female reproductive organs. 4th edition. Lyon (France): The International Agency for research on Cancer; 2014.
16. Fischerova D, Burgetova A. Imaging techniques for the evaluation of ovarian cancer. Best Pract Res Clin Obstet Gynaecol 2014;28:697–720.
17. Stuart GC, Kitchener H, Bacon M, et al. 2010 Gynecologic Cancer InterGroup (GCIG) consensus statement on clinical trials in ovarian cancer: report from the Fourth Ovarian Cancer Consensus Conference. Int J Gynecol Cancer 2011;21:750–5.
18. Grab D, Flock F, Stöhr I, et al. Classification of asymptomatic adnexal masses by ultrasound, magnetic resonance imaging, and positron emission tomography. Gynecol Oncol 2000;77:454–9.
19. Khiewvan B, Torigian DA, Emamzadehfard S, et al. An update on the role of PET/CT and PET/MRI in ovarian cancer. Eur J Nucl Med Mol Imaging 2017;44:1079–91.
20. Bandiera E, Romani C, Specchia C. Serum human epididymis protein 4 and risk for ovarian malignancy algorithm as new diagnostic and prognostic tools for epithelial ovarian cancer management. Cancer Epidemiol Biomarkers Prev 2011;20: 2496–506.

21. Jacobs I, Bast RC Jr. The CA 125 tumour-associated antigen: a review of the literature. Hum Reprod 1989;4:1–12.
22. Holcomb K, Vucetic Z, Miller MC, et al. Human epididymis protein 4 offers superior specificity in the differentiation of benign and malignant adnexal masses in premenopausal women. Am J Obstet Gynecol 2011;205(4):358.
23. Grant P, Sakellis C, Jacene HA. Gynecologic oncologic imaging with PET/CT. Semin Nucl Med 2014; 44:461–78.
24. Brown DL. A practical approach to the ultrasound characterization of adnexal masses. Ultrasound Q 2007;23:87–105.
25. Brown DL, Doubilet PM, Miller FH, et al. Benign and malignant ovarian masses: selection of the most discriminating gray-scale and Doppler sonographic features. Radiology 1998;208:103–10.
26. Reles A, Wein U, Lichtenegger W, et al. Transvaginal color Doppler sonography and conventional sonography in the preoperative assessment of adnexal masses. J Clin Ultrasound 1997;25:217–25.
27. Bharwani N, Reznek RH, Rockall AG. Ovarian Cancer Management: the role of imaging and diagnostic challenges. Eur J Radiol 2011;78:41–51.
28. Hanbidge AE, Lynch D, Wilson SR. US of the peritoneum. Radiographics 2003;23:663–84.
29. Ferrazzi E, Zanetta G, Dordoni D, et al. Transvaginal ultrasonographic characterization of ovarian masses: comparison of five scoring systems in a multicenter study. Ultrasound Obstet Gynecol 1997;10:192–7.
30. Mitchell DG, Javitt MC, Glanc P, et al. ACR appropriateness criteria staging and follow-up of ovarian cancer. J Am Coll Radiol 2013;10:822–7.
31. Gu P, Pan LL, Wu SQ, et al. CA 125, PET alone, PET-CT, CT and MRI in diagnosing recurrent ovarian carcinoma: a systematic review and meta-analysis. Eur J Radiol 2009;71:164–74.
32. Fenchel S, Grab D, Nuessle K, et al. Asymptomatic adnexal masses: correlation of FDG PET and histopathologic findings. Radiology 2002;223:780–8.
33. Kitajima K, Ebina Y, Sugimura K. Present and future role of FDG-PET/CT imaging in the management of gynecologic malignancies. Jpn J Radiol 2014;32: 313–23.
34. Castellucci P, Perrone AM, Picchio M. Diagnostic accuracy of 18F-FDG PET/CT in characterizing ovarian lesions and staging ovarian cancer: correlation with transvaginal ultrasonography, computed tomography, and histology. Nucl Med Commun 2007;28:589–95.
35. Risum S, Høgdall C, Loft A, et al. The diagnostic value of PET/CT for primary ovarian cancer-a prospective study. Gynecol Oncol 2007;105:145–9.
36. Nam EJ, Yun MJ, Oh YT, et al. Diagnosis and staging of primary ovarian cancer: correlation between PET/CT, Doppler US, and CT or MRI. Gynecol Oncol 2010;116:389–94.
37. Semaan A, Munkarah AR, Arabi H, et al. Expression of GLUT-1 in epithelial ovarian carcinoma: correlation with tumor cell proliferation, angiogenesis, survival and ability to predict optimal cytoreduction. Gynecol Oncol 2011;121:181–6.
38. Cho H, Lee YS, Kim J, et al. Overexpression of glucose transporter-1 (GLUT-1) predicts poor prognosis in epithelial ovarian cancer. Cancer Invest 2013;31:607–15.
39. Yamamoto Y, Oguri H, Yamada R, et al. Preoperative evaluation of pelvic masses with combined 18F-fluorodeoxyglucose positron emission tomography and computed tomography. Int J Gynaecol Obstet 2008;102:124–7.
40. Tanizaki Y, Kobayashi A, Shiro M, et al. Diagnostic value of preoperative SUVmax on FDG-PET/CT for the detection of ovarian cancer. Int J Gynecol Cancer 2014;24(3):454–60.
41. De Gaetano AM, Calcagni ML, Rufini V, et al. Imaging of peritoneal carcinomatosis with FDG PET-CT: diagnostic patterns, case examples and pitfalls. Abdom Imaging 2009;34:391–402.
42. Kurokawa T, Yoshida Y, Kawahara K, et al. Expression of GLUT-1 glucose transfer, cellular proliferation activity and grade of tumor correlate with [F-18]-fluorodeoxyglucose uptake by positron emission tomography in epithelial tumors of the ovary. Int J Cancer 2004;109:926–32.
43. Tsukioka M, Matsumoto Y, Noriyuki M, et al. Expression of glucose transporters in epithelial ovarian carcinoma: correlation with clinical characteristics and tumor angiogenesis. Oncol Rep 2007;18:361–7.
44. Karantanis D, Allen-Auerbach M, Czernin J. Relationship among glycolytic phenotype, grade, and histological subtype in ovarian carcinoma. Clin Nucl Med 2012;37:49–53.
45. Valentin L, Ameye L, Savelli L, et al. Adnexal masses difficult to classify as benign or malignant using subjective assessment of gray-scale and Doppler ultrasound findings: logistic regression models do not help. Ultrasound Obstet Gynecol 2011;38:456–65.
46. Fruscio R, Sina F, Dolci C, et al. Preoperative 18F-FDG PET/CT in the management of advanced epithelial ovarian cancer. Gynecol Oncol 2013; 131:689–93.
47. van der Burg ME. Advanced ovarian cancer. Curr Treat Options Oncol 2001;2(2):109–18.
48. Funicelli L, Travaini LL, Landoni F, et al. Peritoneal carcinomatosis from ovarian cancer: the role of CT and [18F]FDG-PET/CT. Abdom Imaging 2010; 35:701–7.
49. Omura GA, Brady MF, Homesley HD, et al. Long-term follow-up and prognostic factor analysis in advanced ovarian carcinoma: the Gynecologic

Oncology Group experience. J Clin Oncol 1991;9: 1138–50.

50. Forstner R, Sala E, Kinkel K, et al. ESUR guidelines: ovarian cancer staging and follow-up. Eur Radiol 2010;20:2773–80.

51. Coakley FV, Choi PH, Gougoutas CA. Peritoneal metastases: detection with spiral CT in patients with ovarian cancer. Radiology 2002;223:495–9.

52. Akin O, Sala E, Moskowitz CS, et al. Perihepatic metastases from ovarian cancer: sensitivity and specificity of CT for the detection of metastases with and those without liver parenchymal invasion. Radiology 2008;248:511–7.

53. Trimbos JB, Vergote I, Bolis G, et al. Impact of adjuvant chemotherapy and surgical staging in early-stage ovarian carcinoma: European Organisation for Research and Treatment of Cancer-Adjuvant ChemoTherapy in Ovarian Neoplasm trial. J Natl Cancer Inst 2003;95(2):113–25.

54. van Meurs HS, Tajik P, Hof MH, et al. Which patients benefit most from primary surgery or neoadjuvant chemotherapy in stage IIIC or IV ovarian cancer? An exploratory analysis of the European Organisation for Research and Treatment of Cancer 55971 randomised trial. Eur J Cancer 2013;49(15):3191–201.

55. Vergote I, Tropé CG, Amant F, et al, European Organization for Research and Treatment of Cancer-Gynaecological Cancer Group, NCIC Clinical Trials Group. Neoadjuvant chemotherapy or primary surgery in stage IIIC or IV ovarian cancer. N Engl J Med 2010;363:943–53.

56. Rauh-Hain JA, Rodriguez N, Growdon WB, et al. Primary debulking surgery versus neoadjuvant chemotherapy in stage IV ovarian cancer. Ann Surg Oncol 2012;19:959–65.

57. Aletti GD, Dowdy SC, Gostout BS, et al. Aggressive surgical effort and improved survival in advanced-stage ovarian cancer. Obstet Gynecol 2006;107: 77–85.

58. Angioli R, Palaia I, Zullo MA, et al. Diagnostic open laparoscopy in the management of advanced ovarian cancer. Gynecol Oncol 2006;100:455–61.

59. Tempany CM, Zou KH, Silverman SG, et al. Staging of advanced ovarian cancer: comparison of imaging modalities-report from the Radiological Diagnostic Oncology Group. Radiology 2000;215:761–7.

60. Michielsen K, Vergote I, Op de Beeck K, et al. Whole-body MRI with diffusion-weighted sequence for staging of patients with suspected ovarian cancer: a clinical feasibility study in comparison to CT and FDG-PET/CT. Eur Radiol 2014;24:889–901.

61. Kurtz AB, Tsimikas JV, Tempany CM, et al. Diagnosis and staging of ovarian cancer: comparative values of Doppler and conventional US, CT, and MR imaging correlated with surgery and histopathologic analysis-report of the Radiology Diagnostic Oncology Group. Radiology 1999;212:19–27.

62. Kitajima K, Murakami K, Yamasaki E, et al. Diagnostic accuracy of integrated FDG-PET/contrast-enhanced CT in staging ovarian cancer: comparison with enhanced CT. Eur J Nucl Med Mol Imaging 2008;35:1912–20.

63. Signorelli M, Guerra L, Pirovano C, et al. Detection of nodal metastases by 18F-FDG PET/CT in apparent early stage ovarian cancer: a prospective study. Gynecol Oncol 2013;131(2):395–9.

64. Yuan Y, Gu ZX, Tao XF, et al. Computer tomography, magnetic resonance imaging, and positron emission tomography or positron emission tomography/computer tomography for detection of metastatic lymph nodes in patients with ovarian cancer: a meta-analysis. Eur J Radiol 2012;81:1002–6.

65. Bristow RE, Giuntoli RL 2nd, Pannu HK, et al. Combined PET/CT for detecting recurrent ovarian cancer limited to retroperitoneal lymph nodes. Gynecol Oncol 2005;99:294–300.

66. Hynninen J, Kemppainen J, Lavonius M, et al. A prospective comparison of integrated FDG-PET/contrast-enhanced CT and contrast-enhanced CT for pretreatment imaging of advanced epithelial ovarian cancer. Gynecol Oncol 2013;131:389–94.

67. Baats AS, Hugonnet F, Huchon C, et al. Prognostic significance of mediastinal 18F-FDG uptake in PET/CT in advanced ovarian cancer. Eur J Nucl Med Mol Imaging 2012;39:474–80.

68. Risum S, Høgdall C, Loft A, et al. Does the use of diagnostic PET/CT cause stage migration in patients with primary advanced ovarian cancer? Gynecol Oncol 2010;116(3):395–8.

69. Dong C, Hemminki K. Second primary neoplasms among 53 159 haematolymphoproliferative malignancy patients in Sweden, 1958-1996: a search for common mechanisms. Br J Cancer 2001;85: 997–1005.

70. De Iaco P, Musto A, Orazi L, et al. FDG-PET/CT in advanced ovarian cancer staging: value and pitfalls in detecting lesions in different abdominal and pelvic quadrants compared with laparoscopy. Eur J Radiol 2011;80(2):e98–103.

71. Nakamura K, Kodama J, Okumura Y, et al. The SUVmax of 18F-FDG PET correlates with histological grade in endometrial cancer. Int J Gynecol Cancer 2010;20:110–5.

72. Konishi H, Takehara K, Kojima A, et al. Maximum standardized uptake value of fluorodeoxyglucose positron emission tomography/computed tomography is a prognostic factor in ovarian clear cell adenocarcinoma. Int J Gynecol Cancer 2014;24: 1190–4.

73. González García B, García Vicente AM, Jiménez Londoño GA, et al. 18F-FDG PET/CT as predictor of tumour biology and prognosis in epithelial ovarian carcinoma. Rev Esp Med Nucl Imagen Mol 2017;36(4):233–40.

74. Lee JW, Cho A, Lee JH, et al. The role of metabolic tumor volume and total lesion glycolysis on ^{18}F-FDG PET/CT in the prognosis of epithelial ovarian cancer. Eur J Nucl Med Mol Imaging 2014;41:1898–906.

75. Chung HH, Kwon HW, Kang KW, et al. Prognostic value of preoperative metabolic tumor volume and total lesion glycolysis in patients with epithelial ovarian cancer. Ann Surg Oncol 2012;19(6):1966–72.

76. Gallicchio R, Nardelli A, Venetucci A, et al. F-18 FDG PET/CT metabolic tumor volume predicts overall survival in patients with disseminated epithelial ovarian cancer. Eur J Radiol 2017;93:107–13.

77. Risum S, Loft A, Engelholm SA, et al. Positron emission tomography/computed tomography predictors of overall survival in stage IIIC/IV ovarian cancer. Int J Gynecol Cancer 2012;2:1163–9.

78. Avril N, Sassen S, Schmalfeldt B. Prediction of response to neoadjuvant chemotherapy by sequential F-18-fluorodeoxyglucose positron emission tomography in patients with advanced-stage ovarian cancer. J Clin Oncol 2005;23:7445–53 [Erratum appears in J Clin Oncol 2005;23(36):9445].

79. Martoni AA, Fanti S, Zamagni C, et al. [18F]FDG-PET/CT monitoring early identifies advanced ovarian cancer patients who will benefit from prolonged neo-adjuvant chemotherapy. Q J Nucl Med Mol Imaging 2011;55:81–90.

80. Vallius T, Peter A, Auranen A, et al. 18F-FDG-PET/CT can identify histopathological non-responders to platinum-based neoadjuvant chemotherapy in advanced epithelial ovarian cancer. Gynecol Oncol 2016;140:29–35.

81. Antunovic L, Cimitan M, Borsatti E, et al. Revisiting the clinical value of 18F-FDG PET/CT in detection of recurrent epithelial ovarian carcinomas: correlation with histology, serum CA-125 assay, and conventional radiological modalities. Clin Nucl Med 2012;37:e184–8.

82. Rew F, Galaal K, Brynt A, et al. Evaluation of follow-up strategies for patients with epithelial ovarian cancer following completion of primary treatment. Cochrane Database Syst Rev 2011;(6):CD006119.

83. Goonewardene TI, Hall MR, Rustin GJ. Management of asymptomatic patients on follow-up for ovarian cancer with rising CA-125 concentrations. Lancet Oncol 2007;8:813–21.

84. Rustin GJ, Nelstrop AE, McClean P, et al. Defining response of ovarian carcinoma to initial chemotherapy according to serum CA 125. J Clin Oncol 1996;1:1545–51.

85. Marcus CS, Maxwell GL, Darcy KM, et al. Current approaches and challenges in managing and monitoring treatment response in ovarian cancer. J Cancer 2014;5:25–30.

86. Low RN, Duggan B, Barone RM, et al. Treated ovarian cancer: MR imaging, laparotomy reassessment, and serum CA-125 values compared with clinical outcome at 1 year. Radiology 2005;235:918–26.

87. Ghosh J, Thulkar S, Kumar R, et al. Role of FDG PET-CT in asymptomatic epithelial ovarian cancer with rising serum CA-125: a pilot study. Natl Med J India 2013;26:327–31.

88. Brunetti JC. Fludeoxyglucose F 18 PET-computed tomography: management changes effecting patient outcome in gynecologic malignancies. PET Clin 2015;10:395–409.

89. Sironi S, Messa C, Mangili G, et al. Integrated FDG PET/CT in patients with persistent ovarian cancer: correlation with histologic findings. Radiology 2004;233:433–40.

90. Suppiah S, Chang WL, Hassan HA, et al. Systematic review on the accuracy of positron emission tomography/computed tomography and positron emission tomography/magnetic resonance imaging in the management of ovarian cancer: is functional information really needed? World J Nucl Med 2017;1:176–85.

91. Evangelista L, Palma MD, Gregianin M, et al. Diagnostic and prognostic evaluation of fluorodeoxyglucose positron emission tomography/computed tomography and its correlation with serum cancer antigen-125 (CA125) in a large cohort of ovarian cancer patients. J Turk Ger Gynecol Assoc 2015; 16:137–44.

92. Pan HS, Lee SL, Huang LW, et al. Combined positron emission tomography-computed tomography and tumor markers for detecting recurrent ovarian cancer. Arch Gynecol Obstet 2011;283:335–41.

93. Bhosale P, Peungjesada S, Wei W, et al. Clinical utility of positron emission tomography/computed tomography in the evaluation of suspected recurrent ovarian cancer in the setting of normal CA-125 levels. Int J Gynecol Cancer 2010;20:936–44.

94. Sala E, Kataoka M, Pandit-Taskar N, et al. Recurrent ovarian cancer: use of contrast-enhanced CT and PET/CT to accurately localize tumor recurrence and to predict patients survival. Radiology 2010;257:125–34.

95. Fulham MJ, Carter J, Baldey A, et al. The impact of PET-CT in suspected recurrent ovarian cancer: a prospective multi-centre study as part of the Australian PET Data Collection Project. Gynecol Oncol 2009;112:462–8.

96. Menzel C, Döbert N, Hamscho N, et al. The influence of CA 125 and CEA levels on the results of (18)F-deoxyglucose positron emission tomography in suspected recurrence of epithelial ovarian cancer. Strahlenther Onkol 2004;180: 497–501.

97. Thrall MM, DeLoia JA, Gallion H, et al. Clinical use of combined positron emission tomography and computed tomography (FDG-PET/CT) in recurrent ovarian cancer. Gynecol Oncol 2007;105:17–22.

98. Risum S, Høgdall C, Markova E, et al. Influence of 2-(18F) fluoro-2-deoxy-D-glucose positron emission tomography/computed tomography on recurrent ovarian cancer diagnosis and on selection of patients for secondary cytoreductive surgery. Int J Gynecol Cancer 2009;19(4):600–4.

99. Mangili G, Picchio M, Sironi S, et al. Integrated PET/CT as a first-line re-staging modality in patients with suspected recurrence of ovarian cancer. Eur J Nucl Med Mol Imaging 2007;34:658–66.

100. Ricke J, Sehouli J, Hach C, et al. Prospective evaluation of contrast-enhanced MRI in the depiction of peritoneal spread in primary or recurrent ovarian cancer. Eur Radiol 2003;13:943–9.

101. Santillan A, Garg R, Zahurak ML, et al. Risk of epithelial ovarian cancer recurrence in patients with rising serum CA-125 levels within the normal range. J Clin Oncol 2005;20(23):9338–43.

102. Peng NJ, Liou WS, Liu RS, et al. Early detection of recurrent ovarian cancer in patients with low-level increases in serum CA-125 levels by 2-[F-18]fluoro-2-deoxy-D-glucose-positron emission tomography/computed tomography. Cancer Biother Radiopharm 2011;26:175–81.

103. Kim S, Chung JK, Kang SB, et al. 18F-FDG PET as a substitute for second-look laparotomy in patients with advanced ovarian carcinoma. Eur J Nucl Med Mol Imaging 2004;31:196–201.

104. Obermair A, Sevelda P. Impact of second look laparotomy and secondary cytoreductive surgery at second-look laparotomy in ovarian cancer patients. Acta Obstet Gynecol Scand 2001;80:432–6.

105. Harter P, Hilpert F, Mahner S, et al. Prognostic factors for complete debulking in first- and second-line ovarian cancer. Int J Gynecol Cancer 2009; 19(Suppl 2):S14–7.

106. Chuang CM, Chou YJ, Yen MS, et al. The role of secondary cytoreductive surgery in patients with recurrent epithelial ovarian, tubal, and peritoneal cancers: a comparative effectiveness analysis. Oncologist 2012;17:847–55.

107. Peng P, Zhu ZH, Zhong ZJ, et al. Benefits of fluorine-18 fludeoxyglucose positron emission tomography in secondary cytoreductive surgery for patients with recurrent epithelial ovarian cancer. Br J Radiol 2015;88(1052):20150109.

108. Hebel CB, Behrendt FF, Heinzel A, et al. Negative 18F-2-fluorodeoxyglucose PET/CT predicts good cancer specific survival in patients with a suspicion of recurrent ovarian cancer. Eur J Radiol 2014;83: 463–7.

109. Morris M, Gershenson DM, Wharton JT, et al. Secondary cytoreductive surgery for recurrent epithelial ovarian cancer. Gynecol Oncol 1989;34:334–8.

110. Segna RA, Dottino PR, Mandeli JP, et al. Secondary cytoreduction for ovarian cancer following cisplatin therapy. J Clin Oncol 1993;11:434.

111. Simcock B, Neesham D, Quinn M, et al. The impact of PET/CT in the management of recurrent ovarian cancer. Gynecol Oncol 2006;103:271–6.

112. You JJ, Cline KJ, Gu CS, et al. (18)F-fluorodeoxyglucose positron-emission tomography-computed tomography to diagnose recurrent cancer. Br J Cancer 2015;112:1737–43.

113. Hillner BE, Siegel BA, Liu D, et al. Impact of positron emission tomography/computed tomography and positron emission tomography (PET) alone on expected management of patients with cancer: initial results from the National Oncologic PET Registry. J Clin Oncol 2008;26:2155–61.

114. Hillner BE, Siegel BA, Shields AF, et al. The impact of positron emission tomography (PET) on expected management during cancer treatment: findings of the National Oncologic PET Registry. Cancer 2009;115:410–8.

115. Musto A, Grassetto G, Marzola MC, et al. Management of epithelial ovarian cancer from diagnosis to re-staging: an overview of the role of imaging techniques with particular regard to the contribution of 18F-FDGPET/CT. Nucl Med Commun 2014;35:588–97.

116. Vargas HA, Burger IA, Goldman DA, et al. Volume-based quantitative FDG PET/CT metrics and their association with optimal debulking and progression-free survival in patients with recurrent ovarian cancer undergoing secondary cytoreductive surgery. Eur Radiol 2015;25:3348–53.

117. Caobelli F, Alongi P, Evangelista L, et al. Predictive value of (18)F-FDG PET/CT in restaging patients affected by ovarian carcinoma: a multicentre study. Eur J Nucl Med Mol Imaging 2016;43(3):404–13.

118. Kim CY, Jeong SY, Chong GO, et al. Quantitative metabolic parameters measured on F-18 FDG PET/CT predict survival after relapse in patients with relapsed epithelial ovarian cancer. Gynecol Oncol 2015;136:498–504.

119. Boers-Sonderen MJ, de Geus-Oei LF, Desar IM, et al. Temsirolimus and pegylated liposomal doxorubicin (PLD) combination therapy in breast, endometrial, and ovarian cancer: phase Ib results and prediction of clinical outcome with FDG-PET/CT. Target Oncol 2014;9:339–47.

120. Partovi S, Kohan A, Rubbert C. Clinical oncologic applications of PET/MRI: a new horizon. Am J Nucl Med Mol Imaging 2014;4:202–12.

121. Queiroz MA, Kubik-Huch RA, Hauser N, et al. PET/MRI and PET/CT in advanced gynaecological tumours: initial experience and comparison. Eur Radiol 2015;25:2222–30.

122. Grueneisen J, Schaarschmidt BM, Heubner M, et al. Implementation of FAST-PET/MRI for whole-body staging of female patients with recurrent pelvic malignancies: a comparison to PET/CT. Eur J Radiol 2015;84:2097–102.

FDG-PET Assessment of Other Gynecologic Cancers

Silvana Faria, MD, PhD*, Catherine Devine, MD, Chitra Viswanathan, MD,
Sanaz Javadi, MD, Brinda Rao Korivi, MD, MPH, Priya R. Bhosale, MD

KEYWORDS

- Positron emission tomography (PET)
- Positron emission tomography/computed tomography (PET/CT) • Endometrial cancer
- Vulvar cancer • Vaginal cancer • Uterine cancer • Uterine sarcoma

KEY POINTS

- PET/computed tomography has value in the preoperative assessment of patients with endometrial, vulvar, and vaginal cancers owing to detection of locoregional lymph nodes and distant metastases.
- PET/computed tomography can monitor response to treatment and detect early recurrent disease of gynecologic malignancies, allowing for prompt and adequate treatment of patients.
- PET/computed tomography imaging plays an important role in the management of patients with endometrial cancer, vulvar and vaginal cancers, and uterine sarcomas.

INTRODUCTION

PET is a noninvasive radiologic modality that images glucose consumption. The ability of PET to detect malignancy relies on the metabolic activity and the rate of glucose use in tumor cells compared with normal cells. Currently, the most commonly used radiotracer for PET imaging is ^{18}F-fluorodeoxyglucose (FDG). FDG is a glucose analogue that is injected into the patient, enters tumor cells, is phosphorylated by hexokinase but does not undergo further glucose metabolism, and becomes trapped within tumor cells. The radioactive decay of FDG by positron emission allows for the spatial localization and detection of active sites of tumor by the PET scanner.[1] When PET is combined with computed tomography (CT) scanning, it allows for the simultaneous anatomic localization and metabolic assessment of sites of disease. During the last decade, PET/CT scanning has advanced tremendously and has become an essential diagnostic tool in the oncologic staging and surveillance of patients with different types of cancer. There is growing evidence supporting the use of PET and PET/CT scanning in gynecologic malignancies. They are already largely used to stage, monitor response to treatment, and detect recurrent disease in patients with cervical and ovarian cancers. This article reviews the usefulness as well as the limitations of PET and mostly PET/CT imaging in patients with endometrial cancer and other gynecologic malignancies, such as vulvar and vaginal cancers and uterine sarcomas.

IMAGING PROTOCOL

Patients must fast for at least 6 hours and avoid vigorous exercise for 24 hours before the study. If diabetic, they are asked to hold their medication or insulin for 6 hours before the study.

All authors have no disclosures.
Department of Diagnostic Radiology, Abdominal Imaging Section, The University of Texas MD Anderson Cancer Center, 1400 Pressler Street, Unit 1473, Houston, TX 77030-4008, USA
* Corresponding author.
E-mail address: SCFaria@mdanderson.org

PET Clin 13 (2018) 203–223
https://doi.org/10.1016/j.cpet.2017.11.006
1556-8598/18/© 2017 Elsevier Inc. All rights reserved.

PET/CT imaging is usually performed 90 minutes after the injection of intravenous FDG, because the half-life of the ^{18}F isotope is 110 minutes. FDG is mainly excreted through the urinary tract, and so patients should empty their bladder before scanning. Activity in normal bowel and in the urinary tract can limit interpretation of PET in gynecologic malignancies.[2] Therefore, technical modifications such as intravenous hydration with concomitant diuresis, continuous bladder irrigation, and mechanical bowel preparation or insertion of a Foley catheter can be performed to limit bowel, bladder, and ureteric activity.

In premenopausal patients, normal endometrial and ovarian FDG uptake changes cyclically with the menstrual cycle. Endometrial activity and activity in uterine fibroids increase during the menstrual and ovulatory phases. Endometriomas and corpus luteal cysts in the ovaries may also be FDG avid.[3] These benign physiologic causes of increased metabolic activity must be taken into consideration during the interpretation of PET/CT images in premenopausal patients to avoid false-positive results. To differentiate physiologic activity from malignancy, repeat imaging can be performed in the early follicular phase of the menstrual cycle. In postmenopausal woman, increased uterine and ovarian FDG uptake is much less likely to indicate a benign process and is usually associated with malignancy.

ENDOMETRIAL CANCER

Endometrial carcinoma is the most common gynecologic malignancy in industrialized nations.[4] Approximately 61,380 new cases are expected in the United States and 10,920 deaths are estimated to occur during 2017.[5] Endometrial carcinoma is more common during the sixth and seventh decades of life, affecting mainly postmenopausal women. However, up to 20% of cases may occur in premenopausal women. Abnormal uterine bleeding, intermenstrual or postmenopausal, is present in more than 80% of cases. The main risk factors for the development of endometrial cancer include increased unopposed estrogen, obesity, nulliparity, diabetes mellitus, Stein-Leventhal syndrome, Lynch syndrome, and tamoxifen therapy.[6] Definitive diagnosis of endometrial cancer is generally made via endometrial biopsy or dilation and curettage.

Traditionally, endometrial carcinomas have been classified based on clinical and endocrine features as type I (the most common type, associated with estrogen excess, obesity, low grade, and a good prognosis) or type II (not estrogen dependent, occurring in older women, and associated with a worse prognosis), as defined by Bokhman or on histopathologic characteristics (endometrioid, serous, or clear cell adenocarcinoma).[7] Correlations have been noted between the subtypes in these 2 classification systems, with type I cancers generally having endometrioid histology and most type II cancers being serous carcinomas. However, most recently, there has been an incorporation of molecular, genomic, and histopathologic features into classification and risk determination of endometrial carcinoma.[8]

Parameters that impact prognosis and survival include the stage of disease at diagnosis, pathologic grade, depth of myometrial invasion, histologic features, lymphovascular invasion, and lymph node status. The tumor typically spreads by myometrial invasion, extension into the cervix, transtubal spread via the fallopian tubes to the ovaries, or transserosal spread to the bladder or bowel.[9]

Endometrial cancer is staged according to the International Federation of Gynecology and Obstetrics (FIGO) system (**Table 1**).[10] Stage I reflects tumor that is confined to the uterine corpus, which is further divided into stage IA (<50% myometrial invasion) and IB (>50% of myometrial invasion). Tumors with cervical stromal invasion are defined as stage II. Stage III represents tumor spread beyond the uterus but not outside the true pelvis, which is further divided into stage IIIA (invading the uterine serosa and/or adnexa), stage IIIB (extending into the parametrium and/or vagina), stage IIIC1 (with pelvic lymph node involvement), and stage IIIC2 (with paraaortic lymph node involvement). Stage IVA includes tumors with extension to the bladder or bowel, and stage IVB tumors have distant metastases. Owing to early symptoms, approximately 75% of women with endometrial cancer are diagnosed with stage I disease. The mean 5-year survival rate for stage I is 85%, for stage II 70%, for stage III 50%, and for stage IV 18%.[11]

MR imaging is considered the most accurate imaging technique for the preoperative assessment of endometrial cancer, particularly regarding the presence and depth of myometrial invasion. PET/CT scanning has little value in detecting early stage disease because most early stage patients have disease confined to the uterus. The reported mean standardized uptake value (SUV) of endometrial cancer is 11.2 ± 5.9 (SD) with maximum SUV (SUV_{max}) ranging from 2.3 to 8.2.[12] Although

Table 1
FIGO staging of endometrial cancer

FIGO Stage	Definition
IA	Tumor confined to the uterus, no invasion or invasion of less than one-half of the myometrial thickness.
IB	Tumor confined to the uterus with invasion equal to or more than one-half of the myometrial thickness.
II	Tumor invades the cervical stroma but does not extend beyond the uterus.
IIIA	Tumor invades the uterine serosa or adnexa.
IIIB	Vaginal and/or parametrial involvement.
IIIC	Metastases to pelvic or paraaortic lymph nodes.
IIIC1	Pelvic lymph node involvement.
IIIC2	Paraaortic lymph node involvement (with or without pelvic nodes).
IVA	Tumor invasion of the bladder and/or bowel mucosa.
IVB	Distant metastases including abdominal metastases and/or inguinal lymph nodes.

Abbreviation: FIGO, International Federation of Gynecology and Obstetrics.

Adapted from Amant F, Mirza MR, Koskas M, et al. Cancer of the corpus uteri. Int J Gynaecol Obstet 2015;131 Suppl 2:S97; with permission.

endometrial cancer shows intense FDG uptake, the added value of PET/CT scanning in initial staging of early stage disease is restricted owing to limited spatial resolution, as well as physiologic uptake of FDG in premenopausal women and in other benign conditions such as endometrial hyperplasia, polyps, adenomyosis, and leiomyomas that can also show metabolic activity.[13] Additionally, because of this wide range of values and dependence of SUV_{max} on various factors such as delay time after radiotracer injection, serum blood glucose, partial volume effects, and differences between scanners and image reconstruction methods, a diagnosis of malignancy cannot be based on SUV measurements alone.[14]

MR imaging can also be used to evaluate extra-uterine disease. However, PET and most recently, PET/CT scanning, have added value in the preoperative assessment of regional and distant metastatic lymph node in patients with endometrial carcinoma. Park and colleagues[15] compared

PET/CT and MR imaging for preoperative detectability of lymph node metastases in 53 patients with endometrial cancer, and found that PET/CT scanning had better sensitivity and specificity (69% and 90%, respectively) than MR imaging (46% and 87%, respectively) for the detection of pelvic lymph node metastases (**Fig. 1**).

In a study comparing diffusion-weighted imaging and PET/CT scanning for preoperative evaluation of pelvic lymph node metastases in uterine cancer, diffusion-weighted imaging showed higher sensitivity (83%) than PET/CT scanning (38%), but lower specificity (51% vs 96%, respectively) and lower accuracy (57% vs 86%, respectively). Based on these findings, the authors concluded that neither diffusion-weighted imaging nor PET/CT scanning were sufficiently accurate to replace lymphadenectomy.[16]

Kitajima and colleagues[17] reported an overall node-based sensitivity of 51%, specificity of 99.8%, and accuracy of 98.7% for the detection of nodal metastases by PET/CT scanning. They also observed that the sensitivity for detecting metastatic nodal lesions varied with size. For lesions 4 mm or less in diameter, sensitivity was low at 13%; for lesions between 5 and 9 mm, sensitivity increased to 67%; and for nodes 10 mm or larger, sensitivity increased to 100%. Other authors also showed that detectability using PET/CT scanning is low for metastatic lymph nodes with a short axis diameter of 6 mm or less.[18] Mayoral and colleagues[19] showed a higher retention index in malignant lymph nodes when compared with inflammatory lymph nodes, suggesting that the use of dual time-point imaging may help to differentiate between inflammatory and malignant lymph nodes, although no statistically significant differences were found.

A prospective multicenter study of 207 patients confirmed that PET/CT scanning has satisfactory accuracy in the detection of pelvic and abdominal lymph node metastases (**Fig. 2**) in patients with high-risk endometrial cancer.[20] In a recent metaanalysis of 13 studies with 861 patients with endometrial cancer, the overall pooled sensitivity and specificity for PET/CT scanning preoperative detection of lymph node metastases were 72% and 94%, respectively.[21] These results suggest that one-fourth of metastatic lymph nodes are still not detected. A possible explanation is that PET/CT scanning may not be able to detect small tumors or micrometastases. However, the combination of sentinel lymph node mapping and PET/CT scanning may reduce the incidence of unnecessary systematic lymphadenectomy, thereby preventing unnecessary complications from this invasive surgical procedure.[22]

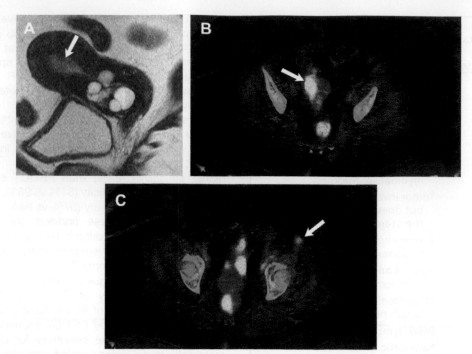

Fig. 1. A 57-year-old woman with endometrial cancer. (A) Preoperative sagittal T2-weighted MR image shows thickened endometrium (arrow). (B) Preoperative PET/computed tomography (CT) axial image showing focal high ^{18}F-fluorodeoxyglucose (FDG) uptake within the endometrium (arrow) corresponding with the primary endometrial cancer. (C) Preoperative PET/CT axial image shows FDG uptake in the left inguinal lymph node (arrow) that was biopsied with confirmation of metastatic disease.

Preoperative primary tumor metabolic parameters such as preoperative SUV_{max} have been associated with more aggressive endometrial tumors and, consequently, with the presence of lymph node metastases and tumor recurrence.[23,24] However, SUV_{max} measurements of endometrial tumors have considerable overlap between low-risk and high-risk groups despite a higher mean SUV_{max} in high-risk groups. Recently, advanced techniques such as whole tumor voxel-by-voxel analysis may allow for decreased operator dependence and capture of more

relevant and comprehensive measures of tumor microenvironment and heterogeneity to be correlated with prognostic features.[25]

As the depth of myometrial invasion increases, so does the likelihood of lymphovascular invasion, with subsequent lymphatic, peritoneal, and hematogenous metastases. PET/CT scanning is highly sensitive and specific (100% and 96%, respectively) for detecting distant metastases in the abdomen and in extraabdominal regions in selected high-risk patients with endometrial carcinoma[26] (Fig. 3).

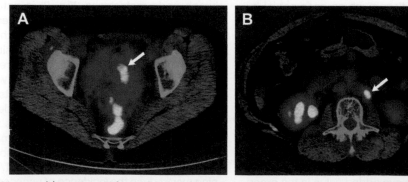

Fig. 2. A 69-year-old woman with grade III endometrioid adenocarcinoma. (A) Preoperative PET/computed tomography (CT) axial image shows focal high ^{18}F-fluorodeoxyglucose (FDG) uptake within the endometrium (arrow) corresponding with the primary endometrial cancer. (B) Preoperative PET/CT axial image shows FDG uptake in the left paraaortic lymph node (arrow) that was biopsied with a confirmation of metastatic disease.

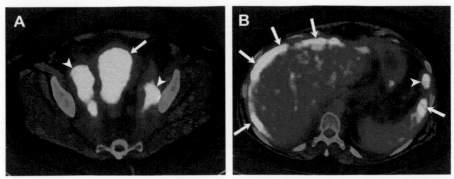

Fig. 3. A 64-year-old woman with high-grade endometrial cancer. (*A*) Preoperative PET/computed tomography (CT) axial image shows distended endometrial cavity by a large heterogeneous mass associated with high ^{18}F-fluorodeoxyglucose (FDG) uptake (*arrow*) corresponding with the primary endometrial cancer. Note the metastatic bilateral pelvic lymph nodes (*arrowheads*). (*B*) Preoperative PET/CT axial image shows FDG uptake in perihepatic and perisplenic peritoneal implants (*arrows*) and in an omental implant (*arrowhead*).

PET/CT scanning also plays a role in the post-treatment surveillance of patients. Approximately 25% to 30% of patients with advanced disease and poor prognosis factors may develop recurrent disease.[27] Early detection of recurrent endometrial cancer with prompt initiation of therapy is believed to affect survival.[28] Posttherapeutic changes can be difficult to differentiate from recurrent disease on CT scanning, because they can have similar morphologic appearances. Viable tumor is more likely to demonstrate hypermetabolism, and thus can be differentiated from posttherapeutic change on PET/CT scanning.

Tumor recurrence usually occurs at an overall median time of 13 months after the primary surgery. The vagina is the most common location for locally recurrent endometrial carcinoma,[29] where the vaginal apex is the site most frequently affected (**Fig. 4**). On PET, recurrent tumor appears as a focal area of increased FDG uptake. In a series of patients analyzed retrospectively by Belhocine and colleagues,[30] PET/CT scanning changed the management in 35% of cases by finding tumor recurrence in 88% of symptomatic patients and in 12% of asymptomatic patients.

Other observed sites of relapse of endometrial cancer include distant lymph nodes, peritoneum, lungs, and liver[29] (**Fig. 5**). In the setting of suspected recurrent disease, PET/CT scanning has a reported sensitivity of 90% to 93%, a specificity

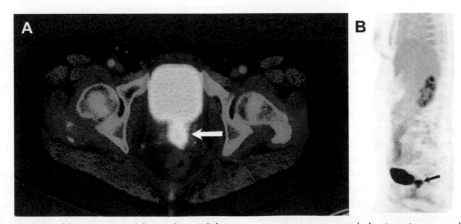

Fig. 4. A 72-year-old woman with endometrial cancer, status post total hysterectomy and salpingo-oophorectomy, returned for a 6-month follow-up evaluation. (*A*) PET/computed tomography (CT) axial image shows focal high ^{18}F-fluorodeoxyglucose (FDG) uptake at the region of the vaginal cuff (*arrow*), suspicious for recurrent disease. (*B*) Sagittal PET maximum intensity projection image shows focal high FDG uptake behind the bladder at the region of the vaginal cuff (*arrow*). PET/CT shows that there were no other sites of recurrent disease. Biopsy confirmed locally recurrent disease in the vaginal cuff. The patient was treated with radiation therapy.

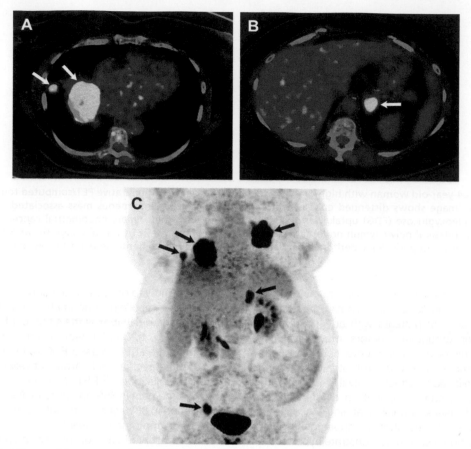

Fig. 5. A 75-year-old woman with endometrial cancer, status post total hysterectomy and salpingo-oophorectomy, returns for an 18-month follow-up evaluation. (*A*) PET/computed tomography (CT) axial image shows focal high ^{18}F-fluorodeoxyglucose (FDG) uptake in lung nodule and mass (*arrows*), suggestive of metastatic disease. (*B*) PET/CT axial image shows focal high FDG uptake in the left adrenal gland (*arrow*), suggestive of metastatic disease. (*C*) Coronal PET maximum intensity projection image demonstrates focal high FDG uptake in the lungs, left adrenal gland, and in a right external iliac lymph node (*arrows*).

of 81% to 100%, an accuracy of 87% to 96%, a positive predictive value (PPV) of 93% to 95%, and a negative predictive value (NPV) of 100%.[31,32] In a recent metaanalysis of 8 studies with 378 patients, the overall pooled sensitivity and specificity for the detection of endometrial cancer recurrence were 95% and 91%, respectively, concluding that PET/CT scanning has an excellent diagnostic performance in the detection of recurrence after endometrial carcinoma surgery with curative intent.[21] Most recently, Kang and colleagues[33] reported an association between the preoperative intratumoral FDG uptake heterogeneity derived from PET/CT scanning and a high tumor recurrence in endometrial cancer. In a study with 29 patients, the metabolic tumor volume was used to predict deep myometrial invasion and lymph node metastases with odds ratios of 7.8 and 16.5, respectively.[34] The metabolic tumor volume also showed a correlation with disease-free survival in a study of 84 patients with endometrial cancer.[35]

The treatment for recurrent endometrial cancer depends on the anatomic location of the recurrence and the presence of a single or multiple recurrent sites. The 5-year cure rate for patients with isolated recurrence at the vaginal apex is reported to be 40% to 60%.[2] PET/CT scanning can be used to exclude or to detect extrapelvic recurrence (see **Fig. 5**). The use of radiotherapy to treat patients with localized recurrence at the vaginal cuff (see **Fig. 4**) who had not received whole pelvic radiation therapy is reported to increase the cure rates to 90%. In some cases, isolated pelvic recurrences can be treated with pelvic exenteration. Patients with systemic disease can be treated with chemotherapy or hormonal therapy.[36]

PET/MR imaging systems have recently been developed, adding the strengths of PET in detecting nodal and distant metastatic disease to the strengths of MR imaging in local staging. PET/MR imaging scanners acquire MR imaging and PET data either simultaneously or sequentially. In a simultaneous acquisition device, the PET and MR imaging scanners are housed in a single gantry, allowing for concurrent imaging of the same body regions simultaneously. In the sequential acquisition device, 2 spatially separate PET and MR imaging scanners are connected by a moving table that reduces changes in patient positioning between successive imaging events. Both devices collect MR imaging and PET datasets in a single imaging session, allowing for fusion image analysis.[37]

It has been shown that fused PET/MR imaging is valuable in the preoperative evaluation of patients with endometrial cancer (**Fig. 6**). Fused contrast-enhanced PET/MR imaging and contrast-enhanced MR imaging detected more primary tumors in comparison with contrast-enhanced PET/CT scanning (96.7% vs 93.3%, respectively).[38] In a direct comparison of fused PET/MR imaging, MR imaging, and PET/CT scan data, PET/MR imaging and MR imaging alone were both more accurate for local staging of endometrial cancer compared with PET/CT imaging (accuracy of 80% vs 60%, respectively).[38] In 1 study comparing PET/CT imaging with simultaneously acquired PET/MR imaging, although both modalities correctly detected all malignant lesions in patients with recurrent tumors of the female pelvis, the diagnostic confidence was significantly higher for PET/MR imaging ($P \le .01$).[39] In an additional

study of 24 patients with suspected tumor recurrence who underwent PET/CT and PET/MR imaging studies, there was a comparable high diagnostic performance between PET/CT and PET/MR imaging with no significant differences (sensitivity, specificity, and accuracy of 82%, 91%, and 84% vs 85%, 87%, and 86%, respectively).[40]

On PET/MR imaging, an increased SUV_{max} and decreased minimum apparent diffusion coefficient on preoperative imaging has been correlated with endometrial cancer having high-risk features. The ratio of the SUV_{max} to the minimum apparent diffusion coefficient was also correlated with greater risk or higher stage tumors.[41] A recent systematic review of the literature suggested that PET/MR imaging is comparable with PET/CT scans in the detection of local lymph node and distant metastases, whereas PET/MR imaging is superior for local staging and determining the local extent of disease.[42]

Future directions for this rapidly developing PET/MR imaging technology include investigation of new PET radiotracers as well as novel MR imaging contrast agents with altered molecular specificity, such as hyperpolarized ^{13}C compounds and superparamagnetic iron oxide particles that, in conjunction with an increase in availability, are likely to make PET/MR imaging a very important tool in the preoperative staging and surveillance of patients with endometrial cancer[43] (**Box 1**).

UTERINE SARCOMAS

Uterine sarcomas are rare gynecologic malignancies representing 3% to 7% of all uterine

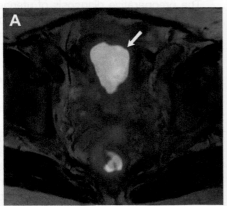 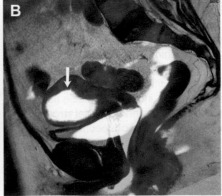

Fig. 6. A 65-year-old woman with intermittent postmenopausal bleeding. (*A*) Axial PET/T2-weighted MR image shows a distended endometrial cavity by a heterogeneous mass associated with high ^{18}F-fluorodeoxyglucose (FDG) uptake (*arrow*). (*B*) Sagittal PET/T2-weighted MR image shows high FDG uptake within an endometrial cavity mass with an maximum standardized uptake value of 18.4 corresponding with the primary endometrial cancer (*arrow*). Note that the tumor is confined to the uterine corpus, but there is more than 50% myometrial invasion (stage IB).

malignant neoplasms and less than 1% of all malignancies from female genital organs. The incidence is 0.4 per 100,000 women.[5]

The mean age at diagnosis is in the sixth to seventh decades of life. Although the majority of cases are seen in postmenopausal women, uterine sarcomas have also been diagnosed in young women.[44] Generally, patients do not have identifiable risk factors. Although uncertain, prior treatment with tamoxifen and previous pelvic irradiation have been reported as potential risk factors. Additionally, studies in soft tissue sarcoma have attributed an increased risk with p53 gene mutations.[45]

Most symptoms are nonspecific and may resemble those associated with the much more common uterine leiomyomas, including abdominal pain, abnormal uterine bleeding, a rapidly enlarged uterine size, or a uterine mass. Some women are asymptomatic. Thus, owing to the absence of specific signs and symptoms, the diagnosis may be incidental when examining the resected hysterectomy specimen.

The histopathologic classification of uterine sarcomas was revised in 2003 by the World Health Organization.[46] Histologic classification of uterine sarcomas is based on the differentiation and growth pattern of the neoplastic cells and their presumed cell of origin. They are referred to as homologous or heterologous. The majority are homologous, which differentiate in ways similar to normal uterine tissues including muscle (leiomyosarcomas), endometrium (endometrial stromal sarcomas), or sarcomas of nonspecific supporting tissue.[47] Historically, uterine carcinosarcoma was classified as a type of sarcoma (malignant mixed Mullerian tumor), but they are now classified as carcinomas owing to their different spreading pattern as a dedifferentiated or metaplastic form of endometrial cancer. There are 3 main subtypes of uterine sarcomas: leiomyosarcoma (the most common), endometrial stromal sarcoma, and adenosarcoma. Uterine sarcomas spread via intra-abdominal, lymphatic, or hematogenous routes.[48]

Recently, a new FIGO classification and staging system has been designed specifically for uterine sarcomas. Briefly, 3 new classifications have been developed: staging for leiomyosarcomas and endometrial stromal sarcomas, staging for adenosarcomas, and staging for carcinosarcomas that continue to be staged as endometrial carcinomas (Table 2).[49] Stage I involves a tumor limited to the uterus, stage II involves a tumor extending to the pelvis, stage III involves a tumor invading abdominal tissues, and stage IV involves a tumor invading the bladder and/or rectum or the presence of distant metastases. Depending on the histology, in leiomyosarcoma and endometrial stromal sarcomas, stage I is divided into 2 categories, IA 5 cm or less, and IB greater than 5 cm. In adenosarcoma, IA is within the endometrium, IB 50% or less myometrial invasion, and IC greater than 50% myometrial invasion. Carcinosarcoma should be staged as endometrial cancer.

Standard treatment includes surgical resection with total hysterectomy and bilateral salpingo oophorectomy. Adjuvant treatment with chemotherapy, hormonal therapy, or radiation therapy may be considered. Routine lymph node dissection is controversial because nodal metastases are infrequent, but should be considered in patients with suspicious lymph nodes or extrauterine disease.[50]

Uterine sarcomas have an aggressive biology and can lead to early spread locally and hematogenously giving distant metastases most commonly to the lungs and liver. The overall 5-year survival rate ranges from 17.5% to 54.7%. Therefore, imaging has a pivotal role in the preoperative mapping of uterine sarcomas to select the best therapeutic strategy.[51]

The preoperative diagnosis of uterine sarcoma is challenging. Imaging studies are performed preoperatively to characterize a uterine mass. However, there is overlap in imaging features between degenerated leiomyomas and sarcomas and, therefore, imaging studies cannot reliably differentiate between uterine sarcoma and other uterine findings. A definite diagnosis can be obtained by tissue sampling.

Ultrasonography is usually the first-line imaging modality for the evaluation of vaginal bleeding and a pelvic mass, and MR imaging, owing to its superior tissue contrast, is an important modality in the characterization of complex pelvic masses. Recently, PET/CT imaging has been used in the evaluation of uterine masses. Uterine sarcomas have been shown to demonstrate high FDG uptake (Fig. 7), but because leiomyomas can uptake FDG, the differentiation between them by PET/CT imaging is crucial. Kusunoki and colleagues[52]

Table 2
FIGO staging of uterine sarcomas

FIGO Stage	Definition
Leiomyosarcomas and endometrial stromal sarcomas	
I	Tumor limited to the uterus
IA	≤5 cm
IB	>5 cm
II	Tumor extends beyond the uterus, within the pelvis
IIA	Adnexal involvement
IIB	Involvement of other pelvic tissues
III	Tumor invades abdominal tissues
IIIA	One site
IIIB	More than 1 site
IIIC	Metastasis to pelvic and/or paraaortic lymph nodes
IV	
IVA	Tumor invades bladder and/or rectum
IVB	Distant metastasis
Adenosarcomas	
I	Tumor limited to the uterus
IA	Tumor limited to endometrium/endocervix with no myometrial invasion
IB	Less than or equal to one-half myometrial invasion
IC	More than one-half myometrial invasion
II	Tumor extends beyond the uterus, within the pelvis
IIA	Adnexal involvement
IIB	Tumor extends to extrauterine pelvic tissue
III	Tumor invades abdominal tissues
IIIA	One site
IIIB	More than one site
IIIC	Metastasis to pelvic and/or paraaortic lymph nodes
IV	
IVA	Tumor invades bladder and/or rectum
IVB	Distant metastasis

Abbreviation: FIGO, International Federation of Gynecology and Obstetrics.
From Prat J, Mbatani. Uterine sarcomas. Int J Gynaecol Obstet 2015;131 Suppl 2:S106; with permission.

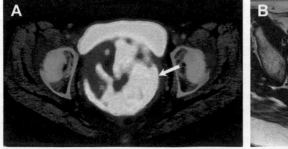
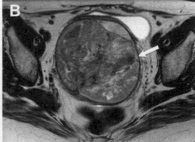

Fig. 7. A 68-year-old woman with a large uterine sarcoma and vaginal bleeding. (A) Preoperative axial PET/computed tomography image shows a large uterine mass with intense ^{18}F-fluorodeoxyglucose uptake and standardized uptake (arrow) value of 16. (B) Axial T1-weighted postcontrast MR image shows a large 8.9 cm uterine mass (arrow) causing mass effect on the posterior bladder wall without frank invasion.

reported a significant difference between the median SUV_{max} for uterine sarcoma and leiomyoma (12 vs 4.1, respectively), and that an SUV_{max} of 7.5 was able to exclude leiomyoma with a sensitivity of 80% and a specificity of 100%. Additionally, the combination of PET/CT imaging and lactate dehydrogenase levels had a sensitivity of 86.6% and a specificity of 100%.[53] The combination of PET with newer radiotracers such as 16α-[^{18}F] fluoro-17β-estradiol, which is an ^{18}F-labeled version of estradiol, the most bioactive type of estrogen, can help in the differential diagnosis between uterine leiomyoma and uterine sarcoma by providing molecular information about estrogen receptor activity in patients when PET/CT scanning results show equivocal or positive FDG uptake.[54]

Uterine sarcomas have a poor prognosis. SUV_{max} can be used to identify highly aggressive tumors in a preoperative setting. Park and colleagues[55] reported that the SUV_{max} was associated with a worse outcome in patients with uterine leiomyosarcoma in a retrospective study of 19 patients. Yamamoto and colleagues[56] reported that the pretreatment tumor FDG/^{18}F-fluoroestradiol ratio is useful for predicting the prognosis of uterine sarcoma with patients, with ratios greater than 2.6 presenting with worse progression-free survival and overall survival.

Owing to their aggressive tumor biology, these tumors may recur within 2 years of initial treatment. Recurrent disease may be seen in about 50% of patients.[57] Large tumor size and high SUV_{max} are risk factors for recurrence. PET is helpful in evaluating suspected recurrent uterine sarcomas, because recurrence can be masked on conventional imaging modalities such as MR imaging and CT scanning by underlying postoperative changes, leading to additional delay in the diagnosis of recurrence. Locoregional pelvic recurrences and paraaortic lymph nodes are frequent locations of recurrent disease (**Figs. 8** and **9**). The most common sites for distant metastatic disease are the lungs and liver[58] (**Figs. 10** and **11**). When compared with CT scanning, PET has been shown to have a better detection rate for extrapelvic recurrence. The sensitivity of PET was 100% compared with 85.7% for CT scanning.[59] In another study of 36 patients, PET or PET/CT scanning had a sensitivity, specificity, accuracy, PPV, and NPV of 92.9%, 100%, 94.4%, 100%, and 80%, respectively, in symptomatic patients. In asymptomatic patients with suspected recurrence, these values were 87.5%, 95.5%, 93.3%, 87.5%, and 95.5%, respectively.[60] PET/CT scanning also is used to monitor response of treatment for metastatic disease

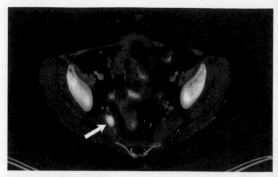

Fig. 8. A 74-year-old woman with uterine leiomyosarcoma, status post hysterectomy. Surveillance PET/computed tomography (CT) was performed 12 months after surgery. Axial PET/CT image shows a metabolically active solid lesion in the right pelvis along the pelvic sidewall (*arrow*) abutting the internal iliac vasculature measuring 2.8 cm in size with a standardized uptake value of 5.8. Biopsy was performed and was diagnostic of metastatic leiomyosarcoma.

in patients with unresectable disease (**Box 2, Fig. 12**).

VULVAR CARCINOMA

Vulvar carcinomas are uncommon gynecologic tumors. In 2017, an estimated 6020 women will be diagnosed with vulvar cancer, and 1150 are expected to die from the disease in the United States.[5] Although vulvar cancer accounts for only 3% to 5% of gynecologic malignancies, it is the most common anogenital cancer in women over the age of 70 years.

Vulvar carcinoma usually occurs in women in the seventh decade of life, and many cases, particularly in younger women, are associated with human papilloma virus infection.[61] Symptoms include a lump in the vulva, thickening of the skin of the vulva, pain, itching, or bleeding. Early stage disease may have no symptoms. The diagnosis is made by physical examination and biopsy. The most common histology of vulvar carcinoma is squamous cell carcinoma. Other rare vulvar malignancies include adenocarcinoma, melanoma, sarcoma, and basal cell carcinoma.

These tumors are usually detected at relatively early clinical stages, without obvious metastases, and are staged according to the FIGO staging system (**Table 3**).[62] Stage I disease includes tumors confined to the vulva or perineum, and is divided into stages IA and IB. Stage IA disease includes lesions 2 cm or less in size with stromal invasion of 1 mm or less. Stage IB includes tumors greater than 2 cm in size or with stromal invasion greater

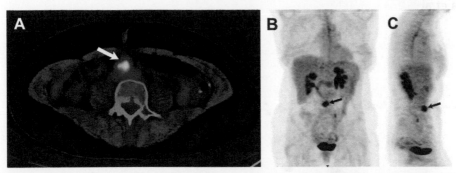

Fig. 9. A 56-year-old woman with uterine leiomyosarcoma, status post hysterectomy. Surveillance PET/computed tomography (CT) was performed 24 months after surgery. (A) Axial PET/CT image shows a metabolically active solid mass (arrow) in the midpelvic region measuring 2.5 cm in size with a standardized uptake value of 4.2. (B) Coronal and (C) sagittal PET maximum intensity projection images show a single metastatic lesion in the pelvic region (arrows). Biopsy was performed and was diagnostic of metastatic leiomyosarcoma.

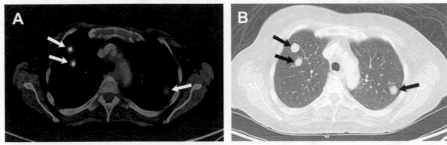

Fig. 10. A 78-year-old woman with uterine leiomyosarcoma, status post hysterectomy. Surveillance PET/computed tomography (CT) was performed 18 months after surgery. (A) Axial PET/CT image shows multiple metabolically active metastatic pulmonary nodules bilaterally (arrows). (B) Axial CT portion of the PET/CT in lung windows shows the metastatic pulmonary nodules (arrows).

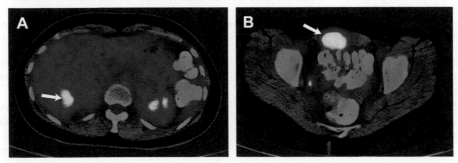

Fig. 11. A 79-year-old woman with uterine leiomyosarcoma, status post hysterectomy. Surveillance PET/computed tomography (CT) was performed 8 months after surgery. (A) Axial PET/CT image shows a metabolically active lesion within the posterior right liver (arrow). (B) Axial PET/CT image shows additional metastatic lesion involving the inferior right rectus abdominis muscle (arrow).

Box 2
Uterine sarcomas: teaching points

- The main subtypes of uterine sarcomas include leiomyosarcoma, endometrial stromal sarcoma, and adenosarcoma.
- Preoperative diagnosis of uterine sarcoma is challenging. The use of new PET radiotracers such as ^{18}F-fluoroestradiol can help to differentiate uterine leiomyoma and uterine sarcoma.

than 1 mm, confined to the vulva or perineum. Stage II disease represents any size tumor with extension to adjacent perineal structures (lower one-third of the urethra, lower one-third of the vagina, anus). Stage III disease is any size tumor with or without extension to adjacent perineal structures with positive inguinofemoral nodes. Stage IIIA is defined as vulvar cancer with 1 or 2 lymph nodes metastases less than 5 mm or a single lymph node metastasis 5 mm or greater. Stage IIIB disease is defined by the involvement of 2 or

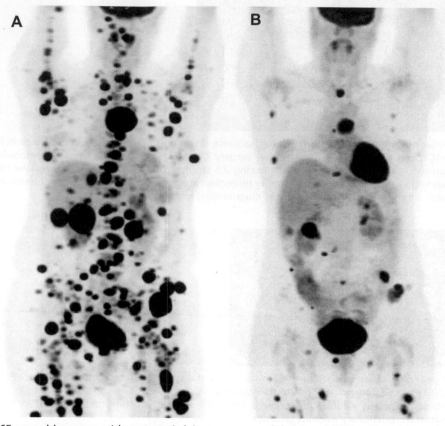

Fig. 12. A 65-year-old woman with metastatic leiomyosarcoma. (*A*) Coronal PET maximum intensity projection (MIP) image shows multiples sites of metastatic disease in the skeleton, soft tissues, muscles, mediastinum, lymph nodes, liver, kidneys, and thyroid gland. (*B*) Follow-up coronal PET MIP image 2 months after treatment with chemotherapy show interval improvement of disease with resolution and interval decrease in size of multiple sites of metastatic disease.

more lymph node metastases 5 mm or greater or 3 or more lymph nodes metastases of less than 5 mm. Stage IIIC disease includes positive lymph nodes with extracapsular spread. Stage IV disease includes tumor of any size with involvement of the pelvic lymph nodes or adjacent structures, or the presence of distant metastatic disease. Stage IVA disease represent tumors that invade other regional structures (upper two-thirds of the ure-thra, upper two-thirds of the vagina), bladder, or rectum, are fixed to pelvic bones, or with inguino-femoral lymph nodes that are fixed or ulcerated. Stage IVB disease includes any distant metastatic disease, including pelvic lymph nodes.

Typical patterns of spread include local invasion and lymphatic dissemination. The vulva primarily drains into the inguinal and femoral lymph nodes ipsilateral to the primary tumor. If the tumor ex-tends to the midline, both right and left inguinal lymph nodes are at risk and can be involved. Vulvar cancer can also spread to the pelvic lymph nodes (external iliac [including obturator], internal iliac, and common iliac) and is considered

metastatic disease. It is rare for pelvic lymph nodes to be involved unless the ipsilateral inguinal nodes are also involved.[63]

Lymph node metastases are the important prog-nostic factor in vulvar cancer. The incidence of nodal metastases in the groin increases with size and depth of invasion. Even superficial tumors 5 mm or less can be associated with lymph node metastases 20% of the time.[64] The presence of lymph node me-tastases decreases the 5-year survival range from 70% to 93% to 25% to 41%.[65] Patients with lymph node metastases also experience recurrence earlier than patients without nodal involvement.

The standard treatment for early squamous cell carcinoma of the vulva with no local or distant metastasis disease has been wide local excision (**Fig. 13**). However, one-third of patients with early stage disease have lymph node metastases and would benefit from inguinal lymphadenec-tomy. Approximately 50% of patients after inguinal lymph node dissection may experience complications including groin wound infections, wound breakdown, lymphedema, and cellulitis.

Table 3
FIGO staging of vulvar cancer

FIGO Stage	Definition
I	Tumor is confined to the vulva or perineum
IA	Tumor ≤2 cm in size with stromal invasion ≤1 mm
IB	Tumor >2 cm in size, or a tumor with stromal invasion >1 mm
II	Any size tumor with extension to adjacent perineal structures
III	Any size tumor with or without extension to adjacent perineal structures with positive inguinofemoral lymph nodes
IIIA	One or 2 lymph nodes metastases <5 mm or a single lymph nodes metastasis ≥5 mm
IIIB	Two or more lymph nodes metastases ≥5 mm or ≥3 lymph nodes metastases <5 mm
IIIC	Positive lymph nodes with extracapsular spread
IV	Tumor of any size with involvement of the pelvic lymph nodes or adjacent structures or distant metastatic disease
IVA	Tumors that invades other regional structures (upper two-thirds of the urethra, upper two-thirds of the vagina), bladder, or rectum, are fixed to pelvic bones, or presence of inguinofemoral lymph nodes that are fixed or ulcerated
IVB	Any distant metastatic disease including pelvic lymph nodes

Abbreviation: FIGO, International Federation of Gynecology and Obstetrics.
From Hacker NF, Eifel PJ, van der Velden J. Cancer of the vulva. Int J Gynaecol Obstet 2015;131 Suppl 2:S77; with permission.

Therefore, noninvasive methods for the pretreatment evaluation of the extent of disease are important.

Radiolabeled colloid in conjunction with a marking dye has been used to map sentinel lymph nodes and provide a landmark for dissection. However, this is less suitable in tumors located in the midline or for very big tumors.[66] In this scenario, PET/CT is useful in the evaluation of inguinal lymph node status in vulvar cancer (**Fig. 14**). Kamran et al,[67] in a study correlating PET/CT imaging with histologically proven vulvar cancer metastatic groin lymph nodes, reported a sensitivity of 50%, specificity of 100%, PPV of 100%, and NPV of 57% in identifying metastatic groin lymph nodes in patients with vulvar cancer. Owing to the low sensitivity, a negative scan result does not preclude surgical resection. Given the high specificity of PET, this study supports the notion that PET/CT imaging can be used for treatment planning preceding surgical staging and to adequately plan preoperative chemoradiation therapy. Furthermore, PET/CT imaging has the potential to identify metastatic disease in pelvic lymph nodes, which can help to prevent extensive groin dissection, where these patients can be treated with definitive chemoradiation[68] (**Fig. 15**).

Lin and colleagues,[69] studying 23 patients with vulvar cancer, concluded that PET/CT imaging can have a positive impact on patient management. A recent study of PET/CT in patients with vulvar cancer reported that preoperative PET/CT changed the therapeutic management in 61.5%,[70] although on PET/CT scanning, inflammatory lymph nodes may also be FDG avid and can result in false-positive results, whereas necrotic lymph nodes may not be metabolically active and can result in false-negative results.

Recently, dual time-point PET/CT scanning has been suggested as a means for detecting metastatic lymph node in gynecologic cancers. Dual time-point PET/CT scanning requires 2 image acquisitions after a single injection of the radiotracer, that is, standard images (1 hour after injection) followed by delayed time point images (2–3 hours after injection) of the body region under assessment. In a prospective study of 33 patients with vulvar cancer comparing dual time-point PET/CT scanning with standard PET/CT scanning, Collarino and colleagues[71] reported a sensitivity of 95.2%, specificity of 75%, NPV of 96.4%, PPV of 69%, and accuracy of 82.5% in detecting metastatic groin lymph nodes in patients with vulvar cancer. They concluded that standard PET/CT scanning has a high sensitivity and NPV, allowing one to predict pathologically negative groin nodes, thereby facilitating the selection of patients suitable for minimally invasive surgery, and that dual time-point PET/CT imaging did not improve the specificity or PPV.

The presence of distant metastases at the initial staging of vulvar cancer is rare, but PET/CT imaging can help in the evaluation of the extent of distant disease. In cases where PET/CT imaging identifies distant metastases, patients are treated with chemotherapy.

Squamous cell carcinoma of the vulva may recur in 30% to 50% of cases within the first 2 years.[72] Although the majority of recurrences are local, one-third occur in the groin (**Fig. 16**). Other distant

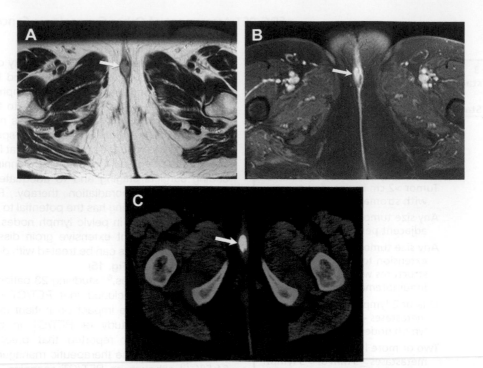

Fig. 13. A 76-year-old woman with vulvar cancer. (*A*) Axial T2-weighted MR image shows a small, polypoid, slightly high signal intensity lesion in the vulva (*arrow*). (*B*) Axial T1-weighted postcontrast image shows enhancement of the vulvar lesion. (*C*) Axial PET/computed tomography image shows a highly ^{18}F-fluorodeoxyglucose-avid vulvar lesion (*arrow*). There were no suspicious lymph nodes or distant metastases. The patient was treated with surgical resection.

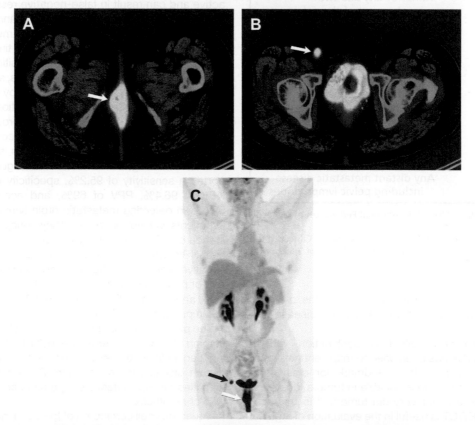

Fig. 14. A 68-year-old woman with vulvar cancer. (*A*) Axial PET/computed tomography (CT) image shows an ^{18}F-fluorodeoxyglucose (FDG)-avid large vulvar mass (*arrow*). (*B*) Axial PET/CT axial image shows an FDG-avid right inguinal lymph node (*arrow*) compatible with metastatic disease. (*C*) Coronal PET maximum intensity projection image shows the FDG-avid mass in the vulvar region (*white arrow*) and a single right inguinal metastatic lymph node (*black arrow*).

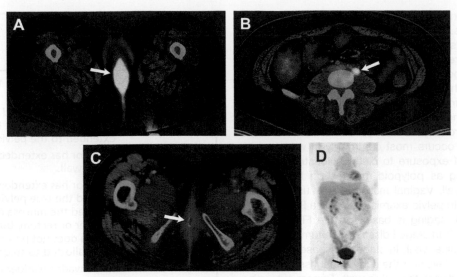

Fig. 15. A 75-year-old woman with vulvar cancer. (*A*) Axial PET/computed tomography (CT) image shows a large ^{18}F-fluorodeoxyglucose (FDG)-avid vulvar mass (*arrow*). (*B*) Axial PET/CT axial image shows an FDG-avid left common iliac lymph node that was biopsied and owing to metastatic disease. (*C, D*) Follow-up axial PET/CT image and coronal PET maximum intensity projection image performed 4 months later show interval decrease in size of the vulvar mass (*arrows*) and of the left common iliac lymph node, consistent with treatment response.

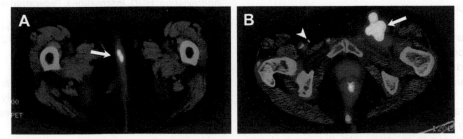

Fig. 16. A 70-year-old woman with vulvar cancer. (*A*) Axial PET/computed tomography (CT) image shows a highly ^{18}F-fluorodeoxyglucose (FDG)-avid lesion corresponding with the primary vulvar cancer (*arrow*). There were no suspicious lymph nodes or distant metastasis. The patient was treated with surgical resection and lymphadenectomy. (*B*) Surveillance PET/CT performed 12 months later shows FDG-avid enlarged recurrent metastatic left inguinal lymph nodes (*arrow*). Note the surgical clips in the right inguinal region from prior lymphadenectomy (*arrowhead*).

sites of recurrent disease include lung, liver, and bone marrow.[73] PET/CT imaging is useful in the detection of groin lymph node metastasis and distant recurrent disease. This consideration is important because reexcision is the therapy of choice for isolated local and regional recurrences with much better outcomes than the distant metastatic disease treated with chemotherapy (**Box 3**).

VAGINAL CANCER

Vaginal cancer is rare and predominantly seen in elderly women, typically beginning in the seventh decade of life. In the United States, approximately 4810 new cases and 1240 deaths are estimated for the year of 2017, where it accounts for less than 3% of all malignant neoplasms of the female genital tract.[5] The risk factors that increase the

patient's lifetime risk are early coitarche, multiple sexual partners, smoking, exposure to diethylstilbestrol in utero, and human papilloma virus infection, and many of them are the same risk factors for cervical cancer.[74] Symptoms include vaginal bleeding or discharge, pain during sexual intercourse, and a lump in the vagina, although 20%

Box 3
Vulvar cancer: teaching points

- Preoperative PET/computed tomography (CT) and dual time-point PET/CT are useful for detecting metastatic pelvic lymph nodes.

- If metastatic pelvic lymph nodes are identified on PET/CT, patients are treated with chemoradiation therapy.

of women may be asymptomatic at the time of diagnosis. These tumors may present as an ulcerated mass, a lobulated soft tissue mass, or circumferential thickening. They can be unifocal or multifocal, and can be present throughout the vagina. There are 2 histologic types of vaginal cancer: squamous cell carcinoma (the most common accounting for nearly 80% of all cases), and adenocarcinoma.[75] Clear cell adenocarcinoma is rare and occurs most commonly in women with history of exposure to diethylstilbestrol in utero, presenting as polypoid masses on the anterior vaginal wall. Vaginal malignancy is usually diagnosed with pelvic examination and a Pap smear.

Clinical staging is based on the FIGO system (**Table 4**).[76] In stage I disease, the tumor is limited to the vaginal wall. In stage II disease, the carcinoma has involved the subvaginal tissue but has not extended to the pelvic wall. Tumors extending to the pelvic wall are classified as stage III disease. Stage IVA disease indicates involvement of adjacent organs, with invasion of the bladder or rectal mucosal layer and/or direct extension beyond the true pelvis. Stage IVB disease includes the presence of distant metastases.

Tumor spread is typically by local invasion, lymphatic dissemination to inguinal and pelvic lymph nodes, and hematogenous spread to the lungs and liver. The lymph node drainage pattern differs depending on the location of tumor. For example, the tumors in the upper one-third of the vagina drain into the internal iliac and external iliac (including obturator) chains, whereas tumors from the lower one-third drain into the inguinal and femoral lymph nodes.[2] Therapy planning in primary vaginal cancer is complex, and treatment strategies are usually based on combined external beam radiation therapy and/or intracavitary or interstitial brachytherapy, often with concurrent chemotherapy. Surgery is usually reserved for patients with in situ or very early stage disease.[77] The

Table 4	
FIGO staging of vaginal cancer	
FIGO Stage	**Definition**
I	The tumor is limited to the vaginal wall.
II	The tumor has involved the subvaginal tissue but has not extended to the pelvic wall.
III	The tumor has extended to the pelvic wall.
IV	The tumor has extended beyond the true pelvis or has involved the mucosa of the bladder or rectum; bullous edema does not permit a case to be allotted to stage IV.
IVA	Tumor invades bladder and/or rectal mucosa and/or direct extension beyond the true pelvis.
IVB	The tumor has spread to distant organs.

Abbreviation: FIGO, International Federation of Gynecology and Obstetrics.
From Hacker NF, Eifel PJ, van der Velden J. Cancer of the vagina. Int J Gynaecol Obstet 2015;131 Suppl 2:S84; with permission.

prognosis depends on the stage of the cancer. The reported 5-year survival is approximately 85% for stage I disease, 78% for stage II disease, and 58% for stages III and IV disease.[78]

Vaginal cancer diagnosis and staging rely primarily on clinical evaluation. Pelvic examination continues to be the most important tool for evaluating the local extent of disease, although it is limited in its ability to detect lymphadenopathy and the extent of tumor infiltration. PET/CT scanning detects the metabolically active tumor (**Fig. 17**) and permits more accurate assessment

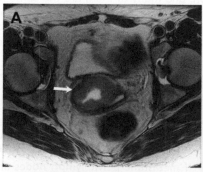 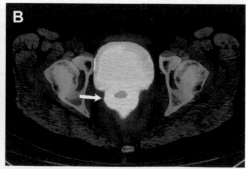

Fig. 17. A 72-year-old woman with vaginal bleeding. (*A*) Axial T2-weighted MR image shows circumferential vaginal wall thickening (*arrow*). (*B*) Axial PET/computed tomography image shows hypermetabolic circumferential vaginal wall thickening corresponding with the primary vaginal carcinoma (*arrow*).

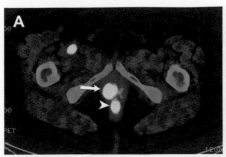
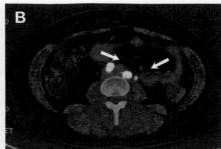

Fig. 18. A 68-year-old woman with vaginal cancer. (*A*) Axial PET/computed tomography (CT) image shows soft tissue fullness involving the right vaginal wall (*arrow*) with avid ^{18}F-fluorodeoxyglucose (FDG) activity and a maximum standardized uptake value of 16, consistent with primary vaginal cancer, along with a hypermetabolic right inguinal lymph node owing to metastatic disease. Also, note the nodular hypermetabolic FDG activity involving the adjacent lower anal canal (*arrowhead*), likely related to anal sphincter contraction. (*B*) Axial PET/CT image shows FDG-avid aortocaval and left paraaortic lymph nodes (*arrows*) owing to metastatic disease.

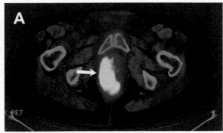
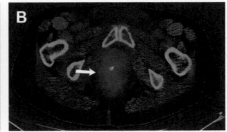

Fig. 19. A 75-year-old woman with a vaginal cancer. (*A*) Axial PET/computed tomography (CT) image shows a large ^{18}F-fluorodeoxyglucose-avid vaginal lesion (*arrow*). (*B*) Follow-up PET/CT image after 4 months of treatment with chemoradiation therapy shows good response of the tumor to treatment (*arrow*).

of nodal involvement and distant metastases. However, very few studies have reported the use of PET/CT imaging in the staging of vaginal cancer.

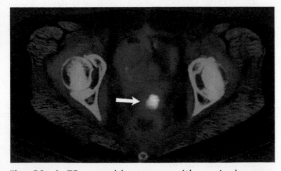

Fig. 20. A 73-year-old woman with vaginal cancer treated with surgical resection. Follow-up axial PET/computed tomography image 14 months later shows soft tissue with hypermetabolic activity at the vaginal cuff (*arrow*), suspicious for locally recurrent disease and no distant metastases. Biopsy confirmed recurrent disease and so the patient was treated with pelvic exenteration.

Lamoreaux and colleagues[79] in a prospective study of 23 patients compared the results of CT with PET, and demonstrated that PET detected all metabolically active primary tumor with a sensitivity of 100% and detected metastatic lymph nodes more often than conventional CT scans. Thus, PET can potentially provide a noninvasive method to diagnose nodal metastases (**Fig. 18**) as well as distant metastases. PET/CT imaging also plays an important role in the treatment planning and monitoring of vaginal cancer (**Fig. 19**). Robertson and colleagues[80] reported a change in patient management in 36% of patients with vaginal cancer after PET/CT.

Box 4
Vaginal cancer: teaching points

- The primary value of PET/computed tomography is in the detection of pelvic lymph nodes metastases and distant metastatic disease.

- The most common tumor of the vagina is metastatic disease.

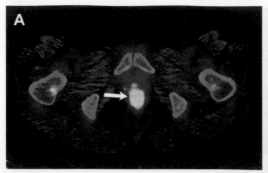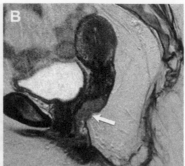

Fig. 21. A 56-year-old woman with anal cancer, status post abdominoperineal resection with omental pedicle flap, presenting with vaginal bleeding. (*A*) Axial PET/computed tomography image shows an ^{18}F-fluorodeoxyglucose-avid lesion (*arrow*) in the lower vagina suspicious for metastatic disease. (*B*) Sagittal T2-weighted MR image shows a mass at the lower vagina that was biopsied and confirmed to be due to metastatic disease from anal cancer.

Vaginal adenocarcinoma, unlike squamous cell carcinoma, commonly affects younger patients (median age, 19 years) and is more likely to metastasize to the lungs and supraclavicular or pelvic lymph nodes.[81] PET/CT imaging is helpful in the detection of distant metastases.

Vaginal cancer can present with recurrent disease in up to 25% of patients at 5 years.[82] Higher stages of disease and a lower and/or posterior tumor location are more likely to recur. In patients with vaginal or cervical cancer who have suspected recurrence after pelvic radiation, PET was found to have a sensitivity of 100% and specificity of 73% in detection of disease in extrapelvic sites.[83] PET can, therefore, be used to identify patients who are candidates for pelvic exenteration for localized recurrence in the pelvis (**Fig. 20**).

Although primary vaginal cancer is rare, the vagina can be a common site of metastatic disease by either direct extension from the cervix, endometrium, or vulva, or by lymphatic or hematogenous spread from colon cancer, renal cell carcinoma, melanoma, or breast cancer[84] (**Box 4, Fig. 21**).

SUMMARY

PET and PET/CT imaging play an important role in the management of gynecologic malignancies. The combination of anatomic and functional imaging has improved sensitivity and specificity compared with conventional imaging. Other advantages of PET/CT include scanning the whole body, evaluation of treatment response, and early detection of recurrent disease. Limitations include the difficulties to assess small lesions as well as the presence of physiologic uptake and false-positive findings in benign disease conditions.

REFERENCES

1. Oldan JD, Patel PS. Positron emission tomography/computed tomography for gynecologic malignancies. Obstet Gynecol Surv 2016;71(9):545–56.
2. Bhosale P, Iyer R, Jhingran A, et al. PET/CT imaging in gynecologic malignancies other than ovarian and cervical cancer. PET Clin 2010;5(4):463–75.
3. Lerman H, Metser U, Grisaru D, et al. Normal and abnormal 18F-FDG endometrial and ovarian uptake in pre- and postmenopausal patients: assessment by PET/CT. J Nucl Med 2004;45(2):266–71.
4. Amant F, Cadron I, Fuso L, et al. Endometrial carcinosarcomas have a different prognosis and pattern of spread compared to high-risk epithelial endometrial cancer. Gynecol Oncol 2005;98(2):274–80.
5. Siegel RL, Miller KD, Jemal A. Cancer statistics, 2017. CA Cancer J Clin 2017;67(1):7–30.
6. Arora V, Quinn MA. Endometrial cancer. Best Pract Res Clin Obstet Gynaecol 2012;26(3):311–24.
7. Bokhman JV. Two pathogenetic types of endometrial carcinoma. Gynecol Oncol 1983;15(1):10–7.
8. Murali R, Soslow RA, Weigelt B. Classification of endometrial carcinoma: more than two types. Lancet Oncol 2014;15(7):e268–78.
9. Sorosky JI. Endometrial cancer. Obstet Gynecol 2012;120(2 Pt 1):383–97.
10. Amant F, Mirza MR, Koskas M, et al. Cancer of the corpus uteri. Int J Gynaecol Obstet 2015; 131(Suppl 2):S96–104.
11. Faria SC, Sagebiel T, Balachandran A, et al. Imaging in endometrial carcinoma. Indian J Radiol Imaging 2015;25(2):137–47.
12. Kitajima K, Murakami K, Kaji Y, et al. Established, emerging and future applications of FDG-PET/CT in the uterine cancer. Clin Radiol 2011;66(4):297–307.
13. Kitajima K, Murakami K, Kaji Y, et al. Spectrum of FDG PET/CT findings of uterine tumors. AJR Am J Roentgenol 2010;195(3):737–43.

14. Viswanathan C, Bhosale PR, Shah SN, et al. Positron emission tomography-computed tomography imaging for malignancies in women. Radiol Clin North Am 2013;51(6):1111–25.

15. Park JY, Kim EN, Kim DY, et al. Comparison of the validity of magnetic resonance imaging and positron emission tomography/computed tomography in the preoperative evaluation of patients with uterine corpus cancer. Gynecol Oncol 2008;108(3):486–92.

16. Kitajima K, Yamasaki E, Kaji Y, et al. Comparison of DWI and PET/CT in evaluation of lymph node metastasis in uterine cancer. World J Radiol 2012;4(5):207–14.

17. Kitajima K, Murakami K, Yamasaki E, et al. Accuracy of integrated FDG-PET/contrast-enhanced CT in detecting pelvic and paraaortic lymph node metastasis in patients with uterine cancer. Eur Radiol 2009;19(6):1529–36.

18. Chang MC, Chen JH, Liang JA, et al. 18F-FDG PET or PET/CT for detection of metastatic lymph nodes in patients with endometrial cancer: a systematic review and meta-analysis. Eur J Radiol 2012;81(11):3511–7.

19. Mayoral M, Paredes P, Domenech B, et al. 18F-FDG PET/CT and sentinel lymph node biopsy in the staging of patients with cervical and endometrial cancer. Role of dual-time-point imaging. Rev Esp Med Nucl Imagen Mol 2017;36(1):20–6.

20. Atri M, Zhang Z, Dehdashti F, et al. Utility of PET/CT to evaluate retroperitoneal lymph node metastasis in high-risk endometrial cancer: results of ACRIN 6671/GOG 0233 trial. Radiology 2017;283(2):450–9.

21. Bollineni VR, Ytre-Hauge S, Bollineni-Balabay O, et al. High diagnostic value of 18F-FDG PET/CT in endometrial cancer: systematic review and meta-analysis of the literature. J Nucl Med 2016;57(6):879–85.

22. Bese T, Sal V, Demirkiran F, et al. The combination of preoperative fluorodeoxyglucose positron emission tomography/computed tomography and sentinel lymph node mapping in the surgical management of endometrioid endometrial cancer. Int J Gynecol Cancer 2016;26(7):1228–38.

23. Ozgu E, Oz M, Yildiz Y, et al. Prognostic value of 18F-FDG PET/CT for identifying high- and low-risk endometrial cancer patients. Ginekol Pol 2016;87(7):493–7.

24. Ghooshkhanei H, Treglia G, Sabouri G, et al. Risk stratification and prognosis determination using (18)F-FDG PET imaging in endometrial cancer patients: a systematic review and meta-analysis. Gynecol Oncol 2014;132(3):669–76.

25. Yankeelov TE, Abramson RG, Quarles CC. Quantitative multimodality imaging in cancer research and therapy. Nat Rev Clin Oncol 2014;11(11):670–80.

26. Picchio M, Mangili G, Samanes Gajate AM, et al. High-grade endometrial cancer: value of [(18)F] FDG PET/CT in preoperative staging. Nucl Med Commun 2010;31(6):506–12.

27. Sohaib SA, Houghton SL, Meroni R, et al. Recurrent endometrial cancer: patterns of recurrent disease and assessment of prognosis. Clin Radiol 2007;62(1):28–34 [discussion: 35–6].

28. Saga T, Higashi T, Ishimori T, et al. Clinical value of FDG-PET in the follow up of post-operative patients with endometrial cancer. Ann Nucl Med 2003;17(3):197–203.

29. Wright JD, Barrena Medel NI, Sehouli J, et al. Contemporary management of endometrial cancer. Lancet 2012;379(9823):1352–60.

30. Belhocine T, De Barsy C, Hustinx R, et al. Usefulness of (18)F-FDG PET in the post-therapy surveillance of endometrial carcinoma. Eur J Nucl Med Mol Imaging 2002;29(9):1132–9.

31. Kitajima K, Murakami K, Yamasaki E, et al. Performance of integrated FDG-PET/contrast-enhanced CT in the diagnosis of recurrent uterine cancer: comparison with PET and enhanced CT. Eur J Nucl Med Mol Imaging 2009;36(3):362–72.

32. Chung HH, Kang WJ, Kim JW, et al. The clinical impact of [(18)F]FDG PET/CT for the management of recurrent endometrial cancer: correlation with clinical and histological findings. Eur J Nucl Med Mol Imaging 2008;35(6):1081–8.

33. Kang SY, Cheon GJ, Lee M, et al. Prediction of recurrence by preoperative intratumoral FDG uptake heterogeneity in endometrioid endometrial cancer. Transl Oncol 2017;10(2):178–83.

34. Husby JA, Reitan BC, Biermann M, et al. Metabolic tumor volume on 18F-FDG PET/CT improves preoperative identification of high-risk endometrial carcinoma patients. J Nucl Med 2015;56(8):1191–8.

35. Shim SH, Kim DY, Lee DY, et al. Metabolic tumour volume and total lesion glycolysis, measured using preoperative 18F-FDG PET/CT, predict the recurrence of endometrial cancer. BJOG 2014;121(9):1097–106 [discussion: 1106].

36. Lin LL, Grigsby PW, Powell MA, et al. Definitive radiotherapy in the management of isolated vaginal recurrences of endometrial cancer. Int J Radiat Oncol Biol Phys 2005;63(2):500–4.

37. Lee SI, Catalano OA, Dehdashti F. Evaluation of gynecologic cancer with MR imaging, 18F-FDG PET/CT, and PET/MR imaging. J Nucl Med 2015;56(3):436–43.

38. Kitajima K, Suenaga Y, Ueno Y, et al. Value of fusion of PET and MRI in the detection of intra-pelvic recurrence of gynecological tumor: comparison with 18F-FDG contrast-enhanced PET/CT and pelvic MRI. Ann Nucl Med 2014;28(1):25–32.

39. Beiderwellen K, Grueneisen J, Ruhlmann V, et al. [(18)F]FDG PET/MRI vs. PET/CT for whole-body staging in patients with recurrent malignancies of

the female pelvis: initial results. Eur J Nucl Med Mol Imaging 2015;42(1):56–65.

40. Grueneisen J, Schaarschmidt BM, Heubner M, et al. Implementation of FAST-PET/MRI for whole-body staging of female patients with recurrent pelvic malignancies: a comparison to PET/CT. Eur J Radiol 2015;84(11):2097–102.

41. Ohliger MA, Hope TA, Chapman JS, et al. PET/MR imaging in gynecologic oncology. Magn Reson Imaging Clin N Am 2017;25(3):667–84.

42. Singnurkar A, Poon R, Metser U. Comparison of 18F-FDG-PET/CT and 18F-FDG-PET/MR imaging in oncology: a systematic review. Ann Nucl Med 2017;31(5):366–78.

43. Bagade S, Fowler KJ, Schwarz JK, et al. PET/MRI evaluation of gynecologic malignancies and prostate cancer. Semin Nucl Med 2015;45(4):293–303.

44. Reed NS. The management of uterine sarcomas. Clin Oncol (R Coll Radiol) 2008;20(6):470–8.

45. Ricci S, Stone RL, Fader AN. Uterine leiomyosarcoma: epidemiology, contemporary treatment strategies and the impact of uterine morcellation. Gynecol Oncol 2017;145(1):208–16.

46. Koh WJ, Greer BE, Abu-Rustum NR, et al. Uterine sarcoma, version 1.2016: featured updates to the NCCN guidelines. J Natl Compr Canc Netw 2015; 13(11):1321–31.

47. D'Angelo E, Prat J. Uterine sarcomas: a review. Gynecol Oncol 2010;116(1):131–9.

48. Prat J, Mbatani. Uterine sarcomas. Int J Gynaecol Obstet 2015;131(Suppl 2):S105–10.

49. Prat J. FIGO staging for uterine sarcomas. Int J Gynaecol Obstet 2009;104(3):177–8.

50. Kapp DS, Shin JY, Chan JK. Prognostic factors and survival in 1396 patients with uterine leiomyosarcomas: emphasis on impact of lymphadenectomy and oophorectomy. Cancer 2008;112(4):820–30.

51. Barral M, Place V, Dautry R, et al. Magnetic resonance imaging features of uterine sarcoma and mimickers. Abdom Radiol (NY) 2017;42(6):1762–72.

52. Kusunoki S, Terao Y, Ujihira T, et al. Efficacy of PET/CT to exclude leiomyoma in patients with lesions suspicious for uterine sarcoma on MRI. Taiwan J Obstet Gynecol 2017;56(4):508–13.

53. Nagamatsu A, Umesaki N, Li L, et al. Use of 18F-fluorodeoxyglucose positron emission tomography for diagnosis of uterine sarcomas. Oncol Rep 2010;23(4):1069–76.

54. Yoshida Y, Kiyono Y, Tsujikawa T, et al. Additional value of 16alpha-[18F]fluoro-17beta-oestradiol PET for differential diagnosis between uterine sarcoma and leiomyoma in patients with positive or equivocal findings on [18F]fluorodeoxyglucose PET. Eur J Nucl Med Mol Imaging 2011;38(10):1824–31.

55. Park JY, Lee JW, Lee HJ, et al. Prognostic significance of preoperative (1)(8)F-FDG PET/CT in uterine leiomyosarcoma. J Gynecol Oncol 2017;28(3):e28.

56. Yamamoto M, Tsujikawa T, Yamada S, et al. 18F-FDG/18F-FES standardized uptake value ratio determined using PET predicts prognosis in uterine sarcoma. Oncotarget 2017;8(14):22581–9.

57. Domenici L, Nixon K, Sorbi F, et al. Surgery for recurrent uterine cancer: surgical outcomes and implications for survival-a case series. Int J Gynecol Cancer 2017;27(4):759–67.

58. Gockley AA, Rauh-Hain JA, del Carmen MG. Uterine leiomyosarcoma: a review article. Int J Gynecol Cancer 2014;24(9):1538–42.

59. Sung PL, Chen YJ, Liu RS, et al. Whole-body positron emission tomography with 18F-fluorodeoxyglucose is an effective method to detect extra-pelvic recurrence in uterine sarcomas. Eur J Gynaecol Oncol 2008;29(3):246–51.

60. Park JY, Kim EN, Kim DY, et al. Role of PET or PET/CT in the post-therapy surveillance of uterine sarcoma. Gynecol Oncol 2008;109(2):255–62.

61. Stehman FB, Look KY. Carcinoma of the vulva. Obstet Gynecol 2006;107(3):719–33.

62. Hacker NF, Eifel PJ, van der Velden J. Cancer of the vulva. Int J Gynaecol Obstet 2015;131(Suppl 2): S76–83.

63. Brincat MR, Muscat Baron Y. Sentinel lymph node biopsy in the management of vulvar carcinoma: an evidence-based insight. Int J Gynecol Cancer 2017;27(8):1769–73.

64. Homesley HD, Bundy BN, Sedlis A, et al. Prognostic factors for groin node metastasis in squamous cell carcinoma of the vulva (a Gynecologic Oncology Group study). Gynecol Oncol 1993;49(3):279–83.

65. Woelber L, Eulenburg C, Choschzick M, et al. Prognostic role of lymph node metastases in vulvar cancer and implications for adjuvant treatment. Int J Gynecol Cancer 2012;22(3):503–8.

66. Viswanathan C, Kirschner K, Truong M, et al. Multimodality imaging of vulvar cancer: staging, therapeutic response, and complications. AJR Am J Roentgenol 2013;200(6):1387–400.

67. Kamran MW, O'Toole F, Meghen K, et al. Whole-body [18F]fluoro-2-deoxyglucose positron emission tomography scan as combined PET-CT staging prior to planned radical vulvectomy and inguinofemoral lymphadenectomy for squamous vulvar cancer: a correlation with groin node metastasis. Eur J Gynaecol Oncol 2014;35(3):230–5.

68. Rogers LJ, Howard B, Van Wijk L, et al. Chemoradiation in advanced vulval carcinoma. Int J Gynecol Cancer 2009;19(4):745–51.

69. Lin G, Chen CY, Liu FY, et al. Computed tomography, magnetic resonance imaging and FDG positron emission tomography in the management of vulvar malignancies. Eur Radiol 2015;25(5):1267–78.

70. Peiró V, Chiva L, González A, et al. Utility of the PET/CT in vulvar cancer management. Rev Esp Med Nucl Imagen Mol 2014;33(2):87–92 [in Spanish].

71. Collarino A, Garganese G, Valdes Olmos RA, et al. Evaluation of dual time point imaging 18F-FDG PET/CT for lymph node staging in vulvar cancer. J Nucl Med 2017;58(12):1913–8.

72. Nooij LS, Brand FA, Gaarenstroom KN, et al. Risk factors and treatment for recurrent vulvar squamous cell carcinoma. Crit Rev Oncol Hematol 2016;106:1–13.

73. Prieske K, Haeringer N, Grimm D, et al. Patterns of distant metastases in vulvar cancer. Gynecol Oncol 2016;142(3):427–34.

74. Creasman WT, Phillips JL, Menck HR. The national cancer data base report on cancer of the vagina. Cancer 1998;83(5):1033–40.

75. Mullins DL, Wilkinson EJ. Pathology of the vulva and vagina. Curr Opin Obstet Gynecol 1994;6(4):351–8.

76. Hacker NF, Eifel PJ, van der Velden J. Cancer of the vagina. Int J Gynaecol Obstet 2015;131(Suppl 2): S84–7.

77. Miyamoto DT, Viswanathan AN. Concurrent chemoradiation for vaginal cancer. PLoS One 2013;8(6): e65048.

78. Frank SJ, Jhingran A, Levenback C, et al. Definitive radiation therapy for squamous cell carcinoma of the vagina. Int J Radiat Oncol Biol Phys 2005; 62(1):138–47.

79. Lamoreaux WT, Grigsby PW, Dehdashti F, et al. FDG-PET evaluation of vaginal carcinoma. Int J Radiat Oncol Biol Phys 2005;62(3):733–7.

80. Robertson NL, Hricak H, Sonoda Y, et al. The impact of FDG-PET/CT in the management of patients with vulvar and vaginal cancer. Gynecol Oncol 2016; 140(3):420–4.

81. Di Donato V, Bellati F, Fischetti M, et al. Vaginal cancer. Crit Rev Oncol Hematol 2012;81(3):286–95.

82. Sardain H, Lavoue V, Laviolle B, et al. Prognostic factors for curative pelvic exenterations in patients with recurrent uterine cervical or vaginal cancer. Int J Gynecol Cancer 2014;24(9):1679–85.

83. Husain A, Akhurst T, Larson S, et al. A prospective study of the accuracy of 18Fluorodeoxyglucose positron emission tomography (18FDG PET) in identifying sites of metastasis prior to pelvic exenteration. Gynecol Oncol 2007;106(1):177–80.

84. Gardner CS, Sunil J, Klopp AH, et al. Primary vaginal cancer: role of MRI in diagnosis, staging and treatment. Br J Radiol 2015;88(1052):20150033.

The Role of PET Imaging in Gynecologic Radiation Oncology

Yuan James Rao, MD, Perry W. Grigsby, MD*

KEYWORDS

- PET • Radiation therapy • Gynecologic oncology • Ovarian cancer • Cervical cancer
- Uterine cancer • Vulvar cancer

KEY POINTS

- Tumor uptake of fluorine-18–fluorodeoxyglucose (FDG) can be visualized by PET imaging, which provides anatomic and volumetric data about the primary tumor and regional disease.
- FDG-PET/computed tomography (CT) is recommended for baseline assessment in cervical cancer and for staging in vulvar and vaginal cancer. It is not used as part of routine staging in ovarian or uterine cancer.
- The authors use FDG-PET/CT in definitive radiation treatment planning for cervical, vulvar, and vaginal cancer.
- FDG-PET/CT should be used to restage any recurrent gynecologic malignancy, and can be helpful in treatment planning for salvage radiation.
- There are published data to support the use of PET in posttreatment evaluation of cervical and vulvar cancer.

INTRODUCTION

Fluorine-18 (^{18}F)-fluorodeoxyglucose (FDG)–PET has become established as a mainstay of oncologic imaging, including in several diseases in gynecologic oncology.[1–3] ^{18}F is a radionuclide that decays by positron emission. The detection of photons resulting from the annihilation of the positron allows for accurate localization of the radioisotope. FDG is a glucose analogue in which ^{18}F replaces the 2'-hydroxyl group. In FDG-PET imaging, this compound is intravenously injected into patients, transported into metabolically active cells by glucose transporters, and trapped by phosphorylation. However, FDG cannot be metabolized by glycolysis because of the absence of the 2'-hydroxyl group and, therefore, persists within

the cell until radioactive decay of ^{18}F, which has a half-life of 109.8 minutes. The combination of a metabolic analogue with an imaging radiotracer allows for the production of clinically relevant imaging identifying metabolically active cells, which includes most tumors. The metabolic information provided by FDG-PET can be enhanced by fusion with anatomic imaging provided by computed tomography (CT), which also allows for attenuation correction. Hybrid FDG-PET/CT scanners are in use at many clinical centers in the United States because of these advantages. Additional advances can potentially be made by combining FDG-PET information with MR imaging, which provides better visualization of soft tissue.[4] A hybrid FDG-PET/MR imaging scanner is now in use at the authors' institution, and they are investigating

Disclosures: The authors report no conflicts of interest or financial disclosures.
Department of Radiation Oncology, Washington University School of Medicine, St Louis, MO 63110, USA
* Corresponding author. Department of Radiation Oncology, Washington University School of Medicine, 4921 Parkview Place, 660 South Euclid Avenue, Campus Box 8224, St Louis, MO 63110.
E-mail address: pgrigsby@wustl.edu

PET Clin 13 (2018) 225–237
https://doi.org/10.1016/j.cpet.2017.11.007

its potential in staging and radiation treatment planning for gynecologic malignancies.[5,6]

There has been significant interest in the role of PET in gynecologic malignancies, and investigators from the authors' institution[1-3] and elsewhere[7-10] have published several review articles on these topics. In this monograph, the authors draw on published reviews, updated clinical guidelines, and recently published original research to describe the current utility of FDG-PET for radiation oncologists who treat gynecologic malignancies. The use of FDG-PET is discussed in the context of staging, radiation treatment planning, and follow-up for each disease site.

UTERINE CANCER

Uterine carcinoma is the most common gynecologic malignancy, with an incidence of 25.4 per 100,000 women; the most common histology is endometrial adenocarcinoma.[11] The National Comprehensive Cancer Network's (NCCN) 2017 guidelines recommend FDG-PET/CT as part of pretreatment staging only if there is suspicion for metastatic disease.[12] Kakhki and colleagues[13] reported a meta-analysis of 16 studies of FDG-PET in staging for endometrial cancer, showing a sensitivity and specificity of 82% and 90%, respectively, for the primary lesion, 72% and 93%, respectively, for lymph nodes, and 96% and 95%, respectively, for distant metastasis. A study evaluating FDG-PET/CT staging in uterine carcinosarcoma found a sensitivity of 100% and specificity of 79% for extrauterine lesions.[14] Similar findings were reported in a meta-analysis evaluating FDG-PET staging of uterine sarcomas.[15]

Uterine endometrial cancer is usually treated by total abdominal hysterectomy and salpingo-oophorectomy, with or without lymph node sampling or dissection. Radiation is given in the adjuvant setting as external radiation and/or vaginal cuff brachytherapy to reduce the risk of recurrence for high-intermediate risk or high-risk disease.[16] The rate of lymph node involvement in uterine endometrial carcinoma can be estimated based on the results of the Gynecologic Oncology Group's protocol 33.[17] This study reported the incidence of nodal disease on lymphadenectomy among patients with clinically stage I endometrial cancer before surgery. In the authors' experience, there is variability among surgeons in whether any nodal dissection or sampling is performed; therefore, FDG-PET/CT can be used to evaluate the nodes if there is a high risk of involvement and if no nodal surgery is performed. Indeed, some groups have suggested that the high positive predictive value (93.3%) of FDG-PET/CT can be used to select the

appropriate extent of surgery.[18] Although the Medical Research Council's efficacy of systematic pelvic lymphadenectomy in endometrial cancer (ASTEC) study found no survival benefit to pelvic lymphadenectomy in endometrial cancer,[19] the absence or presence of pelvic lymph nodes or the number of lymph nodes sampled may inform the adjuvant radiation treatment plan.

FDG-PET/CT is likely not necessary for radiation treatment planning in patients at low risk for recurrence or nodal involvement. However, in patients at high risk of recurrence, FDG-PET/CT may provide additional information to inform treatment planning, especially if no nodes were sampled. Simcock and colleagues[20] reported on the use of postoperative FDG-PET/CT for restaging of patients with high-risk disease for treatment planning. Many of the patients in their high-risk population had disease that was International Federation of Gynecology and Obstetrics (FIGO) 2002 stage IC or greater (86%, 41 of 48), grade 3 (38%, 18 of 48), node positive (31%, 15 of 48) or no node dissection (52%, 25 of 48) or they had lympho-vascular space invasion (65%, 31 of 48). They reported that FDG-PET/CT changed the management in 35% of patients, with modification of the radiation plan in 21% of patients (10 of 48), addition of chemotherapy in 10% patients (5 of 48), or addition of surgery or palliation in a few other patients. Therefore, FDG-PET/CT to inform treatment planning is a reasonable option in this population; if FDG-avid disease is detected, additional treatment, such as radiation boost, addition of chemotherapy, or further surgical resection, can be considered.

FDG-PET should be recommended to evaluate patients with recurrent endometrial cancer who are considered for salvage therapy as shown in **Fig. 1**. Lin and colleagues[21] reported that patients with isolated vaginal recurrence can be cured in greater than 50% of cases, a rate higher than historical reports likely because of the use of FDG-PET in selecting for the patients most likely to benefit from aggressive local therapy. Simcock and colleagues[20] had similar results in their study, which reported that PET found additional disease in 72% of patients with recurrent endometrial cancer and changed management in 36%. An additional situation whereby FDG-PET/CT should be considered is in patients who are medically inoperable and are planned for definitive radiation by brachytherapy alone.[22] FDG-PET/CT can be used to exclude the involvement of pelvic lymph nodes, which would necessitate the addition of external radiation in addition to brachytherapy for definitive radiation.

The NCCN's guidelines allow for the use of FDG-PET/CT as clinically indicated for evaluating

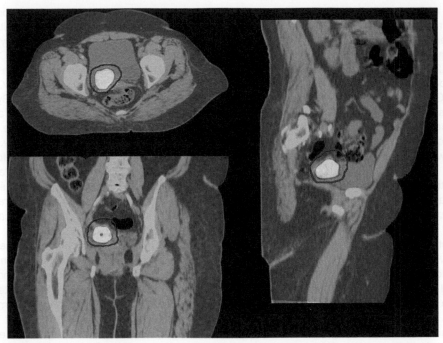

Fig. 1. Use of FDG-PET/CT in restaging and treatment planning for recurrent uterine endometrial cancer. The images are of a patient with a history of FIGO stage IC, grade 2, endometrial adenocarcinoma treated with total abdominal hysterectomy, bilateral salpingo-oophorectomy, and lymph node dissection. She received 36 Gy by vaginal cuff brachytherapy and, unfortunately, developed biopsy-proven vaginal cuff recurrence 4 years later. FDG-PET/CT showed FDG-avid tumor at the vaginal cuff but no lymph nodes or distant disease. The PET was fused with the simulation CT to aid in treatment planning as shown. The red contour shows the clinical target volume encompassing the FDG-avid recurrent tumor, which was treated with intensity-modulated radiation therapy to 60 Gy. The visualization parameters for this image were PET level 10,000 Bq/mL and PET window 20,000 Bq/mL, hot-iron color map, and blended 25% PET and 75% simulation CT in the treatment planning system. These visualization settings are identical in all subsequent images.

recurrent disease.[11] Indeed, a meta-analysis reported by Kadkhodayan and colleagues[23] showed a sensitivity of 96% and specificity of 92% in the recurrent setting. Additionally, the salvage treatment plan changed in 22% to 35% of patients in the evaluated studies because of the FDG-PET findings.

OVARIAN CANCER

Ovarian cancer is the second most common gynecologic malignancy, with an incidence of 12.7 per 100,000 women, and the most common cause of gynecologic cancer death.[24] There is currently no established role for FDG-PET for staging before the treatment of ovarian cancer; it is not routinely recommended by the American College of Radiology's (ACR) 2013 Appropriateness Criteria[25] or the NCCN's 2016 guidelines,[26] although the NCCN does allow FDG-PET/CT for the evaluation of indeterminate ovarian masses. Yuan and colleagues[27] published a meta-analysis of 18 studies, which showed that FDG-PET was more accurate

than CT or MR imaging in the detection of lymph node metastases. Currently, surgery with laparotomy, total abdominal hysterectomy, salpingo-oophorectomy, lymph node dissection, omentectomy, peritoneal cytology, and systematic visualization of the peritoneum and visceral organs is the standard method of staging for ovarian cancer.

In general, the treatment of epithelial ovarian cancer involves maximum surgical cytoreduction followed by platinum-based chemotherapy. The extent of surgical debulking has been associated with survival in a meta-analysis[28]. Additionally, a nomogram has been developed, which incorporates clinical and 5 presurgical FDG-PET/CT imaging factors (diaphragm involvement, ascites, peritoneal carcinomatosis, small bowel mesentery involvement, and tumor uptake ratio) in order to predict the risk of incomplete debulking.[29] Although the use of second-look surgery is controversial, 2 studies have correlated lesions found on PET imaging to direct confirmation by surgery of residual tumor after platinum-based chemotherapy. Rose and colleagues[30] reported in 2001 the results of a prospective study in which all patients had a complete response to the initial therapy except by PET. PET alone (not integrated PET/CT) showed poor potential, with 10% sensitivity and 42% specificity. Sironi and colleagues[31] in 2004 reported more favorable results with integrated FDG-PET/CT in 31 patients and demonstrated a sensitivity and specificity of 78% and 75%, respectively. They reported that the size threshold of a tumor that could be reasonably detected with FDG-PET/CT in this setting was 0.5 cm.

Most patients with epithelial ovarian cancer present with advanced disease disseminated in the peritoneal cavity; therefore, the role of radiation after surgery and chemotherapy is limited. A recent overview of the role of radiation in ovarian cancer has been written by Dr Patricia Eifel.[32] Historically, whole abdominal radiation therapy (WART) was considered after surgery and chemotherapy to reduce the risk of recurrence,[33,34] or for salvage therapy.[35] However, this practice has largely been abandoned due to a high risk of toxicity, most notably bowel obstruction, and a recognition that the maximum tolerable dose of WART was insufficient to provide durable disease control in most patients. However, some subsets of patients may possibly derive a benefit. For instance, a review of 703 patients treated in British Columbia showed no benefit of WART in the patients treated for epithelial ovarian cancer; but there was a disease-specific and overall survival advantage for WART in patients with stage I or II clear cell, endometrioid, or mucinous carcinomas.[36] Another study reported by Hoskins and colleagues[37] in 2012 on 241 patients with clear cell carcinoma replicated these findings, which showed improved survival with WART and chemotherapy compared with chemotherapy alone. Therefore, radiation may still be discussed with selected patients with clear cell carcinoma as adjuvant therapy; this treatment is usually directed at the pelvis and local disease rather than as WART in modern practice. FDG-PET/CT can be considered before adjuvant radiation in this setting to confirm the absence of gross residual disease or disease outside the planned radiation volume.

Recent studies have also suggested that radiation targeted to gross recurrent disease may be effective and a better-tolerated alternative to WART. Brown and colleagues[38] reported in a retrospective study the outcome of 102 patients treated with radiation for localized recurrences of ovarian cancer, and the rate of in-field disease control and survival at 5 years were 71% and 40%, respectively. In the retrospective series from the authors' institution by Chundury and colleagues,[39] they reported the outcomes of intensity-modulated radiation therapy (IMRT) in 33 patients with localized recurrences of ovarian cancer refractory to chemotherapy. The authors used FDG-PET/CT fused to the simulation CT to guide radiation treatment planning in most patients in this study, as shown in **Fig. 2**, with a median dose of 50.4 Gy delivered by IMRT to the FDG-avid lesions. The actuarial 2-year local control and survival were 82% and 63%, respectively, with limited toxicity. Currently, the authors consider radiation therapy for selected patients with localized platinum-resistant ovarian cancer using PET and MR imaging–guided adaptive stereotactic body radiation therapy in the context of a pilot clinical study (ClinicalTrials.gov identifier NCT02582931).

The NCCN's 2016 guidelines endorse the use of FDG-PET/CT in the detection of recurrence after complete response to surgery and chemotherapy.[26] Gu and colleagues[40] reported a meta-analysis of 34 studies in 2009, demonstrating that FDG-PET/CT had the greatest sensitivity (91%) for detecting recurrent disease, whereas cancer antigen 125 had the greatest specificity (93%) compared with other surveillance modalities, which also included CT and MR imaging. Limei and colleagues[41] reported a more recent meta-analysis in 2013 of 29 studies involving 1651 patients, which reported a pooled sensitivity and specificity of 89% and 90%, respectively, for FDG-PET/CT in detecting recurrent ovarian cancer.

CERVICAL CANCER

Cancer of the uterine cervix has an incidence of 7.5 per 100,000 women in the United States[42]; it is the disease in gynecologic oncology in which there are the most data to support the use of FDG-PET/CT in baseline assessment, radiation treatment planning, and follow-up evaluation. The FIGO stage of cervical cancer is a clinical staging system based on physical examination and allows for limited additional imaging, such as urography and chest radiograph. This strict limitation maintains a uniform comparison of FIGO stages between economically mature and developing countries, where cervical cancer is more prevalent but advanced diagnostic tools are often unavailable. Although findings from FDG-PET/CT are not allowed for clinical FIGO staging, they are allowed to develop the treatment plan. Indeed, the NCCN's 2017 guidelines recommend consideration of FDG-PET/CT for the initial evaluation of disease if it is FIGO stage IB2 or higher,[43] whereas the ACR recommends FDG-PET/CT for stage IB1 or higher.[44]

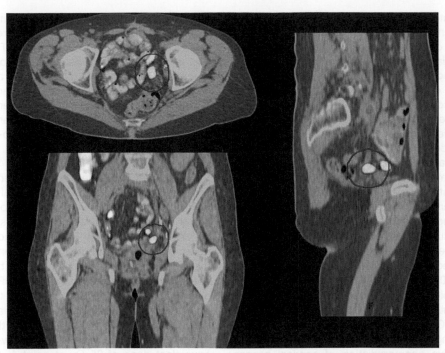

Fig. 2. Use of FDG-PET/CT in restaging and treatment planning for chemotherapy-refractory recurrent ovarian cancer. The patient has a history of FIGO stage IC ovarian adenocarcinoma treated with surgery and platinum-based chemotherapy nearly 10 years previously. The patient has had a long clinical course with multiple recurrences and resections, and the disease was no longer platinum sensitive. FDG-PET/CT was performed for restaging and showed tumor recurrence isolated in the left pelvis without distant metastatic disease. The PET was fused with the simulation CT to aid in treatment planning as shown. The red contour shows the clinical target volume encompassing the FDG-avid recurrent tumor, which was treated with IMRT to 59.2 Gy.

The primary cervical tumor is nearly always FDG avid. PET features, such as maximum standardized uptake value (SUVmax),[45,46] metabolic tumor volume (MTV) as determined by a threshold at 40% of the SUVmax,[47] and tumor heterogeneity[48] have been shown by the authors' group to be associated with prognosis. In particular, the 40% SUVmax volume has been shown to be highly correlated to the size of the tumor in the pathology specimen with a coefficient of determination of 0.951.[49] The 40% SUVmax tumor volume has also been shown to be correlated with the volume of the tumor on diffusion-weighted MR imaging, further supporting the use of this threshold.[50]

Cervical cancer usually spreads to the regional lymph nodes in an orderly fashion: with metastasis to pelvic nodes, followed by para-aortic nodes, followed by supraclavicular nodes, and finally to distant sites. Nodal disease status plays an important role in treatment planning and prognosis; 2 meta-analyses have shown that FDG-PET/CT is more effective than alternative imaging methods, such as CT or MR imaging, in detecting involved lymph nodes.[51,52] These studies report that the pooled sensitivity and specificity of FDG-PET for nodal disease is 82%

and 95%, respectively. Assuming a 27% pretest probability of lymph node metastasis among all patients, a positive finding on PET is estimated to increase the posttest probability to 85% (95% confidence interval 75%–92%). In particular, Grigsby and colleagues[53] in 2001 reported a retrospective study of 101 patients and observed that FDG-PET detected abnormal lymph nodes more often than CT and that FDG-PET findings, especially involvement of para-aortic lymph nodes, were a better predictor of survival than CT findings. These findings were validated in a prospective study of 560 patients reported by Kidd and colleagues[54] in 2010. Lymph node involvement was observed in 47% of patients at diagnosis, and the risk for disease recurrence increased incrementally based on the most distant level of FDG-detected nodal disease. The hazard ratios, compared with a baseline of no FDG-avid nodal disease, were 2.4 for pelvic nodes, 5.9 for para-aortic nodes, and 30.3 for supraclavicular nodes. The SUVmax of pelvic nodes may also be a prognostic biomarker.[55] A prognostic nomogram integrating many of the aforementioned FDG-PET features has been reported by Kidd and colleagues.[56]

The treatment of early stage (FIGO stage IB1 or smaller) tumors may involve surgical resection followed by consideration of adjuvant radiation or chemoradiation if meeting the criteria defined by randomized studies reported by Sedlis and colleagues[57] or Peters and colleagues,[58] respectively. According to the NCCN, FDG-PET/CT can be considered after surgery if para-aortic nodes are identified surgically or if invasive cervical cancer is incidentally found at hysterectomy.[43] Bulky or locally advanced cervical cancer (FIGO stage IB2 or greater) is usually treated with chemoradiation consisting of cisplatin concurrent with external radiation and brachytherapy. This treatment paradigm is supported by randomized trials reporting superior survival with concurrent chemotherapy and no benefit of hysterectomy in this setting as reported in the Radiation Therapy Oncology Group's 90-01 protocol[59] and the study by Landoni and colleagues,[60] respectively.

The authors have extensively investigated FDG-PET/CT image-guided IMRT combined with MR imaging–based high dose rate brachytherapy for definitive chemoradiation of cervical cancer as shown in **Fig. 3**. Details of the authors'

IMRT[3,61] and brachytherapy[62] treatment technique have been published elsewhere. The authors use a pseudo step wedge IMRT technique that is based on their historical use of a central block after 20 Gy to shield the bladder and rectum and to allow for higher doses of brachytherapy aiming to improve local control. Patients receive FDG-PET/CT simulation in the treatment position, and the cervical tumor MTV is auto-contoured based on the 40% SUVmax threshold. The pelvic vessels are contoured from the aortic bifurcation to the medial circumflex femoral artery inferiorly and includes the common iliac, external iliac, internal iliac, and obturator regions. The nodal clinical target volume (CTVnodal) is the vessel contour uniformly expanded by 7 mm and excluding the pelvic bones. The planning target volume (PTV) is the CTVnodal expanded uniformly by 5 mm. The authors typically develop an IMRT plan to deliver 50.4 Gy to the PTV and 20 Gy to the MTV and interdigitate 6 brachytherapy treatments to deliver an additional dose of 39 Gy to the cervical tumor, with a goal of reaching a low-dose rate equivalent dose of 85 Gy at point A. In patients with involved para-aortic nodes on FDG-PET/CT,

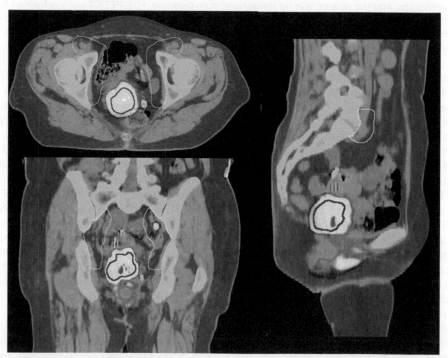

Fig. 3. Use of FDG-PET/CT in baseline assessment and treatment planning for cervical cancer. The images are of a patient with FIGO stage IIIB squamous cell carcinoma of the cervix. FDG-PET/CT for initial assessment showed FDG-avid cervical tumor but no distant disease or lymph nodes (the FDG-avid site lateral to the tumor is due to excreted FDG within the left ureter). FDG-PET/CT was fused with the simulation CT to aid in treatment planning as shown. The red contour shows the MTV defined as the volume greater than or equal to 40% of the SUVmax. The primary cervix tumor was treated to 20 Gy by IMRT and 41.4 Gy by brachytherapy. The cyan volume is the elective nodal clinical target volume, which was treated with IMRT to 50.4 Gy.

the authors deliver extended field radiation up to 60 Gy by IMRT, as supported by a prospective clinical study reported by Esthappan and colleagues.[63] The outcomes of this approach have been reported in a prospective study of 452 patients, which observed that PET-guided IMRT was associated with better overall and cause-specific survival and fewer bowel or bladder complications compared with non–IMRT-treated patients.[64] This treatment approach has, therefore, become the standard practice for definitive treatment of cervical cancer at the authors' institution. The authors have recently begun to routinely acquire hybrid FDG-PET/MR imaging for use in disease detection and treatment planning as shown in **Fig. 4**. MR imaging has superior visualization of soft tissue and may provide additional information to aid in treatment planning. Studies are ongoing to determine the role and benefit of FDG-PET/MR imaging in this setting.

FDG-PET/CT has been associated with prognosis at multiple time points during and after chemoradiation for cervical cancer. Kidd and colleagues[65] and Schwarz and colleagues[66] reported initial prospective and retrospective data supporting the use of FDG-PET/CT in evaluating the treatment response. Most importantly, Schwarz and colleagues[67] reported in 2007 a prospective validation study of this principle involving 92 patients. This study showed that patients with a complete metabolic response at 3 months after treatment had a 3-year progression-free survival of 78%, compared with 33% and 0% for patients with partial response and progressive disease, respectively. A meta-analysis of 20 studies by Chu and colleagues[68] on PET for recurrent cervical cancer reported a pooled sensitivity and specificity of 87% and 97%, respectively, for distant disease and 82% and 98%, respectively, for locoregional disease. The authors routinely

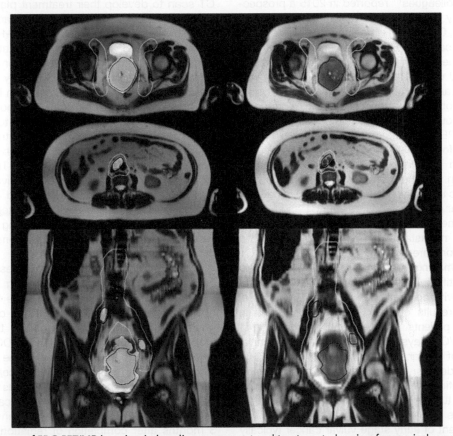

Fig. 4. The use of FDG-PET/MR imaging in baseline assessment and treatment planning for cervical cancer. The images are of a patient with FIGO stage IIB squamous cell carcinoma of the cervix. Diagnostic hybrid FDG-PET and whole-body MR imaging showed involvement of pelvic and para-aortic lymph nodes. The PET and T2-weighted whole-body MR imaging were registered to simulation CT for treatment planning. The red contour shows the cervical metabolic tumor volume defined as the volume greater than or equal to 40% of the SUVmax. The primary cervix tumor was treated to 50.4 Gy by IMRT and 24 Gy by brachytherapy. The cyan volume is the elective CTVnodal, and the magenta volume is the MTV of lymph nodes. The CTVnodal was treated to 50.4 Gy by IMRT.

perform FDG-PET/CT at the 3-month time point or if recurrence is clinically suspected. The NCCN's 2017 guidelines recommend PET in the follow-up period only if recurrence is suspected, although the NCCN's 2016 guidelines allowed for a single PET scan at 3 to 6 months.[43]

VULVAR CANCER

Squamous cell carcinoma of the vulva has an incidence of approximately 2.5 per 100,000 women, and this incidence may be increasing.[69] Although vulvar cancer is a rare disease, recent treatment guidelines and published studies have clarified the role of PET in staging, treatment planning, and follow-up. Cohn and colleagues[70] reported in 2002 a prospective study of 15 patients comparing PET findings before surgery with pathologic results after resection. FDG-PET/CT had a sensitivity of 67%, specificity of 95%, positive predictive value of 86%, and negative predictive value of 86%. Lin and colleagues[71] reported in 2015 a prospective study involving 23 patients imaged with FDG-PET, CT, and MR imaging for primary staging of vulvar cancer. PET was superior in identifying involved pelvic lymph nodes or distant metastasis compared with CT or MR imaging, but there was no significant difference in detecting inguinal lymph nodes. Robertson and colleagues[72] reported in 2016 the outcomes from a retrospective series of 83 FDG-PET/CT studies (65% for vulvar cancer and 35% for vaginal cancer) performed for disease staging in the National Oncologic PET Registry (NOPR). In this important study, PET changed the diagnostic impression in 54% (29 of 54) of patients with vulvar cancer compared with CT and MR imaging alone. FDG-PET/CT detected nodes suspicious for metastasis in 35% (29 of 83) of the studies compared with 11 and 6 studies in CT and MR imaging, respectively. Distant metastasis was identified in 10 cases with FDG-PET and 5 cases with conventional imaging. Furthermore, the PET results changed the treatment plan in 36% of patients. These results suggest that FDG-PET/CT plays an important role in the initial staging of vulvar cancer. Indeed, the NCCN's 2017 guidelines for vulvar cancer recommend consideration of FDG-PET/CT for the initial staging of vulvar tumors greater than 2 cm in size or if metastasis is suspected.

Treatment of early stage vulvar cancer typically involves surgical resection by wide local excision with sampling or dissection of regional lymph nodes or by radical vulvectomy. Radiation therapy is indicated after surgery according to the NCCN's 2017 guidelines for high-risk features, such as involved lymph nodes and positive tumor margins.[73] Patients with other risk factors, such as close margins of less than 8 mm, lympho-vascular space invasion, or depth of invasion as defined by Heaps and colleagues,[74] can also be considered for adjuvant radiation. The NCCN recommends consideration of chemoradiation for patients with multiple involved lymph nodes or a single lymph node with greater than 2 mm metastasis.[73] In contrast to early stage disease, locally advanced vulvar cancer often cannot be treated with primary surgery because of the extent of the tumor or the fact that extensive resection may result in unacceptable toxicity. The recommended treatment is, therefore, usually definitive chemoradiation, with surgery reserved for recurrent or residual disease.[75]

Gaffney and colleagues[76] recently reported guidelines in target delineation in radiation therapy for vulvar cancer, which were generated based on consensus contours drawn by experts in radiation oncology who reviewed data from diagnostic FDG-PET/CT in addition to the simulation CT scan to develop their treatment plans. At the authors' institution, they also plan radiation for vulvar cancer using a simulation FDG-PET/CT as shown in **Fig. 5**. Furthermore, the authors give additional radiation to the FDG-avid primary vulvar tumor using an integrated boost by IMRT as described by Rao and colleagues.[77] In this study, vulvar tumors and regional lymph nodes were treated to a postoperative dose of 50 to 60 Gy or a definitive dose of 60 to 70 Gy. The authors prefer to give an additional radiation dose by brachytherapy in eligible patients after IMRT. The 3-year locoregional control in this retrospective analysis was 89% after adjuvant radiation and 42% after definitive radiation. However, the integration of PET into radiation treatment planning in vulvar cancer varies based on the practitioner; as yet there is no consensus on its role.

The NCCN's posttreatment guidelines for vulvar cancer currently recommend imaging based on symptoms or examination suspicious for recurrence. However, the ACR's 2013 consensus guidelines for vulvar cancer showed that many practitioners would recommend FDG-PET/CT in the follow-up period to assess for the treatment response.[78] Indeed, Rao and colleagues[79] recently reported the clinical outcomes of 21 patients treated with radiation for vulvar cancer who received FDG-PET/CT at a median time of 3 months after completion of radiation. Patients with no evidence of disease on follow-up PET had a 2-year locoregional control and survival of 89% and 100%, respectively, compared with 25% and 42%, respectively, in patients with progressive disease on follow-up PET. These results suggest a role of FDG-PET/CT in the assessment

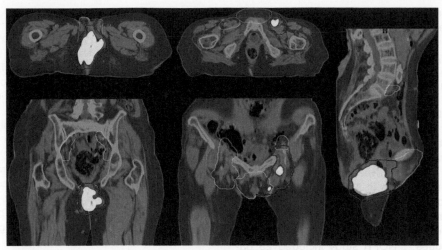

Fig. 5. The use of FDG-PET/CT in staging and treatment planning for vulvar cancer. The images are of a patient with FIGO stage IVA squamous cell carcinoma of the vulva. FDG-PET/CT for initial staging showed FDG-avid vulvar tumor and inguinal lymph nodes but no distant disease. The FDG-PET/CT was fused with the simulation CT to aid in treatment planning as shown. The CTV (CTV 70) around the FDG-avid primary vulvar tumor is shown in red and treated to 70 Gy. The CTV (CTV 66.5) around the FDG-avid inguinal lymph nodes is shown in magenta and treated to 66.5 Gy. The elective volume (CTV 52.5) encompasses the entire vulva as well as the regional nodes, shown in cyan, and was treated to 52.5 Gy. External radiation was delivered by IMRT.

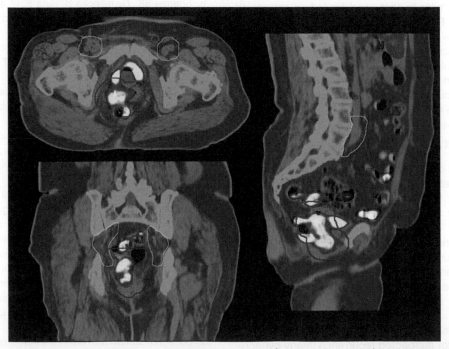

Fig. 6. The use of FDG-PET/CT in staging and treatment planning for vaginal cancer. The images are of a patient with FIGO stage III squamous cell carcinoma of the vagina. FDG-PET/CT for initial staging showed FDG-avid vaginal tumor and no distant disease. The FDG-PET/CT was fused with the simulation CT to aid in treatment planning as shown. The CTV (CTV 66) around the FDG-avid primary vulvar tumor is shown in red and treated to 66 Gy. The elective nodal volume is shown in cyan and was treated to 52.8 Gy. External radiation was delivered by IMRT. Consolidative interstitial brachytherapy to an additional 20 Gy was delivered to the vaginal tumor after completion of external radiation.

of treatment response or surveillance of vulvar cancer after radiation.

VAGINAL CANCER

Vaginal squamous cell carcinoma is rare, with an incidence of approximately 1 per 100,000 women.[80] Currently, data on the role of PET are limited in this disease. Lamoreaux and colleagues[81] analyzed a prospective registry of 23 patients with vaginal cancer and reported that FDG-PET visualized the primary tumor and inguinal lymph nodes in 100% and 35% of the cases, respectively. In contrast, CT visualized the primary tumor and inguinal nodes in 43% and 17% of the cases, respectively. The Robertson and colleagues'[72] NOPR study included 29 patients with vaginal cancer; PET/CT changed the diagnostic impression in 45% of these patients. The authors, therefore, routinely acquire FDG-PET/CT for initial staging. Patients with vaginal squamous cell carcinoma are typically treated with radiation or chemoradiation with a combination of external radiation and brachytherapy to a total dose of 75 to 85 Gy. In the authors' clinic, they use fused FDG-PET simulation or diagnostic images to guide IMRT and/or brachytherapy in a manner similar to that used for vulvar cancer as shown in **Fig. 6**. However, there is currently no consensus or published clinical outcome data on this practice of PET-guided treatment. The Society of Gynecologic Oncologists recommends PET if recurrence of vaginal cancer is suspected, but there is currently no established role of FDG-PET/CT in routine surveillance.[82]

SUMMARY

Published data support the use of FDG-PET/CT in baseline assessment, radiation treatment planning, and follow-up for cervical cancer. It may eventually play a similar role (including staging) for vulvar and vaginal cancers, although more data are needed. There is currently no need to routinely use staging FDG-PET/CT in uterine or ovarian cancer. PET may be helpful for postoperative uterine cancer when there is a high risk of unevaluated nodal involvement or in patients with medically inoperable uterine cancer receiving definitive brachytherapy. FDG-PET/CT should be acquired for suspected recurrence in any gynecologic malignancy and could help guide salvage radiation treatment. Radiation oncologists who treat gynecologic malignancies might improve the outcomes of their patients by incorporating recent guidelines and published data on PET into their practice.

REFERENCES

1. Grigsby PW. Role of PET in gynecologic malignancy. Curr Opin Oncol 2009;21(5):420–4.
2. Haynes-Outlaw ED, Grigsby PW. The role of FDG-PET/CT in cervical cancer: diagnosis, staging, radiation treatment planning and follow-up. PET Clin 2010;5(4):435–46.
3. Speirs CK, Grigsby PW, Huang J, et al. PET-based radiation therapy planning. PET Clin 2015;10(1):27–44.
4. Rosenkrantz AB, Friedman K, Chandarana H, et al. Current status of hybrid PET/MRI in oncologic imaging. Am J Roentgenol 2016;206(1):162–72.
5. Ponisio MR, Fowler KJ, Dehdashti F. The emerging role of PET/MR imaging in gynecologic cancers. PET Clin 2016;11(4):425–40.
6. Bagade S, Fowler KJ, Schwarz JK, et al. PET/MRI evaluation of gynecologic malignancies and prostate cancer. Semin Nucl Med 2015;45(4):293–303.
7. Oldan JD, Patel PS. Positron emission tomography/computed tomography for gynecologic malignancies. Obstet Gynecol Surv 2016;71(9):545–56.
8. Hernandez Pampaloni M, Facchetti L, Nardo L. Pitfalls in [18F]FDG PET imaging in gynecological malignancies. Q J Nucl Med Mol Imaging 2016;60(2):124–38.
9. Sharma SK, Nemieboka B, Sala E, et al. Molecular imaging of ovarian cancer. J Nucl Med 2016;57(6):827–33.
10. Gill BS, Pai SS, McKenzie S, et al. Utility of PET for radiotherapy treatment planning. PET Clin 2015;10(4):541–54.
11. SEER cancer stat facts: endometrial cancer. 2017. Available at: https://seer.cancer.gov/statfacts/html/corp.html. Accessed April 1, 2017.
12. NCCN clinical practice guidelines in oncology: uterine neoplasms. 2017. Available at: https://www.nccn.org/professionals/physician_gls/pdf/uterine.pdf. Accessed April 1, 2017.
13. Kakhki VRD, Shahriari S, Treglia G, et al. Diagnostic performance of fluorine 18 fluorodeoxyglucose positron emission tomography imaging for detection of primary lesion and staging of endometrial cancer patients: systematic review and meta-analysis of the literature. Int J Gynecol Cancer 2013;23(9):1536–43.
14. Lee HJ, Park J-Y, Lee JJ, et al. Comparison of MRI and 18F-FDG PET/CT in the preoperative evaluation of uterine carcinosarcoma. Gynecol Oncol 2016;140(3):409–14.
15. Sadeghi R, Zakavi SR, Hasanzadeh M, et al. Diagnostic performance of fluorine-18-fluorodeoxyglucose positron emission tomography imaging in uterine sarcomas: systematic review and meta-analysis of the literature. Int J Gynecol Cancer 2013;23(8):1349–56.
16. Nout RA, Smit VTHBM, Putter H, et al. Vaginal brachytherapy versus pelvic external beam

radiotherapy for patients with endometrial cancer of high-intermediate risk (PORTEC-2): an open-label, non-inferiority, randomised trial. Lancet 2010; 375(9717):816–23.

17. Creasman WT, Morrow CP, Bundy BN, et al. Surgical pathologic spread patterns of endometrial cancer. A Gynecologic Oncology Group Study. Cancer 1987; 60(8 Suppl):2035–41. Available at: http://www.ncbi. nlm.nih.gov/pubmed/3652025. Accessed March 6, 2017.

18. Signorelli M, Crivellaro C, Buda A, et al. Staging of high-risk endometrial cancer with PET/CT and sentinel lymph node mapping. Clin Nucl Med 2015;40(10): 780–5.

19. ASTEC Study Group, Kitchener H, Swart AMC, Qian Q, et al. Efficacy of systematic pelvic lymphadenectomy in endometrial cancer (MRC ASTEC trial): a randomised study. Lancet 2009;373(9658):125–36.

20. Simcock B, Narayan K, Drummond E, et al. The role of positron emission tomography/computed tomography in planning radiotherapy in endometrial cancer. Int J Gynecol Cancer 2015;25(4):645–9.

21. Lin LL, Grigsby PW, Powell MA, et al. Definitive radiotherapy in the management of isolated vaginal recurrences of endometrial cancer. Int J Radiat Oncol Biol Phys 2005;63(2):500–4.

22. Schwarz JK, Beriwal S, Esthappan J, et al. Consensus statement for brachytherapy for the treatment of medically inoperable endometrial cancer. Brachytherapy 2015;14(5):587–99.

23. Kadkhodayan S, Shahriari S, Treglia G, et al. Accuracy of 18-F-FDG PET imaging in the follow up of endometrial cancer patients: systematic review and meta-analysis of the literature. Gynecol Oncol 2013;128(2):397–404.

24. Siegel R, Ma J, Zou Z, et al. Cancer statistics, 2014. CA Cancer J Clin 2014;64(1):9–29.

25. Mitchell DG, Javitt MC, Glanc P, et al. ACR appropriateness criteria staging and follow-up of ovarian cancer. J Am Coll Radiol 2013;10(11):822–7.

26. NCCN clinical practice guidelines in oncology: ovarian cancer. 2016. Available at: https://www.nccn. org/professionals/physician_gls/pdf/ovarian.pdf. Accessed April 1, 2017.

27. Yuan Y, Gu Z-X, Tao X-F, et al. Computer tomography, magnetic resonance imaging, and positron emission tomography or positron emission tomography/computer tomography for detection of metastatic lymph nodes in patients with ovarian cancer: a meta-analysis. Eur J Radiol 2012;81(5):1002–6.

28. Elattar A, Bryant A, Winter-Roach BA, et al. Optimal primary surgical treatment for advanced epithelial ovarian cancer. Elattar A, ed. Cochrane Database Syst Rev 2011;(8):CD007565.

29. Shim S-H, Lee SJ, Kim S-O, et al. Nomogram for predicting incomplete cytoreduction in advanced ovarian cancer patients. Gynecol Oncol 2015;136(1):30–6.

30. Rose PG, Faulhaber P, Miraldi F, et al. Positive emission tomography for evaluating a complete clinical response in patients with ovarian or peritoneal carcinoma: correlation with second-look laparotomy. Gynecol Oncol 2001;82(1):17–21.

31. Sironi S, Messa C, Mangili G, et al. Integrated FDG PET/CT in patients with persistent ovarian cancer: correlation with histologic findings. Radiology 2004;233(2):433–40.

32. Eifel PJ. Role of radiation therapy. Best Pract Res Clin Obstet Gynaecol 2017;41:118–25.

33. Klaassen D, Shelley W, Starreveld A, et al. Early stage ovarian cancer: a randomized clinical trial comparing whole abdominal radiotherapy, melphalan, and intraperitoneal chromic phosphate: a National Cancer Institute of Canada Clinical Trials Group report. J Clin Oncol 1988;6(8):1254–63.

34. Eifel PJ, Gershenson DM, Delclos L, et al. Twice-daily, split-course abdominopelvic radiation therapy after chemotherapy and positive second-look laparotomy for epithelial ovarian carcinoma. Int J Radiat Oncol Biol Phys 1991;21(4):1013–8. Available at: http://www.ncbi.nlm.nih.gov/pubmed/1917596. Accessed March 6, 2017.

35. Schray MF, Martinez A, Howes AE, et al. Advanced epithelial ovarian cancer: salvage whole abdominal irradiation for patients with recurrent or persistent disease after combination chemotherapy. J Clin Oncol 1988;6(9):1433–9.

36. Swenerton KD, Santos JL, Gilks CB, et al. Histotype predicts the curative potential of radiotherapy: the example of ovarian cancers. Ann Oncol 2011; 22(2):341–7.

37. Hoskins PJ, Le N, Gilks B, et al. Low-stage ovarian clear cell carcinoma: population-based outcomes in British Columbia, Canada, with evidence for a survival benefit as a result of irradiation. J Clin Oncol 2012;30(14):1656–62.

38. Brown AP, Jhingran A, Klopp AH, et al. Involved-field radiation therapy for locoregionally recurrent ovarian cancer. Gynecol Oncol 2013;130(2): 300–5.

39. Chundury A, Apicelli A, DeWees T, et al. Intensity modulated radiation therapy for recurrent ovarian cancer refractory to chemotherapy. Gynecol Oncol 2016;141(1):134–9.

40. Gu P, Pan L-L, Wu S-Q, et al. CA 125, PET alone, PET–CT, CT and MRI in diagnosing recurrent ovarian carcinoma. Eur J Radiol 2009;71(1):164–74.

41. Limei Z, Yong C, Yan X, et al. Accuracy of positron emission tomography/computed tomography in the diagnosis and restaging for recurrent ovarian cancer: a meta-analysis. Int J Gynecol Cancer 2013; 23(4):598–607.

42. SEER cancer stat facts: cervical cancer. 2017. Available at: https://seer.cancer.gov/statfacts/html/ cervix.html. Accessed April 1, 2017.

43. NCCN clinical practice guidelines in oncology: cervical cancer. 2017. Available at: https://www.nccn.org/professionals/physician_gls/pdf/cervical.pdf. Accessed April 1, 2017.

44. Siegel CL, Andreotti RF, Cardenes HR, et al. ACR appropriateness criteria® pretreatment planning of invasive cancer of the cervix. J Am Coll Radiol 2012;9(6):395–402.

45. Xue F, Lin LL, Dehdashti F, et al. F-18 fluorodeoxyglucose uptake in primary cervical cancer as an indicator of prognosis after radiation therapy. Gynecol Oncol 2006;101(1):147–51.

46. Kidd EA, Siegel BA, Dehdashti F, et al. The standardized uptake value for F-18 fluorodeoxyglucose is a sensitive predictive biomarker for cervical cancer treatment response and survival. Cancer 2007; 110(8):1738–44.

47. Miller TR, Grigsby PW. Measurement of tumor volume by PET to evaluate prognosis in patients with advanced cervical cancer treated by radiation therapy. Int J Radiat Oncol Biol Phys 2002;53(2): 353–9. Available at: http://www.ncbi.nlm.nih.gov/pubmed/12023139. Accessed March 7, 2017.

48. Kidd EA, Grigsby PW. Intratumoral metabolic heterogeneity of cervical cancer. Clin Cancer Res 2008;14(16):5236–41.

49. Showalter TN, Miller TR, Huettner P, et al. 18F-fluorodeoxyglucose-positron emission tomography and pathologic tumor size in early-stage invasive cervical cancer. Int J Gynecol Cancer 2009;19(8):1412–4.

50. Olsen JR, Esthappan J, DeWees T, et al. Tumor volume and subvolume concordance between FDG-PET/CT and diffusion-weighted MRI for squamous cell carcinoma of the cervix. J Magn Reson Imaging 2013;37(2):431–4.

51. Selman TJ, Mann C, Zamora J, et al. Diagnostic accuracy of tests for lymph node status in primary cervical cancer: a systematic review and meta-analysis. CMAJ 2008;178(7):855–62.

52. Choi HJ, Ju W, Myung SK, et al. Diagnostic performance of computer tomography, magnetic resonance imaging, and positron emission tomography or positron emission tomography/computer tomography for detection of metastatic lymph nodes in patients with cervical cancer: meta-analysis. Cancer Sci 2010;101(6):1471–9.

53. Grigsby PW, Siegel BA, Dehdashti F. Lymph node staging by positron emission tomography in patients with carcinoma of the cervix. J Clin Oncol 2001; 19(17):3745–9.

54. Kidd EA, Siegel BA, Dehdashti F, et al. Lymph node staging by positron emission tomography in cervical cancer: relationship to prognosis. J Clin Oncol 2010; 28(12):2108–13.

55. Kidd EA, Siegel BA, Dehdashti F, et al. Pelvic lymph node F-18 fluorodeoxyglucose uptake as a prognostic biomarker in newly diagnosed patients with locally advanced cervical cancer. Cancer 2010; 116(6):1469–75.

56. Kidd EA, El Naqa I, Siegel BA, et al. FDG-PET-based prognostic nomograms for locally advanced cervical cancer. Gynecol Oncol 2012;127(1):136–40.

57. Sedlis A, Bundy BN, Rotman MZ, et al. A randomized trial of pelvic radiation therapy versus no further therapy in selected patients with stage IB carcinoma of the cervix after radical hysterectomy and pelvic lymphadenectomy: a gynecologic oncology group study. Gynecol Oncol 1999;73(2):177–83.

58. Peters WA, Liu PY, Barrett RJ, et al. Concurrent chemotherapy and pelvic radiation therapy compared with pelvic radiation therapy alone as adjuvant therapy after radical surgery in high-risk early-stage cancer of the cervix. J Clin Oncol 2000;18(8):1606–13.

59. Morris M, Eifel PJ, Lu J, et al. Pelvic radiation with concurrent chemotherapy compared with pelvic and para-aortic radiation for high-risk cervical cancer. N Engl J Med 1999;340(15):1137–43.

60. Landoni F, Maneo A, Colombo A, et al. Randomised study of radical surgery versus radiotherapy for stage Ib-IIa cervical cancer. Lancet 1997; 350(9077):535–40.

61. Macdonald DM, Lin LL, Biehl K, et al. Combined intensity-modulated radiation therapy and brachytherapy in the treatment of cervical cancer. Int J Radiat Oncol Biol Phys 2008;71(2):618–24.

62. Zoberi JE, Garcia-Ramirez J, Hu Y, et al. Clinical implementation of multisequence MRI-based adaptive intracavitary brachytherapy for cervix cancer. J Appl Clin Med Phys 2016;17(1):5736. Available at: http://www.ncbi.nlm.nih.gov/pubmed/26894342. Accessed March 7, 2017.

63. Esthappan J, Chaudhari S, Santanam L, et al. Prospective clinical trial of positron emission tomography/computed tomography image-guided intensity-modulated radiation therapy for cervical carcinoma with positive para-aortic lymph nodes. Int J Radiat Oncol Biol Phys 2008;72(4):1134–9.

64. Kidd EA, Siegel BA, Dehdashti F, et al. Clinical outcomes of definitive intensity-modulated radiation therapy with fluorodeoxyglucose–positron emission tomography simulation in patients with locally advanced cervical cancer. Int J Radiat Oncol 2010;77(4):1085–91.

65. Kidd EA, Thomas M, Siegel BA, et al. Changes in cervical cancer FDG uptake during chemoradiation and association with response. Int J Radiat Oncol 2013;85(1):116–22.

66. Schwarz JK, Lin LL, Siegel BA, et al. 18-F-fluorodeoxyglucose–positron emission tomography evaluation of early metabolic response during radiation therapy for cervical cancer. Int J Radiat Oncol 2008;72(5):1502–7.

67. Schwarz JK, Siegel BA, Dehdashti F, et al. Association of posttherapy positron emission tomography with tumor response and survival in cervical carcinoma. JAMA 2007;298(19):2289.

68. Chu Y, Zheng A, Wang F, et al. Diagnostic value of 18F-FDG-PET or PET-CT in recurrent cervical cancer. Nucl Med Commun 2014;35(2):144–50.

69. Bodelon C, Madeleine MM, Voigt LF, et al. Is the incidence of invasive vulvar cancer increasing in the United States? Cancer Causes Control 2009;20(9): 1779–82.

70. Cohn DE, Dehdashti F, Gibb RK, et al. Prospective evaluation of positron emission tomography for the detection of groin node metastases from vulvar cancer. Gynecol Oncol 2002;85(1):179–84.

71. Lin G, Chen C-Y, Liu F-Y, et al. Computed tomography, magnetic resonance imaging and FDG positron emission tomography in the management of vulvar malignancies. Eur Radiol 2015;25(5): 1267–78.

72. Robertson NL, Hricak H, Sonoda Y, et al. The impact of FDG-PET/CT in the management of patients with vulvar and vaginal cancer. Gynecol Oncol 2016; 140(3):420–4.

73. NCCN clinical practice guidelines in oncology: vulvar cancer. 2017. Available at: http://www.nccn.org/professionals/physician_gls/pdf/vulvar.pdf. Accessed April 1, 2017.

74. Heaps JM, Fu YS, Montz FJ, et al. Surgical-pathologic variables predictive of local recurrence in squamous cell carcinoma of the vulva. Gynecol Oncol 1990;38(3):309–14.

75. Shylasree TS, Bryant A, Howells RE. Chemoradiation for advanced primary vulval cancer. Cochrane Database Syst Rev 2011;(4):CD003752.

76. Gaffney DK, King B, Viswanathan AN, et al. Consensus recommendations for radiation therapy contouring and treatment of vulvar carcinoma. Int J Radiat Oncol Biol Phys 2016;95(4):1191–200.

77. Rao YJ, Chundury A, Schwarz JK, et al. Intensity modulated radiation therapy for squamous cell carcinoma of the vulva: treatment technique and outcomes. Adv Radiat Oncol 2017;2(2):148–58.

78. Kidd E, Moore D, Varia MA, et al. ACR appropriateness criteria® management of locoregionally advanced squamous cell carcinoma of the vulva. Am J Clin Oncol 2013;36(4):415–22.

79. Rao YJ, Hassanzadeh C, Chundury A, et al. Association of post-treatment positron emission tomography with locoregional control and survival after radiation therapy for squamous cell carcinoma of the vulva. Radiother Oncol 2017;122(3):445–51.

80. Shah CA, Goff BA, Lowe K, et al. Factors affecting risk of mortality in women with vaginal cancer. Obstet Gynecol 2009;113(5):1038–45.

81. Lamoreaux WT, Grigsby PW, Dehdashti F, et al. FDG-PET evaluation of vaginal carcinoma. Int J Radiat Oncol Biol Phys 2005;62(3):733–7.

82. Salani R, Backes FJ, Fung MFK, et al. Posttreatment surveillance and diagnosis of recurrence in women with gynecologic malignancies: Society of Gynecologic Oncologists recommendations. Am J Obstet Gynecol 2011;204(6):466–78.

Non–¹⁸F-2-Fluoro-2-Deoxy-D-Glucose PET/Computed Tomography in Gynecologic Oncology

An Overview of Current Status and Future Potential

Ashwini Kalshetty, Diplomate N. B[a,b],
Sandip Basu, Diplomate N. B[a,b,*]

KEYWORDS

- Gynecologic oncology • FDG • PET/CT • Non-FDG PET/CT

KEY POINTS

- Gynecologic malignancies comprise a heterogeneous group of malignancies of the female reproductive system with diverse clinical courses and prognoses.
- The role of ¹⁸F-2-fluoro-2-deoxy-D-glucose (FDG) PET/computed tomography in various stages of management of gynecologic malignancies is already established.
- In the era of precision medicine and the development of newer therapeutic agents (including targeted therapies), there is a growing need for molecular imaging to address the limitations of FDG through newer PET radiotracers that may be able to aid in personalized management to patients.

INTRODUCTION: POTENTIAL AND SCOPE OF NON-¹⁸F-2-FLUORO-2-DEOXY-D-GLUCOSE PET RADIOTRACERS IN GYNECOLOGIC MALIGNANCIES

Gynecologic malignancies comprise a heterogeneous group of malignancies of the female reproductive system with diverse clinical courses and prognosis. The role of ¹⁸F-2-fluoro-2-deoxy-D-glucose (FDG) PET/computed tomography (CT) in various stages of management of gynecologic malignancies is already established. However, in the era of precision medicine and the development of newer therapeutic agents (including targeted therapies), there is a growing need for molecular imaging to address the limitations of FDG through newer PET radiotracers that may be able to aid in personalized management to patients. The newer molecules, thus, open a gateway of personalized precision medicine with the potential for in vivo immunohistochemistry (IHC) and exploration of the tumor microenvironment with respect to specific biological processes of interest. The scope widens with the introduction of newer therapeutic agents targeting the specific biological pathways. Because mortality from the gynecologic malignancies is on a decreasing trend because of awareness, advancements in medical technology, and new therapeutic agents, the focus has shifted more toward reducing the morbidity and toward palliative care. The limitations of current imaging include the lack of accurate assessment of

[a] Radiation Medicine Centre, Bhabha Atomic Research Centre, Tata Memorial Hospital Annexe Building, Jerbai Wadia Road, Parel, Mumbai 400 012, India; [b] Homi Bhabha National Institute, Mumbai, India
* Corresponding author. Radiation Medicine Centre, Bhabha Atomic Research Centre, Tata Memorial Hospital Annexe Building, Jerbai Wadia Road, Parel, Mumbai 400 012, India.
E-mail address: drsanb@yahoo.com

PET Clin 13 (2018) 239–248
https://doi.org/10.1016/j.cpet.2017.11.008
1556-8598/18/

prognosticators to plan appropriate treatment and of sensitive biomarkers for therapeutic monitoring of newer agents used to treat in advanced disease. The cytostatic effect of most targeted therapies produces a dilemma in assessing the response or monitoring patients because there is minimal change in the parameters detected on conventional imaging, whereas imaging the specific biological processes may help us better understand the internal milieu and open opportunities for the faster development of effective investigational new drugs. The new avenues in metabolomics are promising for monitoring the response with targeted therapy, early identification of chemotherapy resistance, and accurate staging of malignancies.

^{18}F-2-FLUORO-2-DEOXY-D-GLUCOSE: THE SHORTCOMINGS IN GYNECOLOGIC MALIGNANCIES

FDG PET/CT has been commonly used in the management of various malignancies. However, there are few limitations of use of FDG in the management of gynecologic malignancies as described here:

1. A limitation is that due to the nonspecific FDG uptake, one cannot reliably distinguish between benign and malignant primaries. For example, it has low to intermediate sensitivity of 57% to 100% in distinguishing benign and malignant ovarian lesions in premenopausal and postmenopausal women.[1]
2. There is also difficulty in distinguishing residual tumor from inflammatory changes. In cervical cancer, one is able to assess the treatment response only weeks after the inflammatory uptake has subsided. Pyometra is commonly seen in patients with cervical cancer, and inflammatory radiotracer uptake can mimic tumor disease activity.
3. Physiologic FDG uptake in the endometrium, uterine cavity, and ovaries occurs depending on the phase of the menstrual cycle. Similarly, physiologic FDG accumulation is often seen in the bowel and urinary bladder as well as in bladder diverticula.
4. Tiny tumor lesions are difficult to detect, partly because of the spatial resolution, which has implications for the detection of peritoneal metastases.
5. Low FDG accumulation has been reported in mucinous, cystic, and necrotic tumors.
6. There is inaccurate primary tumor (T) staging, whereby one cannot conclusively detect adjacent organ infiltration by the primary tumor.
7. There is occasional difficulty in regional lymph node (N) staging due to nonspecific FDG uptake in reactive lymph nodes.
8. There is limited value in guiding targeted therapeutic agents, such as hormonal agents.
9. There is limited predictive or prognostic value.

OVARIAN CANCER

Ovarian carcinoma is the most fatal gynecologic malignancy, being the fifth most common cause of cancer-related death.[2] Ovarian carcinomas are divided into epithelial and nonepithelial ovarian carcinomas, with epithelial being the most common form. Around 70% to 75% of patients present with advanced disease and have a poor 5-year survival rate (17% for stage IV disease in epithelial ovarian carcinoma). Epithelial ovarian carcinomas (EOCs) are further divided into type I (low grade) and type II (high grade) carcinomas. Type I tumors have a low malignant potential, run an indolent course, and have an identifiable genetic profile. The histopathologies include low-grade serous, endometrioid, mucinous, clear cell, and transitional cell carcinomas. The type II carcinomas, on the other hand, show aggressive behavior and include high-grade serous carcinomas, undifferentiated carcinomas, and carcinosarcomas. Only 15% of patients present with early disease and have a relatively better prognosis. Also, it has been shown that screening for ovarian cancer does not reduce mortality but improves prognosis, suggesting that early detection of metastatic disease may also confer an additional benefit. The pathophysiology of EOC is debated, and the survival rates remain largely unchanged over the past few decades despite increases in the understanding of the molecular, genetic, and clinical profiles. Hence, there seems to be a gap between the current understanding of EOCs and patient outcomes in this area, where research is needed to better understand the microenvironment of the malignancies and their respective behaviors, ultimately helping to achieve better survival outcomes.

FDG PET/CT is widely used in staging and in detecting recurrence of ovarian carcinoma. Contrast-enhanced CT (ceCT) and tumor markers, such as cancer antigen-125 (CA-125) and, more recently, human epididymis protein 4 (HE4), have played an important role in the follow-up of patients with ovarian carcinoma. HE4 is overexpressed in 93% of serous, 100% of endometrioid, and 50% of clear cell ovarian carcinomas and is rarely elevated in mucinous or germ cell tumors. It complements the CA-125 measurement and the follow-up of patients who have negligible or absent pretreatment elevations of CA-125. FDG PET/CT is more sensitive in detecting even small-volume tumors, distant metastases, and assessing disease burden than ceCT or CA-125. Based on preoperative FDG PET/CT, parameters, such as metabolic tumor volume (MTV) of less than 10.1 mL and total lesion glycolysis (TLG) less than 46 mL, are predictive of a good 2-year survival rate in recurrent gynecologic malignancies.[3] However, the limitations of using FDG include its variable uptake, particularly with low uptake noted in type I EOCs, leading to false-negative results; physiologic variation of FDG uptake as in the luteal phase; and physiologic FDG uptake in bowel and urinary excretion, which makes the detection of disease and interpretation difficult. Additionally, the differentiation between benign and malignant lesions based on the pattern of FDG uptake, though reported in some studies, has yet to be reproducible. There is a clear need for more sensitive biomarkers to predict the development or susceptibility to ovarian carcinoma in order to reduce the mortality.

FDG uptake in type I EOCs is low and cannot distinguish benign from malignant lesions conclusively. Unlike FDG, methionine-based radiotracers have been shown to accumulate particularly more in such lesions. One of the earliest studies[4] demonstrated that ^{11}C-methionine differentiates between benign and malignant ovarian carcinomas and histologically poor-grade carcinomas tend to accumulate more radiotracer than well-differentiated ones.

THE METABOLIC PHENOTYPES OF EPITHELIAL OVARIAN CARCINOMAS: THE CHOLINIC PHENOTYPE AND THE LIPOGENIC PHENOTYPE

Although there are many preclinical studies demonstrating the accumulation of choline in EOCs, there have been few clinical studies with very small groups of mixed patient profiles showing variable radiocholine uptake.[5] Bagnoli and colleagues[6] suggested a cholinic phenotype of EOC whereby transformed EOC cells show activation of choline kinase-alpha and phosphatidylcholine-specific phospholipases C and D in the Kennedy pathway with increased accumulation of phosphor-choline metabolites. Similarly, the anabolic enzyme fatty acid synthase (FAS) is also seen to be overexpressed in ovarian cancer cells in many preclinical models, suggesting a so-called lipogenic phenotype. FAS overactivity has been related to platinum resistance and can be assessed by ^{11}C-acetate or ^{18}F-acetate PET-based molecular imaging. Liu and colleagues[7] in 2000 showed ^{11}C-acetate is 76% accurate in diagnosing ovarian cancer. Hence, this suggests exploring [11]C- or ^{18}F-labeled choline and/or acetate in staging of the disease and for metabolic profiling.

The two main treatment protocols in EOCs are either debulking surgery followed by chemotherapy or neoadjuvant chemotherapy followed by debulking surgery and then adjuvant chemotherapy. Systemic chemotherapy is routinely given in advanced ovarian cancer, and almost a third of cases are later detected to demonstrate chemoresistance. Hence, there is an urgent need for early identification of nonresponders to plan therapy in such patient subgroups and to select patients who can largely benefit from chemotherapy.

Most ovarian cancers express estrogen receptor (ER) alpha. van Kruchten and colleagues[8] demonstrated ER alpha expression in vivo, with a sensitivity of 79% and specificity of 100%, with a maximum standardized uptake value (SUVmax) cutoff of 1.8. The role of endocrine therapy is limited in EOCs. Antiestrogen therapy (AET) in platinum-resistant cases may help in achieving stable disease and a longer progression-free survival. AET also offers a less cytotoxic alternative with a comparable/better quality of life in platinum-resistant EOCs. However, a definitive role of this therapy is yet to be established in such cohorts. The 16alpha-^{18}F-fluoro-17beta-estradiol (^{18}F-FES) PET/CT demonstrates ER overexpression in EOCs and, hence, can predict the response to AE as compared with invasive IHC evaluation as reported in a study by Argenta and colleagues[9] in 2013. Overexpression of ER predicts a good response to fulvestrant/AET.[8] However, some studies also state that there is a definitive role of AET irrespective of ER status. **Table 1** summarizes reported clinical studies with non-FDG radiotracers investigated in ovarian cancer.

Chemoresistance is frequently seen in the management of ovarian cancers, leading to a poor prognosis. Preclinical studies exploring the pathways involved in chemoresistance and future targets for therapeutic use are listed later (**Table 2**).

Furthermore, Bagnoli and colleagues[6] have suggested an independent mechanism of chemoresistance in cholinic phenotypes involving intracellular glutathione content. Hence, significant research is needed for exploring the possible mechanisms involved in chemoresistance.

Other preclinical studies for investigating promising cellular targets with PET radiotracers for ovarian cancer are mentioned later (**Table 3**).

CERVICAL CANCER: PRELIMINARY APPLICATION STUDIES WITH ^{11}C-CHOLINE AND 3'-DEOXY-3'-^{18}F-FLUOROTHYMIDINE

Cervical cancer is the fourth most common cancer in women and ranks seventh overall (GLOBOCAN data)[10], with a high incidence and mortality in

Table 1
Non–[18]F-2-fluoro-2-deoxy-D-glucose PET radiotracers used in ovarian cancer: clinical studies

Author/Year/Study Setting	No. of Patients	PET Radiotracer	Final Parameter to Which PET Results Compared	Salient Study Findings
van Kruchten et al,[8] 2015, prospective	15	^{18}F-FES	HPE and IHC	There was an in vivo demonstration of ER alpha receptor status.
Lamberts et al,[11] 2016, prospective	4	[89]Zr-labeled MMOT0530A (antimesothelin antibody)	IHC, treatment response	PET-positive case showed a partial response (1 of 4). There is potential to guide antimesothelin therapy
Pantel et al,[12] 2017, prospective	17	^{18}F-fluoro-thanatrace (FTT)	Autoradiography, immunofluorescent microscopy, IHC	PARP expression and treatment response were predictors of DNA damaging agents.

Abbreviations: HPE, histopathology examination; PARP, poly (ADP-ribose) polymerase.

developing countries.[20] Among the non-FDG PET radiotracers, ^{11}C-choline PET/CT was shown to accurately stage and monitor treatment efficacy in patients with cervical cancer as compared with pelvic MR imaging.[21]

Concurrent chemoradiation is the mainstay therapy for locally advanced cervical cancers. Accurate dose modeling is important in pelvic cancers to deliver a high dose to tumors and to deliver sublethal doses to other structures, especially to ovaries and bone marrow. Various new technologies are continually being investigated toward achieving precise dose models. An adaptive segmentation algorithm based on FDG uptake has

been demonstrated to be accurate,[22] whereas MTV by FDG PET/MR imaging[22,23] has been shown to have potential utility in delineating the gross tumor volume.

Although ^{11}C-choline PET/CT has been used for dose painting in patients with prostate cancer, it has been largely unused in cervical cancer. A study by McGuire and colleagues[24] used 3′-deoxy-3′-^{18}F-fluorothymidine (FLT) uptake in radiotherapy (RT) planning with the intention to reduce hemato-toxicity by sparing pelvic bone marrow. There is a large scope for using such radiotracers in the pretherapy planning setup.

Table 2
Preclinical studies investigating pathways for chemoresistance in ovarian carcinoma: implications for non–[18]F-2-fluoro-2-deoxy-D-glucose molecular PET imaging

Author, Year	PET Radiotracer	Measurement of	Outcome
Perumal et al,[13] 2012	FLT	Thymidine kinase activity	There was PI3K-AKT pathway inhibition, leading to lower proliferation rates, which can be imaged noninvasively.
Bauerschlag et al,[14] 2015	Possible role of FCH	FAS activity	FAS overexpression is related to platinum resistance (lower fluoro-methylcholine uptake in resistant cells); inhibition may result in resensitization and may also be considered for treatment monitoring with bevacizumab + platinum-based chemotherapy.

Abbreviations: FCH, ^{18}F-fluorocholine; FLT, 3′-deoxy-3′-^{18}F-fluorothymidine; PI3K-AKT pathway, phosphatidylinositol 3-kinase (PI3K)/protein kinase B (Akt) signaling pathway.

Table 3
Preclinical studies with promising PET radiotracers in ovarian carcinoma

Author, Year	PET Radiotracer	Target	Important Inferences
Ocak et al,[15] 2015	^{68}Ga-cm09	FR alpha	Can be used for early detection
Sharma et al,[16] 2016	^{89}Zr-B43.13; ^{64}Cu-anti CA-125 mAb	CA-125 in EOC	For the noninvasive delineation of extent of disease and help in treatment planning and treatment monitoring of high-grade serous ovarian cancer
Niu et al,[17] 2009	^{64}Cu-DOTA-trastuzumab	HER2	Treatment monitoring with heat shock protein
Nagengast et al,[18] 2007	^{89}Zr-bevacizumab	VEGFR	In vivo tumor microenvironment and treatment monitoring with bevacizumab
Wu et al,[19] 2007	^{18}F-FPRGD2	Integrin $\alpha_v\beta_3$	Noninvasive quantification of integrin $\alpha_v\beta_3$ expression in vivo

^{68}Ga-cm09 is a radiolabeled albumin-binding folate receptor targeting ligand.

Abbreviations: DOTA, tetra-azacyclododecanetetra-acetic acid; EOC, epithelial ovarian carcinoma; ^{18}F-FPRGD2, ^{18}F-mini-PEG-E(c[RGDyK])$_2$; FR, folate receptor; HER2, human epidermal growth factor receptor 2; mAb, monoclonal antibody; VEGFR, vascular endothelial growth factor receptor; ^{89}Zr-B43.13, ^{89}Zr-DFO(desferrioxamine)-monoclonal antibody-B43.13, which is a radiolabeled anti-CA-125 antibody.

HYPOXIA IMAGING PET RADIOTRACERS IN CERVICAL CANCER: SALIENT RESULTS

Another limitation of FDG is its unrelated uptake in hypoxic areas that are apparent on imaging performed with hypoxia radiotracers. Hypoxia in the intratumoral milieu confers radio resistance, leading to poor outcomes. Hence, identifying hypoxic areas in tumors is especially important in cervical cancer whereby RT is a mainstay treatment modality often used with curative intent. Many studies have been performed with promising results. It was shown that the tumor to muscle uptake ratio of more than 3.2 to 3.5 can serve as a cutoff parameter for distinguishing patients with poor prognosis whereby ^{64}Cu-diacetyl-bis(N4-methylthiosemicarbazone) (^{64}Cu-ATSM), ^{18}F-fluoroazomycin-arabinoside (^{18}F-FAZA), or ^{18}F-fluoroerythronitroimidazole (^{18}F-FETNIM) radiotracers have been used.[25–27] A study by Grigsby and colleagues[28] showed a positive correlation of hypoxia (as measured by ^{60}Cu-ATSM) with overexpression of molecular hypoxia markers like vascular epithelial growth factor, epidermal growth factor receptor (EGFR), cyclooxygenase-2, and carbonic anhydrase 9 in a small number of patients. Additionally, the study also showed poor outcomes in patients with hypoxic tumors. Hence, hypoxia imaging can be included along with FDG PET/CT in the pretherapy assessment for optimal RT planning, dose delivery, and prognostication (**Table 4**).

Additional prospective future targets for PET imaging in cervical cancer are listed later (**Table 5**).

RESPONSE ASSESSMENT IN CERVICAL CANCER

As FDG shows nonspecific uptake in inflammation, response monitoring becomes difficult until inflammation subsides. Hence, to classify the response category, FDG PET/CT should ideally be conducted after the abatement of inflammation (ie, after several weeks). Therefore, there is a need for biomarkers that are robust and can be used early after treatment. A study by Cho and colleagues[31] demonstrated the use of FLT as an early marker for response, as the mean standardized uptake value (SUVmean) decreased as early as 1 to 2 weeks. Also, as mentioned earlier, there was a proportionate reduction documented in the tumor volume and SUV in 5 patients studied with ^{11}C-choline PET/CT.[21]

Non–^{18}F-2-FLUORO-2-DEOXY-D-GLUCOSE PET IN UTERINE MALIGNANCIES: ENDOMETRIAL AND MYOMETRIAL PATHOLOGIES

Studies That Explored Both Endometrial and Myometrial Tumors

^{11}C-methionine PET was able to differentiate between benign endometrial and uterine malignancies (both cervical and endometrial carcinoma) in one of the early studies reported.[32] In this study, uterine carcinoma accumulated more ^{11}C-methionine than the normal endometrium (SUVmean 8.4 vs 4.6), as did poorly differentiated

Table 4
Tumor hypoxia PET imaging in cervical cancer

Author	No. of Patients	PET Radiotracer	Compared with	Outcome
Dehdashti et al,[26] 2008, prospective	38	60Cu-ATSM + FDG	Clinical f/u	Patients with high 60Cu-ATSM uptake (T/M ratio >3.5) showed low progression-free survival, more recurrence, and lower cause-specific survival.
Schuetz et al,[27] 2010, prospective	15	18F-FAZA + FDG	Posttreatment clinical f/u and MR imaging	There was no significant association due to small sample size.
Vercellino et al,[25] 2012, prospective	16	18F-FETNIM + FDG	Osteopontin and FDG	High uptake of 18F-FETNIM was associated with a worse progression-free survival and overall survival.

Abbreviations: 60Cu-ATSM, 60Cu-diacetyl-bis(N[4]-methylthiosemicarbazone); f/u, follow-up; T/M, tumor to muscle.

(grade III)/moderately differentiated (grade II) endometrial carcinomas compared with well-differentiated (grade I) endometrial carcinomas.[32] However, because the study was performed on relatively old technology, there were some limitations. Also, a small sample size confounded the interpretation of disease or conclusively arriving at any criterion or threshold for differentiation. Similar results were obtained by Tsujikawa and colleagues,[33] whereby dual-radiotracer PET with 18F-FES and FDG could aid in the differential diagnosis of uterine tumors. Endometrial carcinoma demonstrated significantly greater SUV-mean for FDG than for 18F-FES (9.6 vs 3.8), whereas patients with endometrial hyperplasia showed significantly higher SUVmean for 18F-FES compared with FDG (7.0 vs 1.7). Patients with leiomyoma showed significantly higher SUVmean for 18F-FES than for FDG (4.2 vs 2.2), whereas patients with sarcoma showed substantially higher uptake for FDG and significantly

lower uptake for 18F-FES compared with those with leiomyoma.

Studies on Non–18F-2-Fluoro-2-Deoxy-D-Glucose PET in Endometrial Pathologies

Endometrial cancer is the sixth most common gynecologic cancer with a lifetime risk of approximately 3% and good 5-year overall survival rate of around 81%. Endometrial carcinomas are conventionally divided into type I and type II tumors whereby type I tumors are low grade, treatment responsive, and potentially curable cancers with low recurrence rates, whereas type II tumors are high grade, have metastatic tendency, and are of a recurrent nature. Type I cancers are usually ER negative, whereas type II cancers tend to be ER positive.

Endometrial carcinomas tend to show relatively increased glucose metabolism, especially in higher tumor grades with a concomitant decrease in ER expression[34]; Tsujikawa and colleagues[35]

Table 5
Prospective future targets with PET radiotracers in cervical cancer: preclinical studies

Author, Year	PET Radiotracer	Target Biologic Pathway	Compared with	Implication
Carlin et al,[29] 2014	18F-HX4, 18F-FMISO, Cu-ATSM, 18F-FAZA	Hypoxia imaging	IHC	Fluorinated nitroimidazoles show uptake comparable with IHC
Eiblmaier et al,[30] 2008	64Cu-DOTA-cetuximab	EGFR expression	IHC	Quantification of EGFR and potential use in treatment of EGFR-positive cancer

Abbreviations: DOTA, tetra-azacyclododecanetetra-acetic acid; 18F-FMISO, 18F-fluoromisonidazole; 18F-HX4, 18F-flortanidazole.

performed dual-radiotracer PET imaging using ^{18}F-FES and FDG to study and differentiate endometrial hyperplasia versus carcinoma and high-risk versus low-risk carcinoma. A cutoff FDG/^{18}F-FES ratio of 0.5 was used to differentiate carcinoma from hyperplasia, whereas that between high-risk and low-risk carcinoma was found to be 2. The same investigators later reported lower ER alpha, and progesterone receptor B (PR-B) expression suggests aggressiveness of the tumor or degree of differentiation.[35] Both of these immunohistochemical parameters correlated well with ^{18}F-FES uptake and the FDG/FES ratio and had allowed differentiation of low-grade lesions (grade 1) from moderately or poorly differentiated carcinoma (grade 2–3). Interestingly, dual-radiotracer PET/CT with ^{18}F-FES and FDG[35] did not have any correlation with the disease stage or with expression of ER beta, Ki-67, or glucose transporter 1 (Table 6).

Thus, ^{18}F-FES PET was found to add incremental value for the management of endometrial malignancies along with FDG PET/CT. The FDG/^{18}F-FES ratio has been shown to be a more sensitive parameter to differentiate the grade of the malignancies or benign lesions from malignant ones.[35]

Studies Exploring Non–[18]F-2-Fluoro-2-Deoxy-D-Glucose PET Radiotracers in Myometrial Tumors: Benign and Malignant Pathologies

FDG uptake is nonspecific in mesenchymal tumors because the fibroids show variable FDG uptake making it difficult to distinguish them from malignant lesions. Similar to the endometrial malignancies, the FDG/^{18}F-FES ratio negatively correlates with leiomyomas and positively correlates with the Ki-67 index.[34,36] Zhao and colleagues[36] studied 47 patients with mesenchymal uterine tumors and found that ^{18}F-FES added to the discrimination between uterine leiomyomas versus uterine sarcomas,[36] especially when FDG

Table 6
Non–[18]F-2-fluoro-2-deoxy-D-glucose PET in endometrial lesions: benign endometrial versus malignant pathologies and differentiation of malignancy grade

Author/Year/ Study Setting	No. of Patients	PET Radiotracer	Final Parameter to Which PET Results Compared	PET Parameter Measured	Salient Findings
Tsujikawa et al,[33] 2008, prospective	38 (endometrial & myometrial combined)	^{18}F-FES & FDG	Histopathology	SUVmean	FDG SUVmean was higher in endometrial carcinoma (FDG/^{18}F-FES: 9.6 vs 3.8). ^{18}F-FES PET SUV was higher in endometrial hyperplasia (^{18}F-FES/FDG: 7.0 vs 1.7)
Tsujikawa et al,[34] 2009, prospective	22	^{18}F-FES & FDG	HPE	SUVmean	A cutoff FDG/^{18}F-FES ratio of 0.5 was used to differentiate carcinoma from hyperplasia, whereas that to differentiate high-risk and low-risk carcinomas was found to be 2.0.
Tsujikawa et al,[35] 2011, prospective	19	^{18}F-FES & FDG	HPE and IHC	SUV, regional FDG to ^{18}F-FES SUV ratio	FDG/^{18}F-FES uptake positively correlated to grades of tumor and was inversely related to ER alpha and PR-B expression.

Abbreviation: HPE, histopathology examination.

Table 7
Non–[18]F-2-fluoro-2-deoxy-D-glucose PET radiotracers in myometrial tumors: differentiation between benign mesenchymal lesions and malignant uterine sarcomas and grading tumor differentiation

Author/Year/ Study Setting	No. of Patients	PET Radiotracer	Final Parameter to Which PET Results Compared	PET Parameter Measured	Important Inferences
Tsujikawa et al,[33] 2008, prospective	38	^{18}F-FES/FDG dual radiotracer PET	HPE	SUVmean	Leiomyomas showed significantly higher SUVmean for ^{18}F-FES than for FDG (4.2 vs 2.2), whereas sarcomas showed the opposite trend.
Zhao et al,[36] 2013, prospective	47	^{18}F-FES + FDG	Postoperative HPE and IHC	FDG/^{18}F-FES ratio	The FDG/^{18}F-FES ratio was significantly higher in uterine sarcomas compared with leiomyomas.
Yoshida et al,[37] 2011, retrospective	24	^{18}F-FES/FDG dual radiotracer PET	Postoperative HPE	FDG/^{18}F-FES ratio	In patients with equivocal or positive FDG uptake, an FDG/^{18}F-FES ratio >2 added incremental value in diagnosis.
Yamane et al,[38] 2012, prospective	15	FLT/FDG	—	SUVmax of both	FLT PET is superior to FDG PET in differentiating malignant tumors from benign leiomyoma. FLT uptake correlated well with Ki-67.

Abbreviation: HPE, histopathology examination.

PET findings were equivocal. In their study, ^{18}F-FES uptake was significantly lower and the FDG uptake and SUV ratio of FDG/^{18}F-FES were significantly higher in uterine sarcomas than in leiomyomas. The ratio demonstrated negative correlations with ER alpha, PR, and PR-B and positive correlation with Ki-67. A similar trend was documented in the previously mentioned study.[35] In a retrospective setting, Yoshida and colleagues[37] examined the role of additional ^{18}F-FES PET in a selected group of 24 patients with equivocal or positive FDG uptake. ^{18}F-FES PET findings confirmed uterine sarcoma in 91.3% of this group.[37]

The other non-FDG radiotracer used in the domain of uterine mesenchymal tumors has been FLT. In a population of 5 patients, Yamane and colleagues[38] observed that FLT can distinguish leiomyomas from leiomyosarcomas better than FDG and that FLT uptake correlates well with Ki-67 (Table 7).

SUMMARY

The use of non–FDG PET radiotracers gives an insight to specific biological pathways and helps in treatment decision-making based on specific therapeutic targets. Basic research is needed for understanding the nuances of ovarian carcinoma and its propensity to be aggressive/recurrent. Clinical research is needed to reduce mortality and improve early detection. Given the availability of a wide array of PET radiotracers, we will be able to study specific biological pathways and offer precision medicine to patients, hoping to decrease morbidity and mortality, which is not possible by only relying on FDG. There is also a necessity to consider whether reclassification of these gynecologic tumors into metabolic or hormonal phenotypes based on PET imaging would help to tailor treatments or to identify high-risk groups.

REFERENCES

1. Rockall AG, Cross S, Flanagan S, et al. The role of FDG-PET/CT in gynaecological cancers. Canc Imag 2012;12:49–65.
2. Key statistics about ovarian cancer. Available at: https://www.cancer.org/cancer/ovarian-cancer/about/key-statistics.html/lovarian. Accessed October 13, 2017.
3. Burger IA, Vargas HA, Donati OF, et al. The value of 18F-FDG PET/CT in recurrent gynecologic malignancies prior to pelvic exenteration. Gynecol Oncol 2013;129(3):586–92.
4. Lapela M, Leskinen-Kallio S, Varpula M, et al. Metabolic imaging of ovarian tumors with carbon-11-methionine: a PET study. J Nucl Med 1995;36(12):2196–200.
5. Torizuka T, Kanno T, Futatsubashi M, et al. Imaging of gynecologic tumors: comparison of (11)C-choline PET with (18)F-FDG PET. J Nucl Med 2003;44(7):1051–6.
6. Bagnoli M, Granata A, Nicoletti R, et al. Choline metabolism alteration: a focus on ovarian cancer. Front Oncol 2016;6:153.
7. Liu R. 31. Clinical application of [C-11]acetate in oncology. Clin Positron Imaging 2000;3(4):185.
8. van Kruchten M, de Vries EFJ, Arts HJG, et al. Assessment of estrogen receptor expression in epithelial ovarian cancer patients using 16α-18F-fluoro-17β-estradiol PET/CT. J Nucl Med 2015;56(1):50–5.
9. Argenta PA, Um I, Kay C, et al. Predicting response to the anti-estrogen fulvestrant in recurrent ovarian cancer. Gynecol Oncol 2013;131(2):368–73.
10. What Are the Key Statistics About Ovarian Cancer? Available at: https://www.cancer.org/cancer/ovarian-cancer/about/key-statistics.html/lovarian. Accessed October 13, 2017.
11. Lamberts LE, van Menke-van der Houven Oordt CW, ter Weele EJ, et al. ImmunoPET with anti-mesothelin antibody in patients with pancreatic and ovarian cancer before anti-mesothelin antibody-drug conjugate treatment. Clin Cancer Res 2016;22(7):1642–52.
12. Pantel A, MaKvandi M, Doot R, et al. A pilot study of a novel poly (ADP-ribose) polymerase-1 (PARP) PET tracer ([[18F]FluorThanatrace) in patients with ovarian carcinoma. J Nucl Med 2017;58(Supplement 1):386.
13. Perumal M, Stronach EA, Gabra H, et al. Evaluation of 2-deoxy-2-18F-fluoro-D-glucose- and 3'-deoxy-3'-18F-fluorothymidine-positron emission tomography as biomarkers of therapy response in platinum-resistant ovarian cancer. Mol Imaging Biol 2012;14(6):753–61.
14. Bauerschlag DO, Maass N, Leonhardt P, et al. Fatty acid synthase overexpression: target for therapy and reversal of chemoresistance in ovarian cancer. J Transl Med 2015;13:146.
15. Ocak M, Gillman AG, Bresee J, et al. Folate receptor-targeted multimodality imaging of ovarian cancer in a novel syngeneic mouse model. Mol Pharm 2015;12(2):542–53.
16. Sharma SK, Sevak KK, Monette S, et al. Preclinical 89Zr Immuno-PET of high-grade serous ovarian cancer and lymph node metastasis. J Nucl Med 2016;57(5):771–6.
17. Niu G, Li Z, Cao Q, et al. Monitoring therapeutic response of human ovarian cancer to 17-DMAG by noninvasive PET imaging with (64)Cu-DOTA-trastuzumab. Eur J Nucl Med Mol Imaging 2009;36(9):1510–9.
18. Nagengast WB, de Vries EG, Hospers GA, et al. In vivo VEGF imaging with radiolabeled bevacizumab in a human ovarian tumor xenograft. J Nucl Med 2007;48(8):1313–9.
19. Wu Z, Li Z-B, Cai W, et al. 18F-labeled mini-PEG spacered RGD dimer (18F-FPRGD2): synthesis and microPET imaging of alphavbeta3 integrin expression. Eur J Nucl Med Mol Imaging 2007;34(11):1823–31.
20. Colombo N, Carinelli S, Colombo A, et al. Cervical cancer: ESMO clinical practice guidelines for diagnosis, treatment and follow-up. Ann Oncol 2012;23(Suppl 7):vii27–32.
21. Sofue K, Tateishi U, Sawada M, et al. Role of carbon-11 choline PET/CT in the management of uterine carcinoma: initial experience. Ann Nucl Med 2009;23(3):235–43.
22. Xu W, Yu S, Ma Y, et al. Effect of different segmentation algorithms on metabolic tumor volume measured on 18F-FDG PET/CT of cervical primary squamous cell carcinoma. Nucl Med Commun 2017;38(3):259–65.
23. Zhang S, Xin J, Guo Q, et al. Comparison of tumor volume between PET and MRI in cervical cancer with hybrid PET/MR. Int J Gynecol Cancer 2014;24(4):744–50.
24. McGuire SM, Jacobson GM, Menda Y, et al. F-18 fluorothymidine (FLT) PET imaging for weekly evaluation of tumor response to chemoradiation therapy in patients with cervical cancer. Int J Radiat Oncol Biol Phys 2011;81(2):S804–5.
25. Vercellino L, Groheux D, Thoury A, et al. Hypoxia imaging of uterine cervix carcinoma with (18)F-FETNIM PET/CT. Clin Nucl Med 2012;37(11):1065–8.
26. Dehdashti F, Grigsby PW, Lewis JS, et al. Assessing tumor hypoxia in cervical cancer by PET with 60Cu-labeled diacetyl-bis(N4-methylthiosemicarbazone). J Nucl Med 2008;49(2):201–5.
27. Schuetz M, Schmid MP, Pötter R, et al. Evaluating repetitive 18F-fluoroazomycin-arabinoside (18FAZA) PET in the setting of MRI guided adaptive radiotherapy in cervical cancer. Acta Oncol 2010;49(7):941–7.

28. Grigsby PW, Malyapa RS, Higashikubo R, et al. Comparison of molecular markers of hypoxia and imaging with (60)Cu-ATSM in cancer of the uterine cervix. Mol Imaging Biol 2007;9(5):278–83.

29. Carlin S, Zhang H, Reese M, et al. A comparison of the imaging characteristics and microregional distribution of 4 hypoxia PET tracers. J Nucl Med 2014; 55(3):515–21.

30. Eiblmaier M, Meyer LA, Watson MA, et al. Correlating EGFR expression with receptor-binding properties and Internalization of 64Cu-DOTA-Cetuximab in 5 cervical cancer cell lines. J Nucl Med 2008; 49(9):1472–9.

31. Cho LP, Kim C, Viswanathan A. Comparison of FLT- and FDG-PET in gynecological cancers. Gynecol Oncol 2015;137:140.

32. Lapela M, Leskinen-Kallio S, Varpula M, et al. Imaging of uterine carcinoma by carbon-11-methionine and PET. J Nucl Med 1994;35(10):1618–23.

33. Tsujikawa T, Yoshida Y, Mori T, et al. Uterine tumors: pathophysiologic imaging with 16alpha-18Ffluoro-17beta-estradiol and 18F fluorodeoxyglucose PET–initial experience. Radiology 2008;248(2): 599–605.

34. Tsujikawa T, Yoshida Y, Kudo T, et al. Functional images reflect aggressiveness of endometrial carcinoma: estrogen receptor expression combined with 18F-FDG PET. J Nucl Med 2009;50(10):1598–604. Available at: http://jnm.snmjournals.org/content/50/10/1598.full.pdf. Accessed August 11, 2017.

35. Tsujikawa T, Yoshida Y, Kiyono Y, et al. Functional oestrogen receptor α imaging in endometrial carcinoma using 16α-^{18}Ffluoro-17β-oestradiol PET. Eur J Nucl Med Mol Imaging 2011;38(1):37–45.

36. Zhao Z, Yoshida Y, Kurokawa T, et al. 18F-FES and 18F-FDG PET for differential diagnosis and quantitative evaluation of mesenchymal uterine tumors: correlation with immunohistochemical analysis. J Nucl Med 2013;54(4):499–506.

37. Yoshida Y, Kiyono Y, Tsujikawa T, et al. Additional value of 16α-18Ffluoro-17β-oestradiol PET for differential diagnosis between uterine sarcoma and leiomyoma in patients with positive or equivocal findings on 18Ffluorodeoxyglucose PET. Eur J Nucl Med Mol Imaging 2011;38(10):1824–31.

38. Yamane T, Takaoka A, Kita M, et al. 18F-FLT PET performs better than 18F-FDG PET in differentiating malignant uterine corpus tumors from benign leiomyoma. Ann Nucl Med 2012;26(6):478–84.

Normal Variants and Pitfalls Encountered in PET Assessment of Gynecologic Malignancies

Jian Q. Yu, MD, FRCPC[a],*, Mohan Doss, PhD, MCCPM[b],
R. Katherine Alpaugh, PhD[c]

KEYWORDS

- PET and PET/CT • FDG PET • Normal variants • Pitfalls • Gynecologic malignancies

KEY POINTS

- The quality of the PET/computed tomography scans is important: consistency in patient preparation and uptake time, glucose level monitoring, and attention to technical details.
- The recognition of normal variations in the female pelvis and the adjacent gastrointestinal tract activity is important.
- The examination and its interpretation must take into consideration treatment effects on the PET/computed tomography scan at time of treatment follow-up.

INTRODUCTION

Integrated PET with computed tomography (PET/CT) has been available since the early 2000s,[1,2] and is commonly used in clinical service for oncological indications, in addition to neurologic and cardiac indications. This technology has enjoyed tremendous growth over the past decade. Other indications for PET/CT are continually evolving. Gynecologic malignancy imaging with PET/CT benefits from the metabolic information of PET overlaid on the CT anatomic localization. Acquisition from the integrated scanner provides data with accurate registration of anatomy and molecular information. However, many physiologic conditions, normal variants, and benign lesions within the pelvis and other areas of the body can cause confusion and uncertainty.

Low ^{18}F-fluorodeoxyglucose (FDG) uptake from the tumor can produce diagnostic challenges resulting in a false-negative result and, therefore, an inaccurate conclusion. This article reviews normal variants and potential pitfalls encountered in the PET assessment of gynecologic malignancies to provide useful information for the referring and reporting physicians.

The most commonly used radiotracer for PET/CT in oncology currently is FDG, a glucose analogue that usually accumulates more in malignant cells in comparison with normal tissues owing to tumor cell elevated glucose transporter molecules and glycolysis. FDG has been studied in the research arena since the 1970s. Its incorporation in the clinical arena began after the Centers for Medicare and Medicaid Services began to provide financial reimbursement in 1998. The clinical

Disclosure Statement: None.
[a] Nuclear Medicine and PET Service, Department of Diagnostic Imaging, Fox Chase Cancer Center, 333 Cottman Avenue, Philadelphia, PA 19111, USA; [b] Department of Diagnostic Imaging, Fox Chase Cancer Center, 333 Cottman Avenue, Philadelphia, PA 19111, USA; [c] Protocol Support Laboratory, Department of Diagnostic Imaging, Fox Chase Cancer Center, 333 Cottman Avenue, Philadelphia, PA 19111, USA
* Corresponding author.
E-mail address: Michael.yu@fccc.edu

PET Clin 13 (2018) 249–268
https://doi.org/10.1016/j.cpet.2017.11.009
1556-8598/18/© 2017 Elsevier Inc. All rights reserved.

indications for use grew rapidly and were aided by the information collected through the National Oncologic PET Registry.

Additional PET radiotracers have been approved over the recent years by the US Food and Drug Administration: ^{11}C-choline for prostate cancer in 2012, ^{68}Ga-DOTATATE for neuroendocrine tumors, and ^{18}F-fluciclovine for prostate cancer in the summer of 2016. However, the mainstay for PET/CT imaging of gynecologic malignancies remains FDG, which is the focus of the current article.

The role of FDG PET/CT continues to change and evolve from initial staging and restaging, to follow-up of treatment response, detection of tumor recurrence, prognosis assessment, and risk stratification.[3–15] Its use has also expanded owing to its use in the planning of external beam radiation therapy.[16–29] There are reports of institutions using FDG PET/CT for surgical planning, especially nodal staging and intraoperative probe guidance for the removal of metastatic implants.[30–41] Imaging the area below the diaphragm involves some special considerations, and it is very important to recognize the artifacts, normal variants, and pitfalls, especially for the female pelvis.[42,43]

In this article, we review the technical aspects of the PET/CT scan in relation to patient preparation, uptake time, and other details; discuss the specific pitfalls related to PET/CT; describe common artifacts and interfering factors; and demonstrate cases of false positives and false negatives encountered during our experience and those noted in literature. We focus our discussions on findings below the diaphragm, and mainly in the pelvis.

TECHNICAL ASPECTS OF THE SCAN TO BE CONSIDERED

Routine PET/CT scanning consists of image acquisition from the base of the skull to the mid-thighs. Standardization of the acquisition technique in the clinical protocol reduces variations during the PET scan procedure and aids in maintaining consistent image quality and reproducibility of semiquantitative measurements such as the standardized uptake value (SUV). Such standardization is crucial for institutions with multiple scanners from different vendors. Uniformity between protocols is also critical for multicenter clinical trials.

We ask all of our patients to fast for at least 4 hours before FDG injection, and we recommend that they perform no strenuous exercise on the day before the scan. Patients who are scheduled early

in the day for PET/CT scanning usually fast overnight. We measure blood glucose levels before radiotracer injection with a glucometer and finger stick. A value of less than 200 mg/dL is considered to be acceptable. Higher glucose levels would cause an altered biodistribution of administered FDG, warranting a repeat of the study. We normally do not use insulin for hyperglycemic patients to avoid obtaining redistribution of FDG to the musculature and lowered sensitivity of lesion detection (Fig. 1).

We use a weight-based (0.07 mCi/lb) dose of FDG with bulk dose from supplier and delivered to each patient by an injector/infusion system. After the injection, all patients would have a waiting/uptake time of 1 hour while reclined in a quiet room, with no talking or walking except to go to the bathroom. Our aim is to perform the scan within 60 ± 10 minutes after FDG injection. For all patients with follow-up scans, we check the previous study's uptake time and maintain the same uptake period ±10 minutes for the follow-up acquisition. It is well-known that tumor FDG uptake increases with time, and so a more delayed scan would lead to higher SUV measurements than an earlier one.[44–47] In one of the recent articles by Weber and colleagues,[48] the variability of repeated measurements of tumor FDG uptake is somewhat greater for multicenter trials than for smaller, single-center studies. The variations in protocol and technical details between sites may play a role accounting for these differences.

At our institution, we generally do not use oral or intravenous contrast material to lower the potential for PET artifacts caused by the high attenuation materials (Fig. 2). Our technologists provide water to the patients and encourage them to drink during the uptake period. All patients void before the scan. Beginning the scan with an empty urinary bladder is even more important for the imaging of gynecologic malignancies. In addition, we do not use furosemide or other diuretics. We normally do not use bladder catheterization for patients or vaginal catheterization, as described in the literature.[49] As a general rule, we acquire PET images in a caudal–cranial direction for gynecologic and colorectal cancer patients to reduce urine accumulation at the time of scanning in the pelvic region.

For our gynecologic patients, we ask them to place their arms up above the head (or on the chest if that is not feasible) to reduce truncation artifacts in the PET scan.[50] For radiation therapy planning scans, we work closely with radiation therapy technologists for positioning, placement of the facial mask, and body marking and

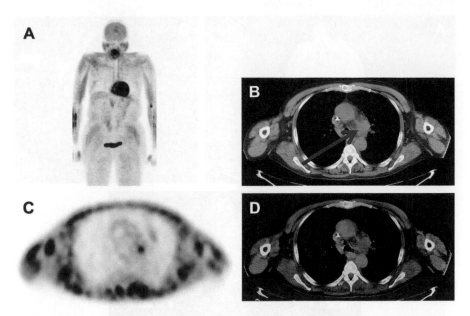

Fig. 1. Muscle redistribution of fludeoxyglucose (FDG). A diabetic patient took an insulin dose shortly before coming to the PET center. The glucose level was normal at 75 mg/dL. The PET maximum intensity projection image demonstrates diffuse FDG activity throughout the muscles (*A*). The aorticopulmonary window lesion is seen on the computed tomography scan (*arrow*) (*B*), but the metabolic activity is low with standard uptake value of only 1.5 (*C*, *D*). We still reported this as highly suspicious disease in the region.

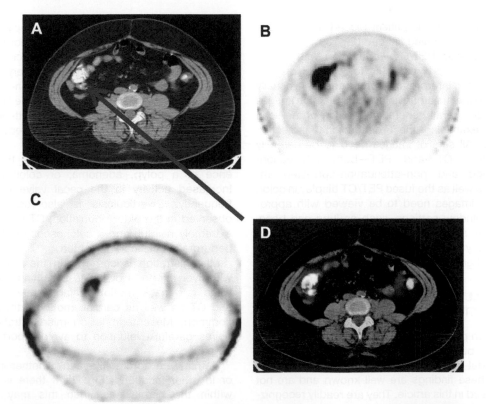

Fig. 2. Artifacts owing to contrast material. There is high-attenuation contrast material (*arrow*) in the ascending colon as seen on a computed tomography scan (*A*). The attenuation-corrected (AC) PET image showed activity in the region (*B*), but the non–attenuation-corrected PET image showed less activity and lower intensity (*C*). The fused image demonstrates some increased activity (*D*), with a certain degree of reconstruction artifact.

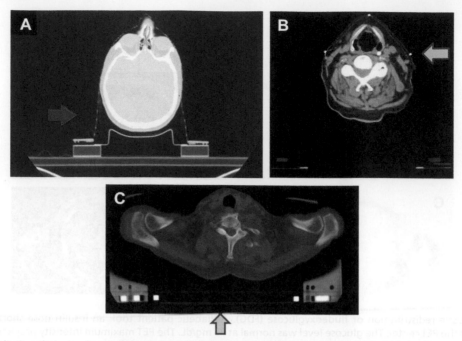

Fig. 3. Radiation therapy planning scan in a patient with head and neck cancer. Facial mask (*arrow*) on computed tomography (CT) image (*A*). Previously placed attenuating markings on face (*arrow*) on CT image (*B*). Hardboard is seen under the body (*arrow*) on CT image (*C*).

contouring, with the patient placed on the radiation therapy planning flat bed (**Fig. 3**).

A dedicated PET/CT workstation with appropriate software is essential for optimal display, viewing, and interpretation of the scan. We usually examine the maximum intensity projection images to get an overall general impression of the scan before examining the 3-dimensional projection images. All sets of images need to be carefully evaluated: CT and PET—both attenuation-corrected and non–attenuation-corrected images, as well as the fused PET/CT display in color. The CT images need to be viewed with appropriate window settings, such as lung and bone, because small and treated lesions would not show any increased radiotracer activity above the background.

NORMAL VARIANTS AND COMMON ARTIFACTS

Common physiologic activity in the upper body includes, but is not limited to, FDG uptake by adenoidal tissues, brown fat, thymus, and muscles. These findings are well-known and are not discussed in this article. They are readily recognizable based on the CT findings in conjunction with the PET/CT fusion image findings.

Metal artifacts are common in patients with prostheses, pacemakers, and insulin pumps (**Fig. 4**).

For gynecologic malignancies, hip replacement artifacts are seen frequently in the senior population. A review of all the images, especially non–attenuation-corrected PET images, is very helpful. If there is no increased activity in the non–attenuation-corrected PET images at all, then the apparent increased radiotracer uptake in attenuation-corrected and fused images are likely reconstruction artifacts (**Fig. 5**).

Focal colonic uptake could indicate the presence of a polyp, adenoma, or colon cancer. Increased activity in the cecal valve is noted frequently. Diverticulosis is also occasionally observed in the older population. CT images are extremely helpful, and a colonoscopy should be performed, if clinically indicated.

Misregistration is common in the lower lung with liver interface owing to breathing artifacts. Head and neck motion artifacts between PET and CT as well as cardiac motion artifacts are common. Mesenteric lesion misregistration requires careful evaluation to avoid report errors (**Fig. 6**).

Hernias are commonly seen, whether inguinal or in other locations (**Fig. 7**). If there is bowel within the hernia sac, then this may reflect some activity. Bladder artifacts and diverticula are less common in women than in men. CT images are very important for anatomic correlation[51] (**Fig. 8**). The activity seen within the

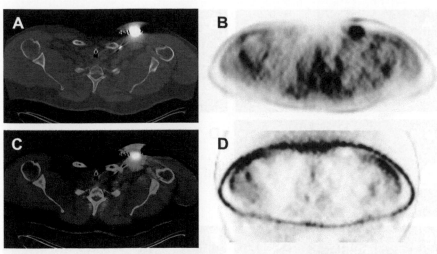

Fig. 4. Metal artifact. The patient has a cardiac pacemaker with metal and associated streak artifact seen on the computed tomography (CT) scan (*A*). There is intense activity in attenuation-corrected (AC) PET image (*B*) and the fused PET/CT image (*C*). However, there is no apparent activity in the non–attenuation-corrected PET image at the pacemaker site (*D*). The increased activity observed in the AC PET image is due to reconstruction artifact.

uterine cavity could be related to the normal menstrual cycle. Clinical correlation and a history should provide a fairly clear explanation (**Fig. 9**). Sometimes, activity is noted in the tampon used during the menstrual period (**Fig. 10**).

Ovarian cysts are common in women of child-bearing age. We have also noted patients with ovarian cysts in different phases of the menstrual cycle. Some of the cysts may reveal increased activity,[52] but a follow-up scan usually shows resolution of the physiologic cyst and/or activity (**Fig. 11**). Transposed ovaries may be in unusual locations,[53] and the activity in the ovaries may be variable during menstrual cycles (**Fig. 12**).

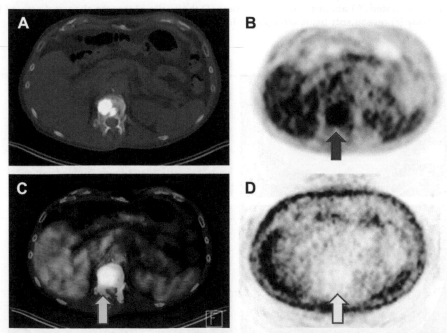

Fig. 5. Cement in spine causing artifact. A 65-year-old patient with high-attenuation cement in the T12 vertebral body predominantly on the right on the computed tomography (CT) image (*A*), related to history of kyphoplasty. There is increased activity (*arrows*) on the attenuation-corrected PET image (*B*) and PET/CT fused image (*C*). However, on the corresponding non–attenuation-corrected PET image (*D*), there is no activity in the region (*arrow*).

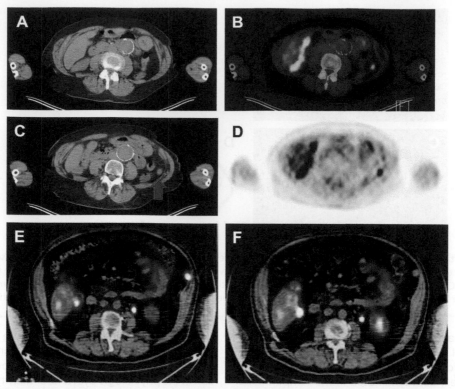

Fig. 6. Motion artifacts. A 75-year-old woman has a mesenteric implant in the left mid abdomen without lesion seen on the computed tomography (CT) image (*A*), but with an increased fludeoxyglucose activity noted on PET/CT image (*B*). However, the soft tissue lesion (*arrow*) is 10 slices away from the site of activity on CT image (*C*) owing to motion of the mesenteric lesion between PET and CT acquisitions. The activity is definitely present in attenuation-corrected PET image (*D*). Another patient has a left mesenteric lesion with mismatch between CT abnormality and associated PET abnormality. PET/CT image (*E*) shows site of intense abnormal activity, but PET/CT image 2 slices away (*F*) reveals soft tissue attenuation lesion with minimal to no activity.

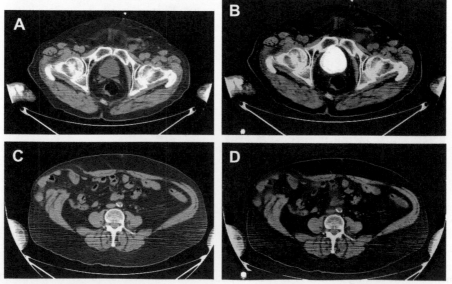

Fig. 7. Two examples of hernias. A left inguinal hernia on a computed tomography (CT) image (*A*). Minimal activity in hernia sac on PET/CT image (*B*) owing to bowel contents. A large right hernia in right anterolateral abdomen on a CT image (*C*). Associated activity in hernia sac on PET/CT image (*D*) owing to bowel contents.

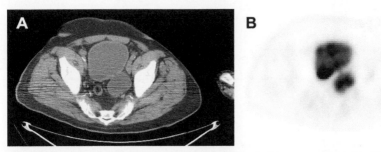

Fig. 8. A large left posterior bladder diverticulum on a computed tomography image (*A*). Associated avid activity is seen on attenuation-corrected PET image owing to excreted fludeoxyglucose (*B*).

Uterine fibroids are commonly seen, with some having increased FDG uptake. In a recent study of 47 patients, fibroids were observed to have highly variable maximum SUV. The maximum SUV is especially higher in younger and premenopausal patients, which may be due to the effects of estrogen on the proliferation of uterine fibroids.[54] However, fibroids are usually not active in postmenopausal women (**Fig. 13**).

Genitourinary tract activity should be evaluated carefully. The ureters can be followed most of the time on CT, and activity is commonly seen in the ureteropelvic junction. CT images should be examined carefully in all the 3 orthogonal projections. When bladder wall thickening is observed, it should be noted in the report. Horseshoe kidney, unusual kidney orientations, and a transplanted kidney can easily be recognized with CT correlation (**Fig. 14**).

Insufficiency fractures in the pelvis related to osteopenia and/or osteoporosis are usually bilateral and typical H-shaped. Associated vertebral fractures in the spine or loss of height of vertebral bodies may be observed. In addition, 1-sided fractures in the sacral region may occur. In such

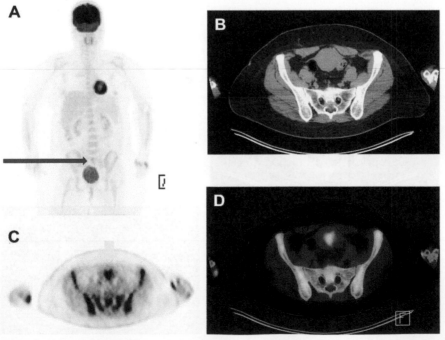

Fig. 9. Activity in uterus owing to menses. A 38-year-old woman with melanoma came for PET/computed tomography (CT) restaging after therapy. There is no abnormal activity in the body except for focal uptake in the pelvis (*arrow*) on coronal maximum intensity projection PET image (*A*). CT image (*B*) through uterus is normal, with focal avid activity (*arrow*) seen in uterine cavity on attenuation-corrected PET image (*C*) and PET/CT image (*D*). The patient stated that she started her menstrual period the day of the scan.

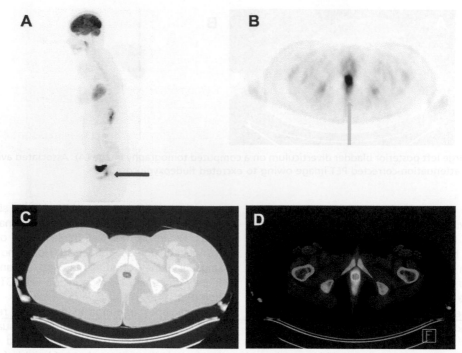

Fig. 10. Activity in a tampon. A 24-year-old woman in the middle of her menstrual period. Increased activity is noted in the pelvis (*arrow*) on sagittal PET maximum intensity projection image (*A*) inferior to the bladder. Attenuation-corrected PET image (*B*) shows the activity (*arrow*) within the vagina. A corresponding computed tomography (CT) image (*C*) demonstrates a predominantly gas attenuation tampon in the vagina (*C*). PET/CT image (*D*) confirms that the activity is localized to the tampon.

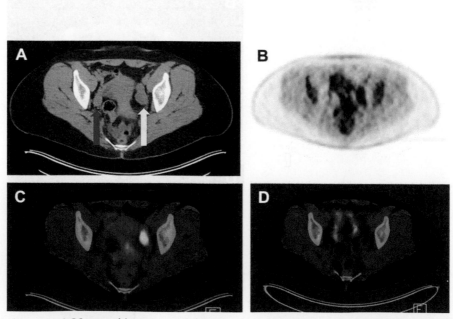

Fig. 11. Ovarian cysts. A 36-year-old woman with breast cancer underwent PET/computed tomography (CT) scans for staging. Cystic structures are present in the adnexa (*arrows*) on the CT image (*A*). There is increased activity on the left (standardized uptake value of 8.4) and no increased activity on the right as seen on attenuation-corrected PET image (*B*) and PET/CT image (*C*). On a follow-up PET/CT study 8 months later (*D*), both cysts are seen to have resolved.

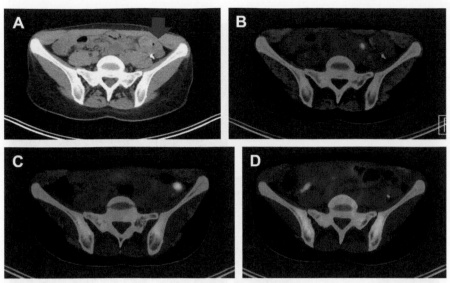

Fig. 12. Transposed ovary in the left pelvis. This is a 31-year-old woman with cervical cancer who is status post total abdominal hysterectomy with ovary transposition in the left pelvis (*arrow*) with surgical clips posterior to the ovary as seen on a computed tomography (CT) image (*A*). There are varying levels of activities in this location on different PET/CT scans (*B–D*) owing to acquisition during different phases of the menstrual cycle.

cases, bone densitometry studies may be recommended (**Fig. 15**).

Neurofibromas and schwannomas are benign nerve sheath tumors. Most are standalone tumors without clinical significance. We have observed a few cases of sacral schwannomas with FDG uptake and stable appearance for many years, and

MR imaging correlation is helpful for tissue characterization (**Fig. 16**).

Urine contamination is not uncommon for senior patients. Careful evaluation with CT in different window settings will help in the reading and interpretation of such contamination (**Fig. 17**).

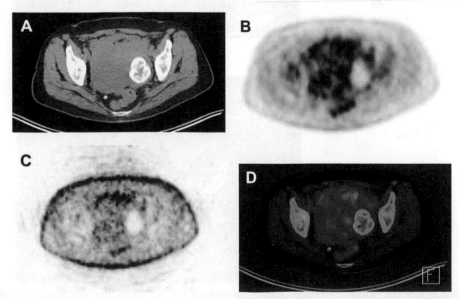

Fig. 13. Fibroid. This is a postmenopausal woman with a calcified fibroid on computed tomography scanning (CT) (*A*). The activity is at the background level for both attenuation-corrected PET image (*B*), non–attenuation-corrected PET image (*C*), and PET/CT image (*D*).

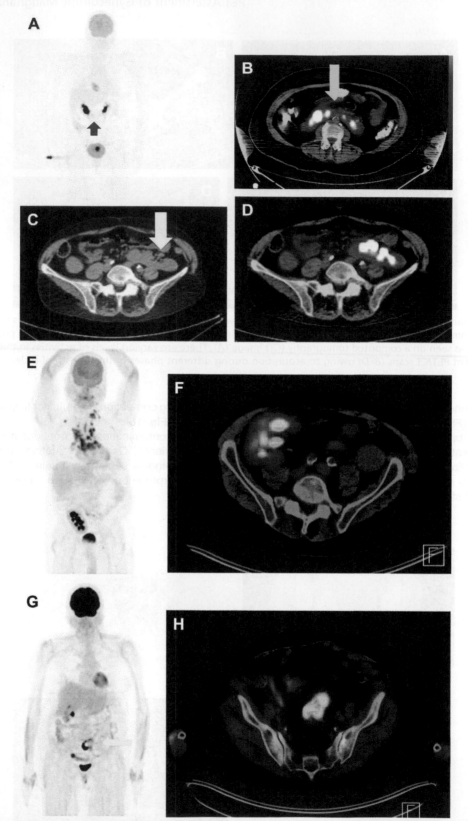

Fig. 14. Unusual kidneys. Horseshoe kidney (*arrows*) on coronal PET maximum intensity projection (MIP) image (*A*) and PET/computed tomography (CT) image (*B*). Malrotated left kidney (*arrow*) on CT image (*C*) and PET/CT image (*D*) in a different patient. Transplanted kidney in right pelvic on coronal PET MIP image (*E*) and PET/CT image (*F*) in a different patient with metastatic lung cancer in thorax. Ptotic pelvic left kidney (*arrow*) on coronal PET MIP image (*G*) and PET/CT image (*H*) in a different patient.

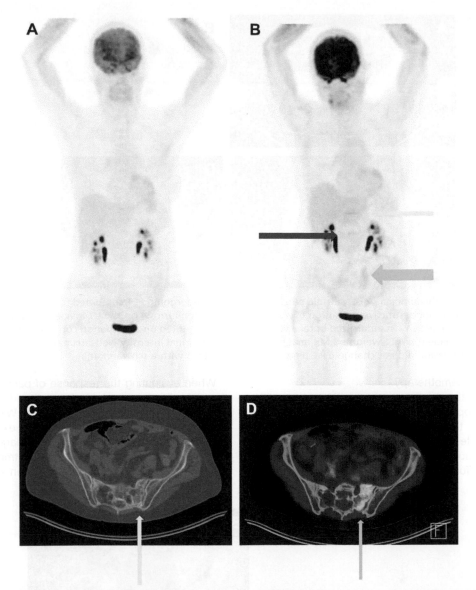

Fig. 15. Insufficiency fractures. A 72-year-old woman with cervical cancer who is on therapy. There is no abnormal activity seen on coronal PET maximum intensity projection image (*A*). On a follow-up PET scan 1 year later (*B*), there is linear activity in the left sacrum (*thick arrow*) along with multiple levels of increased activity in several vertebral bodies (*thin arrows*) corresponding with vertebral compression fractures. A fracture line is seen in the left sacral ala (*arrow*) on a computed tomography (CT) scan. (*C*) Associated increased activity (*arrow*) is seen on PET/CT image (*D*). Bone densitometry subsequently demonstrated presence of osteoporosis.

THERAPY FOLLOW-UP WITH PET

FDG PET/CT scanning is commonly used for posttreatment surveillance, and is very useful for the early detection of tumor recurrence.[55–59] Recognizing the pattern of uptake for different kinds of therapies is extremely important, and helps in differentiating active neoplastic disease from posttherapy changes. Listed are some of the common FDG-avid findings after treatment.

1. Postoperatively
   a. Infection, inflammation
   b. Granuloma, surgical wound
   c. Foreign material related: talc, prosthesis
   d. Surgical site tumor recurrence, usually late
2. After radiation therapy[60]
   a. In the thorax: pneumonitis, myocarditis, esophagitis
   b. In the abdomen and pelvis: hepatitis, enterocolitis
   c. Inflammation in treatment portal configuration

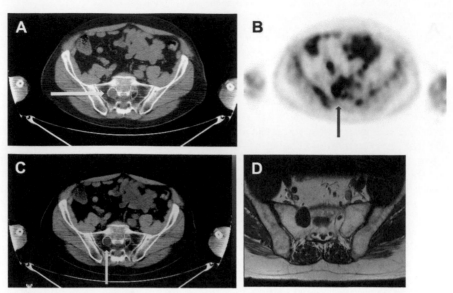

Fig. 16. Sacral schwannoma. A 65-year-old patient with cancer undergoing PET/computed tomography (CT) evaluation. There is nondestructive expansion of a right sacral foramen (*arrow*) on the CT image (*A*) with an associated increase in activity (standardized uptake value of 3.5; *arrow*) noted on attenuation-corrected PET image (*B*) and PET/CT image (*C*). A T1-weighted MR image (*D*) shows a low signal intensity well-circumscribed lesion in this location. This lesion did not change over time, and was consistent with a schwannoma.

3. After chemotherapy
   a. In the thorax: pneumonitis, myocarditis, esophagitis, thymic rebound
   b. In the abdomen and pelvis: hepatitis, enterocolitis
4. After supportive therapy
   a. Diffuse bone marrow activation

When evaluating the response of patients after therapy, all images need to be analyzed carefully to avoid potential misinterpretations. We had a recent patient with pelvic sarcoma. On examining the maximum intensity projection images, she seems to be stable between pretreatment and posttreatment scans, with similar lesion volumes

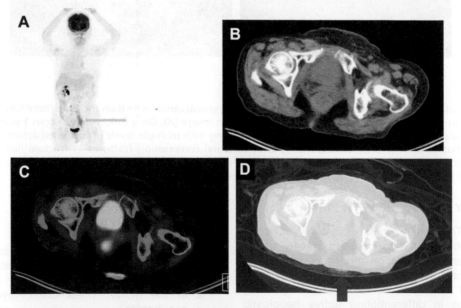

Fig. 17. Urine contamination. Activity is seen in the left pelvis on coronal PET maximum intensity projection image (*arrow*) (*A*) without corresponding abnormality on the computed tomography (CT) image (*B*). PET/CT image (*C*) reveals that the activity is located along the left posterior skin surface of the pelvis. CT image (*D*) shows a corresponding absorbent material/diaper (*arrow*).

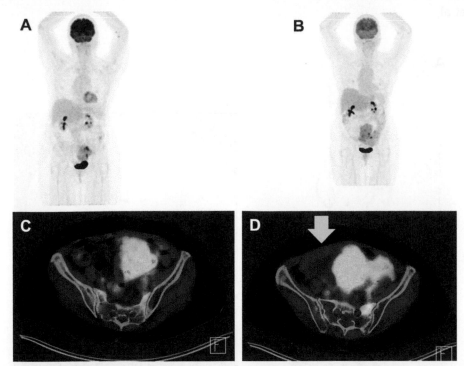

Fig. 18. Sarcoma for follow-up scans. Coronal PET maximum intensity projection images of a patient with pelvic sarcoma before (A) and after (B) therapy show stable appearing activity in a left pelvic lesion. PET/computed tomography (CT) image before therapy (C) demonstrates activity in tumor (C). However, a PET/CT image after therapy (D) reveals new large non–fludeoxyglucose-avid cystic changes (arrow) along the right aspect of the tumor. A subsequent CT scan performed 3 months later (not shown) demonstrated further enlargement of the cystic component owing to tumor progression.

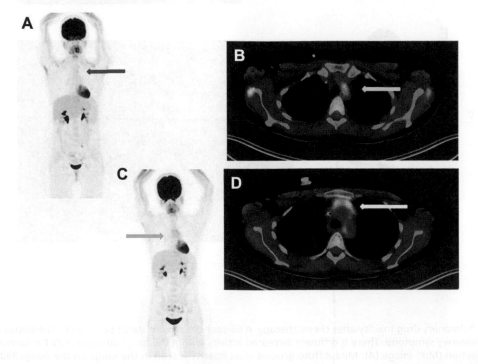

Fig. 19. Thymic rebound after therapy. A 30-year-old woman with multiple pelvic lesions. There is a focus of fludeoxyglucose uptake (arrows) in the high left paratracheal region owing to brown fat on a coronal PET maximum intensity projection (MIP) image (A) and PET/computed tomography (CT) image before treatment. (B) There is new, diffusely increased activity in the anterior mediastinum (arrows) along with increased thymic soft tissue on coronal PET MIP image (C) and PET/CT image (D) at 12 weeks after therapy, consistent with posttreatment thymic rebound.

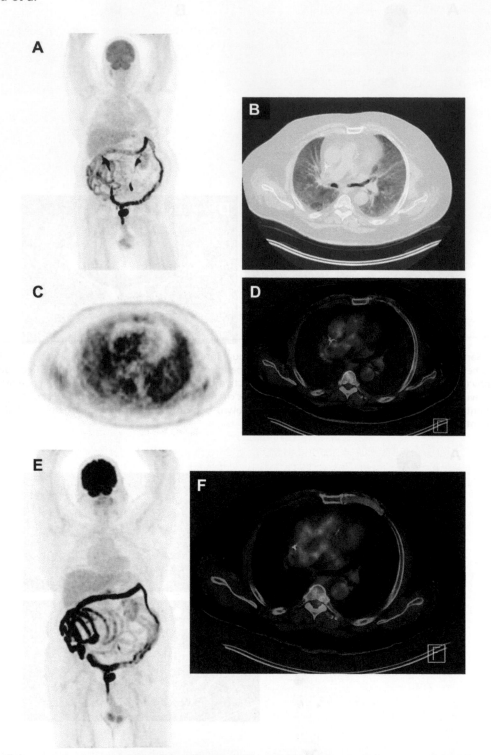

Fig. 20. Pulmonary drug toxicity after chemotherapy. A 66-year-old patient status post recent chemotherapy now with pulmonary symptoms. There is diffusely increased activity within the lungs on coronal PET maximum intensity projection (MIP) image (*A*). Mild diffuse ground glass opacity is seen in the lungs on the computed tomography (CT) image (*B*). Corresponding diffuse activity is seen in the lungs on attenuation-corrected PET image (*C*) and PET/CT image (*D*). A follow-up scan 4 months later showed interval resolution of these abnormalities on coronal PET MIP image (*E*) and PET/CT image (*F*). The patient's symptoms had also resolved by this time.

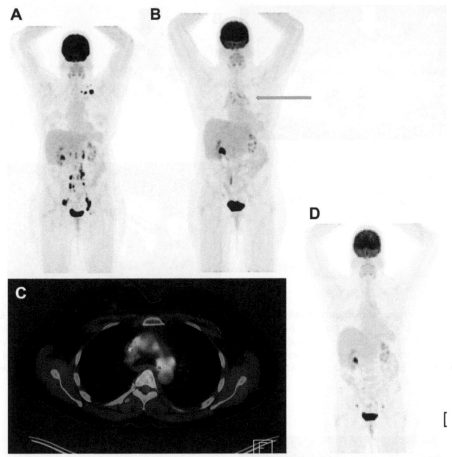

Fig. 21. Posttherapy sarcoidlike reaction changes in the thorax in a 50-year-old woman with endometrial cancer. Multiple active lesions are seen in the abdomen, pelvis, and supraclavicular nodes on baseline coronal PET maximum intensity projection (MIP) image (*A*). Coronal PET MIP image (*B*) 4 months posttherapy shows interval tumor response with minimal disease remaining in the pelvis, but with new symmetric activity seen in the hilar and mediastinal lymph nodes (*arrow*). A PET/computed tomography (CT) image (*C*) shows that the fludeoxyglucose avid lymph nodes are normal in size (*C*). Coronal PET MIP image (*D*) an additional 4 months later reveals interval resolution of activity within the mediastinal and hilar lymph nodes, confirming an inflammatory etiology.

and SUVs. However, there is a significantly larger size for the posttreatment pelvic mass with a markedly larger cystic component (**Fig. 18**).

Thymic uptake is common in the pediatric and young adult population as a physiologic finding. It is also frequently seen owing to "flare-up" after therapy (**Fig. 19**). Isolated mediastinal and hilar nodes could indicate reactive or inflammatory changes, especially if the nodes have been stable over time.[61]

Lung uptake might also be inflammatory, owing to drug toxicity or to sarcoidlike reaction after immunosuppression from the therapy. We had a patient with diffusely increased activity after chemotherapy and subsequent recovery (**Fig. 20**). Another patient showed increased activity in multiple small mediastinal nodes after therapy and subsequent recovery over time in the chest (**Fig. 21**).

Esophageal uptake after treatment is more diffuse owing to reactive changes, and usually involves the entire length of the esophagus.

Foreign body retention after surgery or other interventional procedure has been reported.[62–65] Postprocedural changes require a comprehensive clinical history investigation and attention to all details (**Fig. 22**).

There are always technological limitations, even for modern machines. A lesion with a size below the machine's resolution may potentially be interpreted as falsely negative, with a follow-up scan subsequently showing the lesion (**Fig. 23**).

Many gynecologic malignancies are mucinous or cystic, containing only a small component of solid tissue or cells, such that the metabolic activity is often low[66] (**Fig. 24**). For those patients, the usefulness of PET is limited as a follow-up tool.

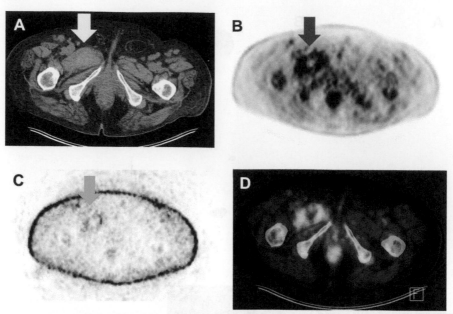

Fig. 22. Right inguinal postprocedural changes from an inferior vena caval (IVC) filter placement. A 60-year-old man with history of esophageal cancer. There is a hyperattenuating hematoma (*arrow*) in the right proximal thigh musculature on the computed tomography (CT) image (*A*). There is associated increased activity (*arrow*) peripherally in this region on the attenuation-corrected PET image (*B*). The non–attenuation-corrected PET image (*C*) and the PET/CT image (*D*) also demonstrate increased activity in this location. Additional history revealed recent placement of an IVC filter.

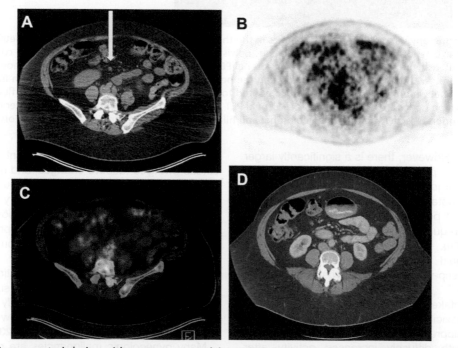

Fig. 23. Tiny mesenteric lesion without apparent activity on PET. A 53-year-old woman with endometrial cancer is status post total abdominal hysterectomy-bilateral salpingo-oophorectomy. There is a subcentimeter mesenteric lesion (*arrow*) on the computed tomography (CT) image (*A*) without apparent activity seen above background levels on the attenuation-corrected PET image (*B*) or PET/CT image (*C*). A follow-up contrast-enhanced CT (*D*) obtained 5 months later demonstrated lesion stability.

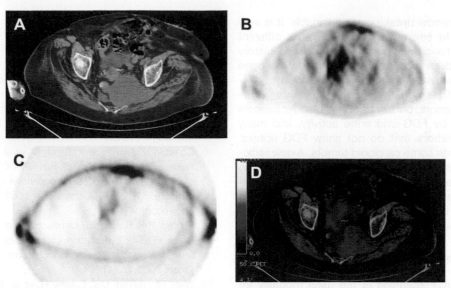

Fig. 24. Mucinous ovarian cancer. An 84-year-old woman with ovarian cancer. Cystic lesions with small solid components are seen in the pelvis on the computed tomography (CT) image (*A*). There is minimal associated activity seen on attenuation-corrected PET image (*B*), non–attenuation-corrected PET image (*C*), and PET/CT image (*D*) in the predominantly cystic lesion in the left pelvis, although some increased activity is seen within solid components predominantly in the right pelvis.

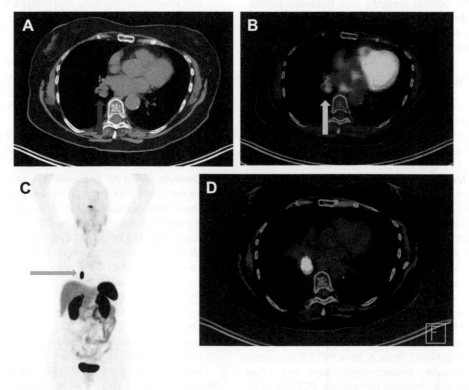

Fig. 25. Variable PET radiotracer uptake of carcinoid tumor. A 68-year-old woman with a small lesion posterior to the right hilum (*arrow*) owing to a carcinoid tumor as seen on a computed tomography (CT) image (*A*). PET/CT scan with fludeoxyglucose shows minimal activity in the soft tissue lesion (*arrow*). (*B*) 68Ga-DOTATATE coronal PET maximum intensity projection image (*C*) and PET/CT image (*D*) show avid activity (standardized uptake value of 97.3) associated with the lesion (*arrow*).

Bone marrow uptake can be variable. It is very common to see reactive marrow after different therapies have been administered. Clinical history and a pattern of diffuse distribution in the bone marrow are useful for study interpretation.

Other false-negative findings include slow-growing tumors, urinary tract and bladder cancers obscured by FDG-avid urine activity, and many indolent tumors that do not show FDG uptake, such as with some carcinoid tumors. A new radiotracer was approved by the US Food and Drug Administration in the summer of 2016 for neuroendocrine tumor imaging: ^{68}Ga-DOTATATE. This is useful for the detection of somatostatin receptor–rich neuroendocrine tumors (**Fig. 25**).

SUMMARY

FDG PET/CT scanning is the main modality for cancer detection, staging, restaging, response assessment, and assessment of prognosis. The usefulness of PET/CT imaging for other indications has increased over the past decades. By recognizing the normal variants and potential pitfalls, we can better use this powerful tool to provide useful information for patients and referring physicians.

REFERENCES

1. Wechalekar K, Sharma B, Cook G. PET/CT in oncology–a major advance. Clin Radiol 2005; 60(11):1143–55.
2. Townsend DW, Beyer T, Blodgett TM. PET/CT scanners: a hardware approach to image fusion. Semin Nucl Med 2003;33(3):193–204.
3. Nakamura K, Kodama J, Okumura Y, et al. The SUVmax of 18F-FDG PET correlates with histological grade in endometrial cancer. Int J Gynecol Cancer 2010;20(1):110–5.
4. Alessi A, Martinelli F, Padovano B, et al. FDG-PET/CT to predict optimal primary cytoreductive surgery in patients with advanced ovarian cancer: preliminary results. Tumori 2016;102(1):103–7.
5. Amit A, Beck D, Lowenstein L, et al. The role of hybrid PET/CT in the evaluation of patients with cervical cancer. Gynecol Oncol 2006;100(1):65–9.
6. Amit A, Schink J, Reiss A, et al. PET/CT in gynecologic cancer: present applications and future prospects-a clinician's perspective. PET Clin 2010; 5(4):391–405.
7. Amit A, Schink J, Reiss A, et al. PET/CT in gynecologic cancer: present applications and future prospects–a clinician's perspective. Obstet Gynecol Clin North Am 2011;38(1):1–21, vii.
8. Bollineni VR, Ytre-Hauge S, Bollineni-Balabay O, et al. High diagnostic value of 18F-FDG PET/CT in endometrial cancer: systematic review and meta-analysis of the literature. J Nucl Med 2016;57(6): 879–85.
9. Bourguet P, Hitzel A, Houvenaeghel G, et al. 2005 monitoring report: use of positron emission tomography with fluorodeoxyglucose in the management of patients with breast cancer, ovarian cancer, and uterine cancer. Gynecol Obstet Fertil 2006;34(5): 437–59 [in French].
10. Chastan M, Manrique A, Baron M, et al. Prognostic value of pretherapeutic 18F-FDG PET/CT in cancer of the uterine cervix: a retrospective study of 53 patients. Gynecol Obstet Fertil 2010;38(4):244–9 [in French].
11. Brooks RA, Rader JS, Dehdashti F, et al. Surveillance FDG-PET detection of asymptomatic recurrences in patients with cervical cancer. Gynecol Oncol 2009;112(1):104–9.
12. Wahl RL, Javadi MS, Eslamy H, et al. The roles of fluorodeoxyglucose-PET/computed tomography in ovarian cancer: diagnosis, assessing response, and detecting recurrence. PET Clin 2010;5(4):447–61.
13. Xu B, Ma J, Jiang G, et al. Diagnostic value of positron emission tomography (PET) and PET/computed tomography in recurrent/metastatic ovarian cancer: a meta-analysis. J Obstet Gynaecol Res 2017; 43(2):378–86.
14. Yoo J, Choi JY, Moon SH, et al. Prognostic significance of volume-based metabolic parameters in uterine cervical cancer determined using 18F-fluorodeoxyglucose positron emission tomography. Int J Gynecol Cancer 2012;22(7):1226–33.
15. Prakash P, Cronin CG, Blake MA. Role of PET/CT in ovarian cancer. AJR Am J Roentgenol 2010;194(6): W464–70.
16. Salem A, Salem AF, Al-Ibraheem A, et al. Evidence for the use PET for radiation therapy planning in patients with cervical cancer: a systematic review. Hematol Oncol Stem Cell Ther 2011;4(4):173–81.
17. Barrett OC, McDonald AM, Lee Burnett O 3rd, et al. Mesorectal node metastasis from gynecological cancer in the era of 3D conformal pelvic radiation therapy and intensity modulated radiation therapy. Pract Radiat Oncol 2016;6(6):402–4.
18. Bjurberg M, Kjellen E, Ohlsson T, et al. Prediction of patient outcome with 2-deoxy-2-[18F]fluoro-D-glucose-positron emission tomography early during radiotherapy for locally advanced cervical cancer. Int J Gynecol Cancer 2009;19(9):1600–5.
19. Brar H, May T, Tau N, et al. Detection of extraregional tumour recurrence with 18F-FDG-PET/CT in patients with recurrent gynaecological malignancies being considered for radical salvage surgery. Clin Radiol 2017;72(4):302–6.
20. Caroli P, Fanti S. PET/CT and radiotherapy in gynecological cancer. Q J Nucl Med Mol Imaging 2010; 54(5):533–42.

21. Chung HH, Kwon HW, Kang KW, et al. Preoperative [F]FDG PET/CT predicts recurrence in patients with epithelial ovarian cancer. J Gynecol Oncol 2012; 23(1):28–34.

22. Chung HH, Lee I, Kim HS, et al. Prognostic value of preoperative metabolic tumor volume measured by (1)(8)F-FDG PET/CT and MRI in patients with endometrial cancer. Gynecol Oncol 2013;130(3):446–51.

23. Du XL, Jiang T, Sheng XG, et al. PET/CT scanning guided intensity-modulated radiotherapy in treatment of recurrent ovarian cancer. Eur J Radiol 2012;81(11):3551–6.

24. Ghooshkhanei H, Treglia G, Sabouri G, et al. Risk stratification and prognosis determination using (18)F-FDG PET imaging in endometrial cancer patients: a systematic review and meta-analysis. Gynecol Oncol 2014;132(3):669–76.

25. Lazzari R, Cecconi A, Jereczek-Fossa BA, et al. The role of [(18)F]FDG-PET/CT in staging and treatment planning for volumetric modulated Rapidarc radiotherapy in cervical cancer: experience of the European Institute of Oncology, Milan, Italy. Ecancermedicalscience 2014;8:405.

26. Risum S, Loft A, Engelholm SA, et al. Positron emission tomography/computed tomography predictors of overall survival in stage IIIC/IV ovarian cancer. Int J Gynecol Cancer 2012;22(7):1163–9.

27. Simcock B, Narayan K, Drummond E, et al. The role of positron emission tomography/computed tomography in planning radiotherapy in endometrial cancer. Int J Gynecol Cancer 2015;25(4):645–9.

28. Vargo JA, Kim H, Choi S, et al. Extended field intensity modulated radiation therapy with concomitant boost for lymph node-positive cervical cancer: analysis of regional control and recurrence patterns in the positron emission tomography/computed tomography era. Int J Radiat Oncol Biol Phys 2014; 90(5):1091–8.

29. Zhao Q, Feng Y, Mao X, et al. Prognostic value of fluorine-18-fluorodeoxyglucose positron emission tomography or PET-computed tomography in cervical cancer: a meta-analysis. Int J Gynecol Cancer 2013; 23(7):1184–90.

30. Signorelli M, Guerra L, Buda A, et al. Role of the integrated FDG PET/CT in the surgical management of patients with high risk clinical early stage endometrial cancer: detection of pelvic nodal metastases. Gynecol Oncol 2009;115(2):231–5.

31. Barranger E, Kerrou K, Petegnief Y, et al. Laparoscopic resection of occult metastasis using the combination of FDG-positron emission tomography/computed tomography image fusion with intraoperative probe guidance in a woman with recurrent ovarian cancer. Gynecol Oncol 2005;96(1):241–4.

32. Bese T, Sal V, Demirkiran F, et al. The combination of preoperative fluorodeoxyglucose positron emission tomography/computed tomography and sentinel lymph node mapping in the surgical management of endometrioid endometrial cancer. Int J Gynecol Cancer 2016;26(7):1228–38.

33. Cohn DE, Hall NC, Povoski SP, et al. Novel perioperative imaging with 18F-FDG PET/CT and intraoperative 18F-FDG detection using a handheld gamma probe in recurrent ovarian cancer. Gynecol Oncol 2008;110(2):152–7.

34. Crivellaro C, Signorelli M, Guerra L, et al. Tailoring systematic lymphadenectomy in high-risk clinical early stage endometrial cancer: the role of 18F-FDG PET/CT. Gynecol Oncol 2013;130(2):306–11.

35. Ferrandina G, Petrillo M, Restaino G, et al. Can radicality of surgery be safely modulated on the basis of MRI and PET/CT imaging in locally advanced cervical cancer patients administered preoperative treatment? Cancer 2012;118(2):392–403.

36. Frumovitz M, Ramirez PT, Macapinlac HA, et al. Anatomic location of PET-positive aortocaval nodes in patients with locally advanced cervical cancer: implications for surgical staging. Int J Gynecol Cancer 2012;22(7):1203–7.

37. Fruscio R, Sina F, Dolci C, et al. Preoperative 18F-FDG PET/CT in the management of advanced epithelial ovarian cancer. Gynecol Oncol 2013; 131(3):689–93.

38. Gemer O, Eitan R, Gdalevich M, et al. Integration of PET/CT into the preoperative evaluation of patients with early cervical cancer does not decrease the proportion of patients with positive lymph nodes found after surgery. Int J Gynecol Cancer 2014; 24(8):1461–5.

39. Gouy S, Morice P, Narducci F, et al. Nodal-staging surgery for locally advanced cervical cancer in the era of PET. Lancet Oncol 2012;13(5):e212–20.

40. Lopez-Lopez V, Cascales-Campos PA, Gil J, et al. Use of (18)F-FDG PET/CT in the preoperative evaluation of patients diagnosed with peritoneal carcinomatosis of ovarian origin, candidates to cytoreduction and hipec. A pending issue. Eur J Radiol 2016; 85(10):1824–8.

41. Risum S, Hogdall C, Markova E, et al. Influence of 2-(18F) fluoro-2-deoxy-D-glucose positron emission tomography/computed tomography on recurrent ovarian cancer diagnosis and on selection of patients for secondary cytoreductive surgery. Int J Gynecol Cancer 2009;19(4):600–4.

42. Wang X, Koch S. Positron emission tomography/computed tomography potential pitfalls and artifacts. Curr Probl Diagn Radiol 2009;38(4):156–69.

43. Robbins J, Kusmirek J, Barroilhet L, et al. Pitfalls in imaging of cervical cancer. Semin Roentgenol 2016;51(1):17–31.

44. Nogami Y, Banno K, Irie H, et al. Efficacy of 18-FDG PET-CT dual-phase scanning for detection of lymph node metastasis in gynecological cancer. Anticancer Res 2015;35(4):2247–53.

45. Mavi A, Urhan M, Yu JQ, et al. Dual time point 18F-FDG PET imaging detects breast cancer with high sensitivity and correlates well with histologic subtypes. J Nucl Med 2006;47(9):1440–6.

46. Mayoral M, Paredes P, Domenech B, et al. 18F-FDG PET/CT and sentinel lymph node biopsy in the staging of patients with cervical and endometrial cancer. Role of dual-time-point imaging. Rev Esp Med Nucl Imagen Mol 2017;36(1):20–6.

47. Xiu Y, Bhutani C, Dhurairaj T, et al. Dual-time point FDG PET imaging in the evaluation of pulmonary nodules with minimally increased metabolic activity. Clin Nucl Med 2007;32(2):101–5.

48. Weber WA, Gatsonis CA, Mozley PD, et al. Repeatability of 18F-FDG PET/CT in advanced non-small cell lung cancer: prospective assessment in 2 multicenter trials. J Nucl Med 2015;56(8):1137–43.

49. Ucak Semirgin S, Basoglu T, Atmaca Saglik B, et al. Diagnostic value of additional 18F-FDG PET/CT imaging using a vaginal catheter in patients with paravaginal malignant lesions. Nucl Med Commun 2016; 37(12):1260–6.

50. Sureshbabu W, Mawlawi O. PET/CT imaging artifacts. J Nucl Med Technol 2005;33(3):156–61 [quiz: 63–4].

51. Roman-Jimenez G, Crevoisier RD, Leseur J, et al. Detection of bladder metabolic artifacts in (18)F-FDG PET imaging. Comput Biol Med 2016;71:77–85.

52. Bacanovic S, Stiller R, Pircher M, et al. Ovarian hyperstimulation and oocyte harvesting prior to systemic chemotherapy-a possible pitfall in 18F-FDG PET/CT staging of oncologic patients. Clin Nucl Med 2016;41(8):e394–6.

53. Chung HH, Kang WJ, Kim JW, et al. Characterization of surgically transposed ovaries in integrated PET/CT scan in patients with cervical cancer. Acta Obstet Gynecol Scand 2007;86(1):88–93.

54. Ma Y, Shao X, Shao X, et al. High metabolic characteristics of uterine fibroids in 18F-FDG PET/CT imaging and the underlying mechanisms. Nucl Med Commun 2016;37(11):1206–11.

55. Oh D, Huh SJ, Park W, et al. Clinical outcomes in cervical cancer patients treated by FDG-PET/CT-based 3-dimensional planning for the first brachytherapy session. Medicine 2016;95(25):e3895.

56. Chung HH, Kim SK, Kim TH, et al. Clinical impact of FDG-PET imaging in post-therapy surveillance of uterine cervical cancer: from diagnosis to prognosis. Gynecol Oncol 2006;103(1):165–70.

57. Han EJ, Park HL, Lee YS, et al. Clinical usefulness of post-treatment FDG PET/CT in patients with ovarian malignancy. Ann Nucl Med 2016;30(9):600–7.

58. Nishiyama Y, Yamamoto Y, Kanenishi K, et al. Monitoring the neoadjuvant therapy response in gynecological cancer patients using FDG PET. Eur J Nucl Med Mol Imaging 2008;35(2):287–95.

59. O'Connor OJ, Prakash P, Cronin CG, et al. PET/CT in the imaging of ovarian cancer. Front Biosci (Elite edition) 2013;5:141–53.

60. Papadopoulou I, Stewart V, Barwick TD, et al. Post-radiation therapy imaging appearances in cervical carcinoma. Radiographics 2016;36(2):538–53.

61. Onal C, Oymak E, Findikcioglu A, et al. Isolated mediastinal lymph node false positivity of [18F]-fluorodeoxyglucose-positron emission tomography/computed tomography in patients with cervical cancer. Int J Gynecol Cancer 2013;23(2):337–42.

62. Kwon YS, Gwack JY, Im KS, et al. Foreign body reaction from anti-adhesion material during follow-up of gynaecological malignancies: mimicking local recurrence. Aust N Z J Obstet Gynaecol 2016; 56(4):403–7.

63. Chen MY, Ng KK, Ma SY, et al. False-positive fluorine-18 fluorodeoxy-D-glucose positron emission tomography imaging caused by retained gauze in a woman with recurrent ovarian cancer: a case report. Eur J Gynaecol Oncol 2005;26(4):451–3.

64. Imperiale L, Marchetti C, Salerno L, et al. Nonabsorbable suture granuloma mimicking ovarian cancer recurrence at combined positron emission tomography/computed tomography evaluation: a case report. J Med Case Rep 2014;8:202.

65. Yu JQ, Milestone BN, Parsons RB, et al. Findings of intramediastinal gossypiboma with F-18 FDG PET in a melanoma patient. Clin Nucl Med 2008;33(5):344–5.

66. Tanizaki Y, Kobayashi A, Shiro M, et al. Diagnostic value of preoperative SUVmax on FDG-PET/CT for the detection of ovarian cancer. Int J Gynecol Cancer 2014;24(3):454–60.

Quantitative Assessment of Gynecologic Malignancies

Sarthak Tripathy, MBBS, Girish Kumar Parida, MD,
Rakesh Kumar, MD, PhD*

KEYWORDS

- FDG • PET/CT • Standardized uptake value • Metabolic tumor volume • Total lesion glycolysis
- Gynecologic malignancies

KEY POINTS

- PET imaging for oncology has advanced rapidly in last couple of decades.
- The ability to image pathophysiologic processes much before there are discernible anatomic abnormalities makes it an ideal modality for imaging.
- The most important radiotracer used for the imaging is ^{18}F-fluorodeoxyglucose.

INTRODUCTION

PET imaging for oncology has advanced rapidly in last couple of decades. The ability to image pathophysiologic processes much before there are discernible anatomic abnormalities makes it an ideal modality for imaging. The most important radiotracer used for the imaging is ^{18}F-fluorodeoxyglucose (FDG). Evaluation of gynecologic malignancies with PET/computed tomography (CT) is an ongoing process and much of the significant work has been done with cervical, ovarian, and endometrial malignancies. FDG PET/CT scanning has been found to be superior to conventional imaging modalities in staging, restaging, and response assessment in many cases, with the additional advantage of quantifying tumor burden. However, the major limitation is the possibility of false-negative results, in some cases owing to high bladder activity secondary to predominant renal excretion of FDG. To overcome this limitation, some institutes follow the imaging protocol with a bladder catheter in situ. In this protocol,

there remains the possibility of urinary activity interference. Besides this, the additional risk of urinary tract infection is also there. So, in our institute, postdiuretic images of the pelvis are taken separately after 3 to 4 times of voiding.

In this review, we discuss the role of PET as quantitative imaging in the assessment of gynecologic malignances. Our discussion is limited to carcinomas of the cervix, endometrium, and ovary, because there is little literature regarding other gynecologic malignancies.

CERVICAL CANCER

Cervical cancer is the third most common malignancy affecting females, and is one of the leading causes of cancer-related death worldwide.[1] Major risk factors include human papilloma virus infection, an increased number of sexual partners, smoking, and early age of first coitus, with human papilloma virus infection exposure being most common. Clinically, patients complain of postcoital bleeding with menorrhagia and metrorrhagia

No funding received from any organization for this study.
The authors declare that there is no conflict of interest.
Department of Nuclear Medicine, All India Institute of Medical Sciences, New Delhi 110029, India
* Corresponding author. Diagnostic Nuclear Medicine Division, Department of Nuclear Medicine, All India Institute of Medical Sciences, Ansari Nagar, New Delhi 110029, India.
E-mail address: rkphulia@hotmail.com

PET Clin 13 (2018) 269–288
https://doi.org/10.1016/j.cpet.2017.11.010

being the most common signs. Cervical cancer is staged in accordance with International Federation of Gynecology and Obstetrics (FIGO) staging. Early stage disease (stages I and IIA) are treated with surgery, whereas advanced stages undergo radiation therapy or concurrent chemoradiotherapy. The most important prognostic factors include tumor size, parametrial invasion, and lymph nodal involvement, with lymph node metastases being the single most important prognostic factor.[2] Lymphatic spread of disease is more common than hematogenous spread, with common iliac and paraaortic lymph nodes being the most common draining stations. Hematogenous spread accounts for just 5% of the cases, and is most commonly to lungs, liver, and bone marrow.[3]

PET/Computed Tomography with ^{18}F-fluorodeoxyglucose in the Evaluation of Primary Lesions

Imaging modalities that play a crucial role in diagnosis and management planning include ultrasound (US), CT, MR imaging, and PET/CT scanning. For localization of the initial lesion in the cervix, MR imaging has been found to be superior owing to better soft tissue resolution among all the modalities. US examination, wither transrectal or transvaginal, can be of benefit in detecting parametrial and urinary bladder invasion, as well as in evaluation of hydronephrosis.[4,5] Various studies over the last few years have shown that FDG PET/CT scanning can have a deep impact ranging from pretreatment planning to response assessment to chemotherapeutic regimens.

MR imaging has been considered as the reference standard for evaluation of primary lesions in the cervix (T staging) because of better soft tissue contrast resolution, which can be superior in identification of parametrial extension and other adjacent soft tissue structures with greater accuracy.[6] PET/CT scanning usually has a role to play in the assessment of involved lymph nodes in cases of cervical cancer. The pattern of lymph node involvement includes pelvic, paraaortic, and then supraclavicular lymph node spread. FDG PET/CT scanning provides a noninvasive imaging modality for the assessment of lymph nodes in such cases and helps to prevent an unnecessary procedure of lymphadenectomy. The sensitivity, specificity, positive predictive value (PPV), negative predictive value (NPV), and accuracy to detect metastasis at the nodal level are 51.1%, 99.8%, 85.2%, 98.9%, and 98.7%, respectively, and 50%, 90.9%, 66.7%, 83.3% and 80.0%, respectively, at the patient level.[7] In another study by Leblanc and colleagues,[8] PET/CT scanning had a sensitivity, specificity, PPV, and NPV of 33.3%, 94.2%, 53.8%, and 87.5%, respectively, to detect microscopic lymph node metastasis in 125 locally advanced stage IB to IVA patients with cervical cancer who had a negative result on CT scanning and MR imaging. Similarly, in one of the other studies in 65 stage IB to IVA patients who had normal studies on morphologic imaging for paraaortic lymphadenopathy, the sensitivity, specificity, PPV, and NPV of PET/CT scans were 36%, 96%, 71%, and 83%, respectively.[9] PET/CT scanning has been shown to be more accurate than CT scanning and MR imaging for lymph nodal assessment; the accuracy for CT scanning and MR imaging is about 43% and 86%, respectively.[10–12] The low accuracy of CT scanning and MR imaging in detecting metastatic lymph nodes can be attributed to the fact that normal sized lymph nodes can contain micrometastatic disease and enlarged lymph nodes can be inflammatory in nature. However, the pooled sensitivity and specificity of PET/CT scanning for detecting metastatic lymph nodes at the patient level are 82% and 95%, respectively, and at the regional or nodal level 54% and 97%, respectively. Similarly, the pooled sensitivity and specificity for CT scanning at the patient level are 50% and 92%, respectively, and at the nodal level 52% and 92%, respectively, whereas those of MR imaging at the patient level are 56% and 91%, respectively, and at the nodal level 38% and 97%, respectively.[13] Left supraclavicular lymph node involvement has been found in about 5% of the patients with cervical cancer.[14] However, the frequency of left supraclavicular lymph node involvement ranges from 4% to 35% in patients with biopsy-proven paraaortic lymph node metastases.[15,16] The PPV of detecting abnormal supraclavicular lymph node metastases in patients with cervical cancer on FDG PET/CT scanning has been reported to be as high as 100%.[17] Using the metabolic semiquantitative functional imaging parameter, namely, the maximum standardized uptake value (SUV_{max}), FDG PET had a sensitivity, specificity, PPV, NPV, and accuracy of 74.4%, 78.6%, 95.5%, 33.3%, and 75%, respectively, to detect metastasis in supraclavicular lymph nodes with an SUV_{max} of greater than 3.[18] Apart from the SUV_{max}, a metabolic tumor volume (MTV) of less than 60 cm^3 in primary cervical lesions has been associated with better overall survival (OS) and progression-free survival (PFS) as compared with an MTV of greater than 60 cm^3.[19]

It has been observed that the serum squamous cell carcinoma antigen (SCC-Ag) had a statistically significant association with lymph node metastasis ($P = .0373$).[20] However, there was no correlation observed between the SUV_{max} of the primary tumor and the SCC-Ag ($r^2 = -0.57$). In this study of 82 patients with biopsy-proven cervical malignancy, it was seen that an SUV_{max} of greater than 11.2 of primary tumor along with pelvic lymphadenopathy and higher SUV_{max} plus higher serum SCC-Ag (>6.4 ng/nL) were the 2 most significant variables that predicted a worse prognosis ($P = .0099$ and $P = .0020$, respectively).

When compared with the imaging modalities in detecting lymph node metastases, FDG PET/CT scanning has been found to be superior, although surgical pathology remains the reference standard for staging and is irreplaceable. The sensitivity to detect pelvic and paraaortic lymph node metastases were 53% and 25%, respectively, when compared with the pathology of stage IA to IIA cervical malignancy patients.[21] In another study by Margulies and colleagues,[22] it was shown that PET/CT scanning has a low sensitivity in detecting pelvic lymph nodes. When compared with diffusion-weighted MR imaging in the preoperative evaluation of patients with cervical cancer, PET/CT scanning had a lower sensitivity compared with diffusion-weighted MR imaging (38.9% vs 83.3%, respectively, at the nodal level; 44.4% vs 88.9%, respectively, at the patient level), but a higher specificity (96.3% vs 51.2%, respectively, at the nodal level; 93.8% vs 43.8%, respectively, at the patient level) to detect lymph node metastases.[23] The false-negative rate in detection of paraaortic lymph node metastases has been around 11% to 22%, which prompts the inclusion of paraaortic lymphadenectomy as an integral part of surgical staging in patients with locally advanced cervix cancer.[22,24] Semiquantitative parameters such as MTV and total lesion glycolysis (TLG) were associated significantly with nodal metastases in patients with early stage cervical cancer, although the same could not be said about the SUV_{max} (**Fig. 1**).[25]

PET/Computed Tomography with ^{18}F-fluorodeoxyglucose in Distant Metastases

PET/CT scanning, being a whole-body evaluation modality, has superiority in detecting distant metastases to lungs, liver, bone marrow, and any other viscera from any malignancy as early as possible. PET/CT scanning has been reported to have a sensitivity, specificity, and accuracy of 100%, 90%, and 94%, respectively, for evaluating distant metastases.[26] Disseminated disease has been detected in up to 17% of the patients by PET/CT scanning alone.[27] PET has been shown to have higher sensitivity than CT scanning ($P = .004$), higher specificity than MR imaging ($P = .04$), and high overall accuracy compared with both the modalities in detecting bone marrow metastasis in patients with FIGO stage III or IV

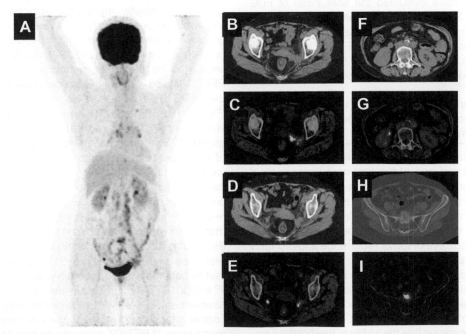

Fig. 1. A 66-year-old woman was diagnosed with cervical cancer, and is undergoing evaluation for disease extent. Coronal maximum intensity projection PET image with fluorodeoxyglucose (FDG) is shown in (A). Axial FDG PET/computed tomography images show a metabolically active soft tissue mass lesion involving the cervix with extension to the left lateral pelvic wall (B, C) along with FDG-avid metastases to bilateral pelvic lymph nodes (D, E), retroperitoneal lymph nodes (F, G), and the S1 vertebra (H, I).

disease, or positive lymph node metastasis and suspected recurrent disease.[28]

PET/Computed Tomography with ^{18}F-fluorodeoxyglucose in Treatment Planning

MR imaging has been found to be superior in delineating the local extent of disease owing to better soft tissue contrast resolution, but FDG PET/CT scanning has been found to be superior in detecting nodal and distant metastases. This difference has significant implications in locally advanced malignancies because it can potentially lead to alterations in radiation therapy fields or can change the management altogether to chemotherapy or concurrent chemoradiotherapy.[29,30] In early stage disease, cervical cancer tumor diameter measured by pretreatment FDG PET significantly correlates with the pathologic tumor diameter ($P<.0001$).[31] Gross tumor volume (GTV) on FDG PET/CT scanning correlates more with the pathologic volume than the GTVs based on CT scanning and MR imaging. Ciernik and colleagues[32] reported a change of GTV of more than 25% based on PET/CT scanning in 56% of solid tumor cases, along with a change in treatment plan from curative to palliative in 16% of cases. FDG PET/CT scan-guided intensity-modulated radiation therapy has also been useful in providing the highest radiation doses to the targeted sites with sparing of normal tissues.[33] Lin and colleagues[34] have evaluated the usefulness of FDG PET for 3-dimensional brachytherapy treatment planning in patients with cervical cancer using the GTV parameters. Thus, FDG PET can improve the isodose tumor coverage while sparing the critical organs, such as the urinary bladder and rectum.

PET/Computed Tomography with ^{18}F-fluorodeoxyglucose in the Assessment of Treatment Response

The evaluation of the response to chemotherapeutics has been one of the foremost indications of PET/CT scanning in cervical cancer. The assessment of response also gains significance, given that it is not only helpful in determining the effectiveness of the chemotherapeutic agents, but also is predictive of tumor recurrence and mortality in patients with cervical cancer.[35,36] Posttreatment changes and tumor recurrence can sometimes be indistinguishable on conventional imaging, but this problem has been solved largely with the advent of PET/CT scanning.[37,38] In addition, PET/CT scanning has the ability to predict the functional disease status before morphologic disease changes.[39] The use of semiquantitative parameters such as SUV_{max} has been well-documented in the evaluation of the assessment of response

and prognosis.[40] The optimal timing to obtain FDG PET/CT scanning to assess for treatment response is at least 6 weeks after surgery and 3 months after completion of concurrent chemoradiation therapy (CCRT).[41] A ratio of SUV_{max} at posttherapy to SUV_{max} at pretherapy of less than 0.33 correlated with tumor pathologic response (area under the curve [AUC] of 0.955; $P<.001$) and a 35% improvement in 6-month PFS ($P = .004$) in patients with advanced stage (IB2 to IVA) cervical cancer.[42] FDG PET/CT scanning has also been used to assess response during the ongoing treatment process.[43] In a study by Kidd and colleagues,[44] where FDG PET/CT scans were performed before treatment, at weeks 2 and 4 of treatment with concurrent chemoradiotherapy, and 3 months after completing chemoradiation therapy, nonresponders had higher SUV_{max}, larger MTV, and greater tumor heterogeneity compared with responders. Pretreatment and week 4 posttreatment were considered as the best time points for evaluating response using SUV_{max}, tumor heterogeneity, and MTV. FDG PET/CT scanning was found to be superior to MR imaging for calculating the midtreatment percent volume reduction ($P = .024$).[45] In another study, Lin and colleagues[46] found a significant tumor volume reduction evaluated by FDG PET within 20 days of starting chemoradiation treatment. The metabolic response determined by FDG PET was categorized into 3 groups: complete metabolic response, partial metabolic response, and progressive disease. Progressive disease (hazard ratio [HR], 32.57; 95% confidence interval [CI], 10.22–103.82) has been shown to be the most significant predictor for PFS.[36] Based on the response assessment by the FDG PET/CT scan to radiotherapy, OS ($P<.0001$), PFS ($P<.0001$), and cause-specific survival rates ($P<.0001$) can be calculated for the 3 groups.[47] Siva and colleagues[48] reported a study of 105 patients where posttherapy FDG PET scans were done in patients with stage IB to III cervical cancer treated with chemoradiation therapy, and found that patients with partial metabolic response had distant failure 36-fold higher than that in patients with complete metabolic response ($P<.0001$). Also, patients with partial a metabolic response had nodal failure 51-fold higher than that in patients with complete metabolic response ($P = .0061$). FDG PET has a limited role in response assessment in early stage patients with cervical cancer after surgery owing to the low tumor recurrence rates.[49] PET/CT scanning as well as MR imaging are not suitable modalities to detect residual disease for patients with locally advanced cervical cancer who have been selected for radical surgery after neoadjuvant treatment (Fig. 2).

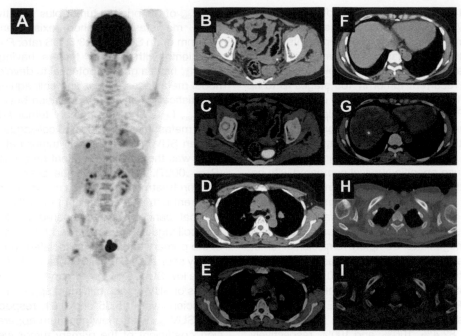

Fig. 2. A 58-year-old woman with known cervical cancer, status post chemotherapy and radiation therapy, undergoing evaluation for suspected tumor recurrence. Coronal maximum intensity projection PET image with fluorodeoxyglucose (FDG) is shown in (A). Axial FDG PET/computed tomography images reveal metabolically active metastatic disease involving left perirectal (B, C), right internal mammary lymph node (D, E), liver (F, G), and right humeral head (H, I).

PET/Computed Tomography with 18F-fluorodeoxyglucose in Restaging and Prognostication

FDG PET/CT scanning has been very useful in detecting locoregional recurrence and distant metastases with high diagnostic accuracy. Early detection of recurrence in cervical malignancy is associated with improved survival rates.[50] The sensitivity, specificity, and accuracy of PET/CT scanning to detect suspected tumor recurrence in patients with cervical cancer has been reported to be 90.3%, 81.0%, and 86.5%, respectively.[51] The patient-level sensitivity, specificity, accuracy, PPV, and NPV of FDG PET/CT scanning to detect local recurrence at the primary site are 93%, 93%, 93%, 86%, and 96%, respectively, as reported by Mittra and colleagues,[52] whereas the patient-level sensitivity, specificity, PPV, NPV, and accuracy to detect distant metastases were 96%, 95%, 95%, 96%, and 95%, respectively. These results were validated in other studies, such as that by Chung and colleagues,[53] where FDG PET/CT findings were able to change the management in patients in 24.2% of patients. In the meta-analysis performed by Chu and colleagues[54] in the evaluation of diagnostic accuracy of the patients with cervical cancer, the pooled sensitivity and specificity to detect local recurrence were 82% (95% CI, 0.72%–0.90%) and 98% (95% CI, 0.96%–0.99%), respectively, whereas those to detect distant metastasis were 87% (95% CI, 0.80%–0.92%) and 97% (95% CI, 0.96%–0.98%), respectively. Apart from changing the management in patients with recurrent cervical cancer, FDG PET/CT findings were also able to predict the disease-free survival (DFS) rate. Patients with negative PET/CT findings had a 2-year DFS rate of 85.0% as compared with 10.9% in those with positive PET/CT findings (P = .002).[53] In the study by Bjurberg and colleagues,[55] PET detected more metastatic sites compared with CT scanning in 56% of patients. PET had high impact (ie, it led to a change or withholding of treatment in 33% of patients), and medium impact (ie, it altered the planned procedure, treatment dose, or mode of delivery in 22% of patients). The intention of treatment was changed in 30% of patients. FDG PET/CT findings have also been used in planning for pelvic exenteration in patients with recurrent cervical cancer by excluding extrapelvic metastatic disease. In these cases, MTV significantly correlated with OS (P<.001) and PFS (P = .001), whereas TLG correlated with OS (P = .022). The AUC to detect pelvic organ and pelvic sidewall invasion has been reported to be 0.74 to 0.91 in various studies.[56–58] FDG PET/CT scanning can be used to detect tumor recurrence in asymptomatic patients as well as patients with increasing tumor markers. Brooks and colleagues[58] evaluated the ability of FDG PET to detect recurrent tumor in 103 stages IB to IIB patients treated with definitive chemoradiation therapy. PET/CT scanning was able to detect 9 tumor recurrences in 78 asymptomatic patients. Also, patients with asymptomatic recurrences detected by FDG PET had a significantly better 3-year cause-specific survival compared with patients with symptomatic recurrences confirmed by FDG PET ($P = .09$). Recurrence is often detected biochemically by elevation of tumor markers such as the SCC-Ag and carcinoembryonic antigen after complete remission of tumor. PET/CT scanning had greater accuracy in the setting of SCC-Ag elevation (100%) than in the setting of carcinoembryonic antigen elevation (66.7%; $P = .0169$).[59] Also, PET/CT scanning showed a sensitivity, specificity, PPV, and NPV of 83.3%, 82.4%, 100%, and 100%, respectively, to detect tumor recurrence. PET was able to detect recurrence in patients when the SCC-Ag was greater than 2 ng/mL and when no disease was evident by conventional methods.[60]

PET/CT scanning can predict the prognosis in patients with cervical cancer in addition to the treatment response assessment. Prognostic factors in patients with cervical cancer include age, tumor size, tumor stage, histologic type, lymph node involvement, vessel invasion, parametrial involvement, and lymphovascular space invasion, with lymph node involvement being the most important.[61–64] PET-derived metabolic parameters such as SUV_{max}, MTV, and TLG as well as PET response are predictors of patient outcome. In the pretreatment evaluation, the degree of FDG uptake in the primary tumor site correlated with the clinical outcome, where high FDG uptake is associated with a poor clinical outcome.

In poorly differentiated cervical tumors, the SUV_{max} was highest (12.23) when compared with well-differentiated cervical tumors (8.58). However, it was not found to be statistically significant.[65] Nakamura and colleagues,[66] in their study of 52 patients with cervical cancer, showed that there were significant correlations between the SUV_{max} of the primary tumor and tumor maximum size ($P = .027$) and the presence of lymph node metastasis ($P = .039$). A high SUV_{max} of the primary tumor (≥ 15.6) plus lymph node metastasis (a short axis diameter of >10 mm with an SUV_{max} of ≥ 3.5) were significant predictors for poor prognosis when compared with a low SUV_{max} of the primary tumor (<15.6) or a high

SUV_{max} of the primary tumor plus negative lymph node metastasis (a short axis diameter of <10 mm or an SUV_{max} of 3.5; OS rate; $P = .0211$).

Patients with primary tumors having a high SUV_{max} have a greater potential to develop lymph nodal metastases. Yilmaz and colleagues[67] found a statistically significant correlation between high SUV_{max} (≥ 13.5) of the primary tumor and lymph node metastatic rate. Kidd and colleagues[40] found that an SUV_{max} of a cervical tumor before treatment was the only independent prognostic factor ($P = .0027$). Prognostic value between SUV_{max} from pretreatment PET/CT scanning and minimum apparent diffusion coefficient from MR imaging in cervical cancer were compared by Nakamura and colleagues,[68] who showed that high SUV_{max} of the primary tumor was associated with a significantly shorter DFS ($P = .0171$) and OS ($P = .0367$) than a low SUV_{max} of the primary tumor. The cutoff values of SUV_{max} and minimum apparent diffusion coefficient were 15.55 and 0.61, respectively. A high SUV_{max} with a low minimum apparent diffusion coefficient of the primary tumor were independent predictive factors for DFS and OS ($P = .003$ and .0036, respectively).

Other independent risk factors that predicted disease recurrence were preoperative SUV_{max} of primary tumor (HR, 1.178; 95% CI, 1.034–1.342), age (HR, 0.87; 95% CI, 0.772–0.980), and parametrial involvement (HR, 27.974; 95% CI, 1.156–677.043).[69] The SUV_{max} of primary cervical cancer and the change in SUV_{max} after treatment is associated with disease recurrence and survival time. This finding has been demonstrated by Xue and colleagues,[70] who reported a significant difference of 5-year DFS in patients with an SUV_{max} of less than 10.2 and of 10.2 or greater ($P = .0289$). Kidd and colleagues[71] in a study of 287 stage IA2 to IVB patients with cervical cancer also demonstrated that the SUV_{max} was an independent predictor for death ($P = .0027$). The 5-year OS was shown to be significantly different among the 3 patient groups, that is, an SUV_{max} of 5.2 or less, an SUV_{max} of greater than 5.2, and an SUV_{max} of 13.3 or less, and an SUV of greater than 13.3. The SUV_{max} also correlated with pelvic recurrence ($P = .0232$), cause-specific survival ($P = .0126$), and OS ($P = .0119$).

In addition, the SUV_{max} was correlated with persistent residual tumor burden 3 months after completion of the chemoradiation treatment ($P = .0472$). Lee and colleagues[72] demonstrated that patients with a high SUV_{max} (≥ 13.4) of primary tumor had significantly lower DFS than patients with a low SUV_{max} ($P = .021$). In this study, a high SUV_{max} was an independent predictor for disease recurrence in patients treated with surgery with or without adjuvant therapy ($P = .0207$). Oh and colleagues[73] demonstrated the use of FDG PET/CT scanning performed before treatment, during CCRT at 4 weeks, and 1 month after CCRT. They showed that the percentage change in SUV_{max} of the primary cervical tumor between pretreatment PET/CT scanning and during CCRT PET/CT scanning of 59.7% or greater predicted a complete response on post-CCRT PET/CT scanning ($P<.001$). They also showed that a percentage change in SUV_{max} of 60% or greater and post-CCRT response were independent predictors for PFS ($P = .045$ and $.012$, respectively). Pan and colleagues[20] reported that a higher pretreatment SUV_{max} of primary tumor of 11.2 or greater with pelvic lymph node metastasis was a significant predictor for worse OS ($P = .0099$). Also, the higher pretreatment SUV_{max} along with higher serum SCC-Ag of 6.4 or greater was a significant predictor for poor OS ($P = .0020$) in patients with cervical squamous cell carcinoma. Various studies have demonstrated the usefulness of the volume-based parameters in determining the prognosis in patients with cervical cancer. Miller and colleagues[19] demonstrated that the patients with a tumor volume of greater than 60 cm^3 had a worse PFS ($P = .007$) and OS ($P = .003$) than patients with a tumor volume 60 cm^3 or less. Tumor volumes were significant predictors of PFS and OS. Patients with a tumor volume of 60 cm^3 or less and negative lymph nodes had a significantly better PFS ($P = .01$) than patients with a tumor volume of greater than 60 cm^3 and/or positive lymph nodes. Some studies also reported that age and an MTV of 23.4 mL or greater were independent predictive factors of DFS in patients with stage IB to IIA cervical cancer treated primarily with radical hysterectomy.[74]

Yoo and colleagues[75] reported that prognostic factors in various patients with cervical cancer include age, cell type, disease stage, primary tumor size, lymph node status on PET, lymph node status on CT/MR imaging, treatment modalities, SUV_{max}, average SUV, MTV, and TLG, and of all these factors plus lymph node status on PET ($P<.001$) and TLG ($P<.05$) were independent predictive factors for DFS or PFS. Maharjan and colleagues[76] reported that the SUV_{max}, which indicates the aggressiveness of the tumor, is the most prognostic factor for PFS in recurrent cervical cancer. Lymph node status is the most important prognostic factor in patients with cervical cancer, and the degree of the FDG uptake in the lymph nodes is of predictive value in determining prognosis. Yen and colleagues[77] demonstrated that an SUV_{max} of paraaortic lymph nodes of 3.3 of greater was an independent predictor for OS

($P = .012$) whereas a FIGO stage of III or greater is an independent predictor for relapse-free survival ($P = .008$) and OS ($P = .008$). Patients with an SUV_{max} of paraaortic lymph nodes of 3.3 or greater, or a FIGO stage of III or higher had a significantly worse recurrence-free survival (HR, 4.52; 95% CI, 1.73–11.80) and OS (HR, 6.04; 95% CI, 1.97–18.57) than patients with an SUV_{max} of greater than 3.3 and a FIGO stage of II or lower. Narayan and colleagues[78] reported that adenocarcinoma histology (HR, 3.08; $P = .001$), FIGO stage (HR, 1.73; $P = .002$), and positive nodes (HR, 2.24; $P = .002$) were independent predictors for OS.

Akkas and colleagues,[79] in a study of 58 inoperable patients with stage IIB to IVB cervical cancer who were treated with chemoradiation therapy, found that the SUV_{max} of the pelvic and paraaortic lymph nodes correlated with persistent disease and is one of the independent prognostic factors for persistent disease, OS, and DFS. Nakamura and colleagues,[80] in a retrospective study of 80 patients with cervical cancer who underwent PET/CT scans before radiotherapy or any chemotherapy, found that the DFS and OS rates of patients with a high lymph node SUV_{max} was significantly lower than those of patients exhibiting low lymph node SUV_{max} ($P = .003$ and $P = .019$, respectively). A lymph node SUV_{max} of greater than 2.1 was found to be the most appropriate cutoff value for predicting tumor recurrence (AUC, 0.779; sensitivity, 80.0%; specificity, 64.8%). A lymph node SUV_{max} cutoff value set at 2.225 or higher provides an AUC of 0.761, sensitivity of 80.0%, and specificity of 63.3% for survival. The high SUV_{max} of lymph nodes was an independent prognostic factor for DFS ($P = .0231$) and OS ($P = .0146$). Preoperative FDG uptake in pelvic lymph nodes has also been associated with recurrent cervical cancer.[81] An SUV_{max} of lymph nodes of 2.36 or greater was significantly associated with a better PFS (HR, 15.20; $P<.001$). An SUV_{max} of lymph nodes (HR, 4.447; 95% CI, 1.379–14.343) and parametrial invasion (HR, 6.728; 95% CI, 1.497–30.235) have been considered to be independent prognostic factors for disease recurrence.

The SUV_{max} of the pelvic lymph nodes has been considered to be the only independent factor for risk of pelvic disease recurrence ($P = .0035$).[82] A high SUV_{max} of pelvic lymph nodes is associated with an increased risk of persistent disease after therapy ($P = .0025$) and an increased risk of persistent disease in pelvic lymph nodes ($P = .0003$). An increased SUV_{max} of pelvic lymph nodes correlated with poor disease-specific survival ($P = .023$) and OS ($P = .0378$). Chung and colleagues[53] demonstrated the value of posttreatment FDG PET/CT scanning in predicting the prognosis where an SUV_{max} of 5.25 or greater is associated with a poor OS ($P = .001$). Patients with positive PET/CT scanning for recurrence had worse 5-year PFS ($P<.0001$) and OS ($P = .0015$) compared with those with a negative PET/CT scanning. Ho and colleagues[83] emphasized on the usefulness of FDG PET/CT scanning by analyzing the SUV_{max} in 31 patients with cervical cancer with supraclavicular lymph node recurrence. Patients with an SUV_{max} of lymph node between 4.3 and 8.0 had significantly better OS than patients with SUV_{max} of lymph node less than 4.3 or greater than 8 ($P = .004$). Also, patients with limited supraclavicular lymph node recurrence by FDG PET had better 3-year OS rates than patients with disease extension beyond the supraclavicular lymph nodes ($P = .031$).

In another study, Sharma and colleagues[84] reported that FDG uptake predicts outcome in recurrent cervical cancer after radiation therapy. Patients with an SUV_{max} of greater than 5.8 had significant lower 1-year PFS than in patients with an SUV_{max} of less than 5.8 ($P = .01$). In a metaanalysis study by Zhao and colleagues[85] to determine the association between FDG PET/CT or PET findings and survival outcomes, it was concluded that positive pretreatment FDG PET findings were associated with poor event-free survival (pooled HR, 2.681; 95% CI, 2.059–3.490) and OS (pooled HR, 2.063; 95% CI, 1.023–4.158). Posttreatment FDG PET significantly predicted event-free survival (pooled HR, 2.030; 95% CI, 1.537–2.681) and OS (pooled HR, 2.322; 95% CI, 1.485–3.630).

ENDOMETRIAL CANCER

Endometrial cancer is the most common invasive gynecologic malignancy and is associated with a favorable prognosis as compared with the other gynecologic malignancies.[86] More than 70% of cases are diagnosed in an early stage owing to the appearance of early symptoms and signs such as vaginal spotting and bleeding.[87] Almost 25% of the patients involve premenopausal women with major risk factors, including unopposed estrogen, nulliparity, anovulation, and polycystic ovarian syndrome.[88] Because the majority of the cases can be detected in an early stage (stage I), it is associated with a good prognosis, with an estimated overall 5-year survival rate of 80% to 90% for stage I disease, 70% to 80% for stage II disease, and 20% to 60% for stage III to IV disease.[89,90]

Surgical staging is the reference standard and is performed by exploratory laparotomy, total abdominal hysterectomy, and bilateral salpingo-oophorectomy with associated lymphadenectomy in high-risk cases. Of the various factors affecting prognosis, the extent of myometrial invasion, degree of cervical involvement, and involvement of pelvic and paraaortic lymph nodes result in a poor prognosis. Patients with more than 50% of myometrial invasion have a 7-fold greater risk of pelvic and paraaortic lymph node involvement.[91] Risk stratification, and thereby shift in management regimes, is a challenge for treating physicians, because this group of patients is mostly postmenopausal, which can flare up serious comorbidities.

PET/Computed Tomography with ^{18}F-fluorodeoxyglucose in Localized Tumor Evaluation

FDG PET/CT scanning has a very limited role in this subset of gynecologic malignancy, with US examination and MR imaging remaining the imaging modalities for initial evaluation. Metabolic imaging can predict the histologic grade of the tumor by using the semiquantitative parameter SUV_{max}, which forms the basis of its use in the preoperative assessment of endometrial carcinoma. Various studies have found a significant correlation between SUV_{max} and the grade of malignancy. In a study of 268 patients, Antonsen and colleagues[92] showed that a high SUV_{max} corresponds with a high grade in the primary tumor and also has a statistically significant correlation with various prognostic factors, such as myometrial invasion, cervical involvement, and lymph node involvement. The SUV_{max} was higher in patients with stage IB than with stage IA disease, and similarly in stage III or IV than in stage I or II disease. The SUV_{max} was significantly higher in patients with myometrial invasion of more than 50% as compared with those with less than 50%, cervical involvement compared with no cervical involvement, and lymph node involvement compared with no lymph node involvement. The best cutoff for SUV_{max} was found to be 11.0 in accurately predicting high stage, greater than 50% myometrial invasion, degree of cervical involvement, and lymph node involvement.[92] The sensitivity, specificity, PPV, NPV, and accuracy of detecting lymph node metastases on FDG PET/CT scanning were 75.0%, 92.7%, 60.0%, 96.2%, and 90.5%, respectively.[92] In a similar study, Torizuka and colleagues[93] differentiated between greater than 50% and less than 50% myometrial invasion correctly in 19 out of 22 patients by using a cutoff SUV_{max} of 12. Nakamura and colleagues[94] and Lee and colleagues[95] in separate studies were even able to find a positive correlation between SUV_{max} and histologic grade. The SUV_{max} can also have an impact upon the OS and DFS of endometrial cancer patients, with an SUV_{max} of greater than 12.7 having a statistically significant lower DFS than with a low SUV_{max}.[96] Apart from SUV_{max}, other parameters that have been used for assessing the tumor burden include MTV and TLG. Liu and colleagues,[97] in a study of 15 patients with stage IVB endometrial cancer, found that total body MTV ($P = .010$) and TLG ($P = .011$) were highly collinear (Pearson's correlation coefficient 0.978 with $P<.001$), apart from being the independent prognostic variable. This study postulated that in stage IVB, MTV, and TLG were more significant semiquantitative factors for prognostication than the SUV_{max}. Patients with an MTV value of greater than 450 mL and a TLG of greater than 2700 g had a drastically reduced survival of 2 months as compared with 47 months in patients below these cutoff values.[97] The prognostic significance of MTV was reiterated in other studies also where the HR for DFS were 7.22 and 5.36 for the SUV_{max} and MTV, respectively.[98] In a metaanalysis by Ghooshkhanei and colleagues,[99] the pooled sensitivity and specificity of SUV_{max} for differentiation between low-risk (endometrioid histology, grades I–II, myometrial invasion < 50%) and high-risk patients were 74% and 46%, respectively. Of all of the semiquantitative metabolic imaging parameters like SUV_{max}, mean SUV, TLG, and MTV, MTV showed the highest AUC of 0.77 in predicting deep myometrial invasion and 0.88 for detecting lymph node metastases.[100] An MTV cutoff of 20 mL yielded an odds ratio (OR) of 7.8 (95% CI, 3.2–19.1; $P = .001$) for deep myometrial invasion, whereas an MTV cutoff of 30 mL yielded an OR of 16.5 (95% CI, 3.4–80.3; $P = .001$) for lymph node metastases.

When adjusting for preoperative biopsy results suggesting high risk (nonendometrioid subtype or endometrioid grade 3), an MTV cutoff of 20 mL yielded an OR of 7.3 (95% CI, 2.9–18.3; $P = .001$) for deep invasion and an MTV cutoff of 30 mL yielded an OR of 10.9 (95% CI, 2.1–55.3, $P = .005$) for lymph node metastases.[100] Over the last decade or so, FDG PET has gradually replaced conventional imaging modalities like CT scanning and MR imaging in preoperative lymph node assessment, owing to low accuracy of CT scanning and MR imaging.[101,102] The sensitivity of FDG PET has been low in lymph node assessment, although the specificity approaches close to 98%.[103] This implies that FDG PET/CT scanning has a tremendous role in saving patients from unnecessary incisions. FDG PET/CT scanning has its own limitations, including high false-positive rates

in cases of inflammatory lymph nodes and an inability to detect lymph node metastasis of less than 1 cm in size owing to poor spatial resolution. However, it can be helpful in cases such as in obese patients where lymphadenectomy cannot be performed after performing the primary hysterectomy. In detecting extrauterine metastatic lesions other than retroperitoneal lymph nodes, FDG PET/CT scanning has a sensitivity of 83.3%, compared with 66.7% for CT/MR imaging, whereas the specificity of all of the modalities approaches 100%.[104] FDG PET/CT scanning has been shown to be sensitive in detecting metastatic disease in the pouch of Douglas and ovaries that were otherwise not seen on CT/MR imaging. Based on the available studies, the sensitivity and specificity for the detection of the primary lesions were 81.8% (77.9%–85.3%) and 89.8% (79.2%–96.2%), respectively; for lymph node staging were 72.3% (63.8%–79.8%) and 92.9% (90.6%–94.8%), respectively; and for distant metastasis detection were 95.7% (85.5%–99.5%) and 95.4% (92.7%–97.3%), respectively.[105] However, the sensitivity of detection of lesions widely varies according to the size of the lesion, with sensitivity of 93.3% for lesions greater than 10 mm, 66.7% for lesions 5 to 9 mm, and 16.7% for lesions less than 4 mm.[106]

PET/Computed Tomography with ^{18}F-fluorodeoxyglucose in the Detection of Recurrence

FDG PET/CT scanning has a potential role for the detection of early tumor recurrence in patients with endometrial cancer. Patients usually complain of vaginal spotting in cases of recurrence, because tumor recurrence usually occurs at the vaginal apex. Functional indices such as SUV_{max}, MTV, and TLG can be important factors to predict recurrence of endometrial cancer. Using an MTV cutoff value of 17.15 mL, the AUC is 0.679 ($P<.022$) and that of using a TLG cutoff value of 56.43 g the AUC is 0.661 ($P<.047$).[107] More so, in a study by Shim and colleagues,[107] a lower MTV (HR, = 1.010; 95% CI, = 1.002–1.018; $P = .010$) and lower TLG (HR, = 1.001; 95% CI, = 1.000–1.002; $P = .024$) were associated with longer DFS. FDG PET/CT scanning has a significant role to play in the detection of tumor recurrence, because morphologic imaging modalities are limited by postoperative and postirradiation changes that are present, potentially requiring invasive tissue sampling to differentiate between the radiation necrosis or fibrosis and sites of tumor recurrence. PET/CT scanning can differentiate between tumor recurrence and radiation necrosis and often spare patients from invasive procedures. Belhocine and colleagues[108] suggested that FDG PET/CT scanning can significantly detect recurrence in asymptomatic patients as well as in symptomatic patients and, thus, can have a significant impact on treatment regimens. Overall, FDG PET/CT scanning is found to have a sensitivity of 93% to 100% and a specificity of 78% to 93% in the detection of tumor recurrence.[108–110] The PPV and NPV in recurrence detection range from 85% to 95% and 90% to 100%, respectively.[111] Moreover, FDG PET/CT scanning had a clinical impact in 73.1% of posttherapy surveillance cases and 57.1% in salvage therapy cases, much more than that in staging cases where it only accounted for 22% of clinical impact in decision making (**Fig. 3**).[111]

OVARIAN MALIGNANCIES

Ovarian malignancies are the second most common gynecologic malignancy and account for approximately 3% of all gynecologic malignancies. It has the highest mortality rate among all gynecologic malignancies.[86] Risk factors for ovarian cancer include postmenopausal age, nulliparity, early menarche, late menopause, and family history. By the time the disease is accurately diagnosed, it has progressed to an advanced stage in the majority of cases. Classical signs and symptoms include abdominal pain and menstrual irregularities, whereas in advanced stages, dyspnea can also occur owing to an increase in intraabdominal pressure from ascites. Histologically, about 90% of the tumors have epithelial cell origin and the remaining 10% have stromal, germ, or mixed cell origin. The standard treatment of choice includes optimal tumor debulking surgery followed by adjuvant chemotherapy with platinum-based compounds.[112]

The preliminary workup for staging ovarian cancers includes a regular physical and pelvic examination along with serum tumor marker levels (CA-125). However, surgery is the mainstay for staging ovarian cancers. Imaging studies in this context include CT, MR imaging, and FDG PET/CT examinations.[113] Around three-quarters of cases are diagnosed at an advanced stage (FIGO stage III or IV) owing to lack of specific signs and symptoms at an early stage.[114] Ovarian cancer usually spreads into the peritoneal cavity. Tumor cells directly spread through penetration of the ovarian capsule and spread into the contiguous organs such as the contralateral ovary, uterus, fallopian tubes, peritoneum, and distant organs such as the lungs and liver. Tumor cells can often be seen as peritoneal implants in the right paracolic gutter, subcapsular surface of the liver,

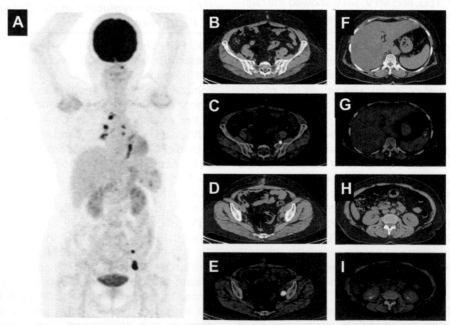

Fig. 3. A 63-year-old woman with known endometrial cancer, status post hysterectomy and chemotherapy, undergoing disease surveillance. Coronal maximum intensity projection PET image with fluorodeoxyglucose (FDG) is shown in (*A*). Axial FDG PET/computed tomography images demonstrate metabolically active metastatic disease involving left internal iliac lymph nodes (*B, C*), left external iliac lymph nodes (*D, E*), spleen (*F, G*), and retroperitoneal lymph nodes (*H, I*).

greater omentum, and left paracolic gutter. This peritoneal carcinomatosis is mostly seen in serous papillary carcinoma and poorly differentiated adenocarcinoma.[115,116] Peritoneal carcinomatosis may also result in pleural involvement through transdiaphragmatic spread.[117] Lymphatic and hematogenous spread is rare in ovarian malignancies. Lymph node involvement commonly occurs with serous papillary carcinoma, and the lymph nodes that are commonly involved include pelvic, paraaortic, supraclavicular nodes.[118] The liver is the most common site of hematogenous involvement followed by the lungs and pleura.[118]

PET/Computed Tomography with 18F-fluorodeoxyglucose in the Initial Evaluation

Preoperative staging for ovarian malignancies is performed using imaging methods such as US, CT, and MR imaging, followed by surgical staging at laparotomy. With the advent of functional imaging over the past 2 decades, there has been a paradigm shift in the diagnosis and management of various oncological conditions. FDG PET/CT imaging is quantitatively evaluated by parameters such as the SUV_{max} and MTV.[119] Glucose metabolism increases in malignant cells as compared with benign cells. This metabolism is the underlying basis of using FDG PET/CT scanning in various malignancies, because it can provide useful information regarding the disease burden that is metabolically active. The most definitive role for FDG PET/CT scanning in patients with ovarian cancer is for surveillance and detecting recurrence in those who have completed primary therapy but have shown a rising trend in CA-125 levels.

PET/CT scanning has a very limited role in diagnosis of the malignant ovarian lesions. When it comes to the initial diagnosis, surgical staging is irreplaceable. One of the main reasons that FDG PET/CT scanning is not used routinely in the initial diagnosis includes high rates of false-positive and false-negative results for evaluating ovarian masses. In premenopausal women, most ovarian masses show increased FDG uptake, but more often than not are benign. Common benign causes of focal increased FDG uptake in the ovaries include normal ovulating ovaries, ovarian torsion, hemorrhage, and corpus luteal cysts.[120–126] Physiologic FDG uptake in the ovaries is usually observed in the late follicular to early luteal phases.[127] The uptake in these cases is mostly unilateral.[128] Thus, menstrual history is mandatory for evaluating any focal FDG uptake in the ovaries of premenopausal women. In postmenopausal women, Lerman and colleagues[129] found that increased ovarian uptake was not noted without the presence of any known gynecologic malignancy. Biochemical correlation with serum CA-125 levels is advised in postmenopausal adnexal mass evaluation, because 97% of such cases are found to be malignant when the serum levels are elevated.[130] Apart from the physiologic conditions, most of the benign ovarian masses such as cystadenoma, endometrioma, hydrosalpinx, cholesterol granuloma, abscess, and thecoma show an increased FDG uptake.[131] In the study of 103 patients by Rieber and colleagues,[131] PET scans showed no incremental value over US and MR imaging in the evaluation of suspicious adnexal lesions when it was confirmed by histopathology. In another series of 101 patients, PET or MR imaging in combination with US examination improved diagnostic accuracy but could not exclude malignancy.[132] These findings were from earlier studies, when the hybrid technology of PET fused with CT scanning for attenuation correction and anatomic localization had not come into routine practice. However, in the postfusion imaging era of PET/CT scans, studies have shown that FDG PET/CT scanning is better for preoperative staging as well as for detecting metastases (15.8% more than radiologic staging) and unexpected tumors (in 3.7% of cases)[133] when compared with other conventional imaging modalities. On the basis of SUV_{max} to discriminate between benign and malignant ovarian lesions, PET/CT scanning was found to have a sensitivity of 87% and specificity of 100% using a cutoff value of greater than 3 as malignant and less than 2.7 as benign.[134] Risum and colleagues[135] evaluated the role of FDG PET/CT scanning in 101 postmenopausal women, and found that the specificity of this modality increases when correlation with CA-125 levels is made. In such cases, FDG PET/CT scanning was 100% sensitive and 92% specific for differentiating malignant and benign or borderline tumors. FDG PET/CT scanning can be falsely negative in small, necrotic, mucinous, and low-grade neoplasms.[136] Although PET/CT scanning is a promising modality for the evaluation of adnexal masses suspicious on US examination, high rates of false positives and false negatives remain one of the reasons for its limited use in this context.

Surgical laparotomy remains the reference standard for initial staging of ovarian cancers.[137] The goal of preoperative (clinical) staging of ovarian cancer is (1) the confirmation of a malignant adnexal mass and exclusion of a primary tumor in the gastrointestinal tract or pancreas, whose metastatic spread might mimic primary ovarian cancer; (2) assessment of tumor burden and mapping of the distribution of metastases; and (3) diagnosis of other possible complications, such as bowel obstruction and hydronephrosis.[138] The early diagnosis of peritoneal spread in malignant disease is essential to prevent unnecessary laparotomies and to select patients in whom complete cytoreduction is feasible. FDG PET/CT scanning can play an important role when compared with the CT and MR imaging in accurate localization of tiny peritoneal implants along with assessing their metabolic status. On PET/CT scanning, peritoneal carcinomatosis can appear as distinctively nodular lesion or can follow a diffuse infiltrative pattern.[139] Sometimes, nodules may coalesce to form large masses and coat the abdominal viscera.[140] Proper assessment of tumor burden can be helpful in avoiding unnecessary laparotomies. One of the important factors for suboptimal cytoreduction includes peritoneal deposits in the large bowel mesentery, which can be detected by PET/CT scanning with higher sensitivity and thus help in prognostication.[141] Thus, PET/CT scanning in the detection of peritoneal deposits has been a useful tool as compared with CT scanning owing to better sensitivity and also high sampling error rates of peritoneal biopsy.[142,143] PET/CT scanning has been found to increase the pretreatment staging accuracy to 75% as compared with 55% based on CT scanning alone (**Fig. 4**).[114]

PET/Computed Tomography with ^{18}F-fluorodeoxyglucose for Residual, Recurrent, and Metastatic Disease

Ovarian malignancies are associated with a relapse rate of 60% to 70% within 2 years after a satisfactory primary therapy.[144] Traditionally, the reference method for the detection of recurrence in ovarian carcinoma is measurement of serum CA-125 levels, which has a PPV of close to 100%.[145,146] Recurrence as well as progression based on sequential CA-125 measurements has been reported by the Gynecologic Cancer Intergroup.[147] However, CA-125 levels cannot localize the exact sites of tumor recurrence. Also, the NPV of CA-125 is close to 50%.[148] CA-125 is neither specific for ovarian cancer nor sensitive for small volume disease, and approximately 20% of all ovarian cancers do not show any increase in levels of CA-125.[149] After a rising trend in CA-125 levels, CT scanning is advised to look for tumor recurrence sites. The pooled sensitivity of CT scanning for the detection of recurrence is 79% and the specificity is 84%.[150] The corresponding values for FDG PET/CT scanning were 91% and 88%, respectively.[150]

PET/CT scanning could be useful in the diagnosis of tumor recurrence by detecting small peritoneal deposits, metastatic lesions outside of the

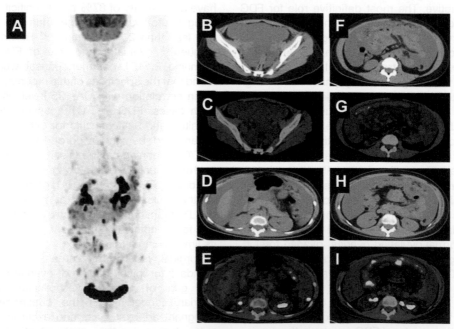

Fig. 4. A 26-year-old woman with known ovarian cancer, undergoing staging assessment. Coronal maximum intensity projection PET image with fluorodeoxyglucose (FDG) is shown in (*A*). Axial FDG PET/computed tomography images show metabolically active ill-defined solid and cystic lesions in the adnexal regions (*B, C*), peritoneal and omental implants (*D, E*), and omental caking (*F–I*).

abdomen and pelvis in suspected stage IV disease, or newly involved lymph nodes.[151] In terms of detecting peritoneal and omental implants, PET/CT scanning can detect tumor lesions as small as approximately 1 cm.[152] The presence of metastatic lymph nodes is an important prognostic factor in ovarian cancer cases. In a metaanalysis involving 882 patients, PET/CT scanning emerged as a more accurate modality for the detection of metastatic lymph nodes when compared with CT and MR imaging.[153] PET/CT scanning was able to diagnose 70% of metastatic lymph nodes and 97% of negative lymph nodes correctly. The pooled sensitivity and specificity for PET/contrast-enhanced CT scanning were 84.4% and 97.4%, respectively.[153] In the setting of suspected recurrence or rising CA-125 levels, FDG PET/CT scanning was found to have a sensitivity of 96% (P<.001) as compared with those of US examination (66%) and CT scanning (81%).[154] In one of the largest metaanalysis involving 1651 patients, the AUC for detecting recurrent versus nonrecurrent ovarian cancer was

found to be 0.9445.[155] No other modality performed as well as PET/CT scanning in this regard, where MR imaging had a very low accuracy rate of approximately 36% as well as a low sensitivity for detecting tumor implants of less than 2 cm.[152] It has also been observed that the PET/CT findings precede those of CT alone by 6 months, and PET/CT scanning can alter the management of recurrent ovarian cancer cases in up to 60% of patients.[156,157] Thus, PET/CT scanning helps to optimize the selection of patients with recurrent ovarian cancer for surgical treatment when conventional imaging modalities are inconclusive or negative (Fig. 5).

PET/Computed Tomography with ^{18}F-fluorodeoxyglucose for Response Assessment to Therapy

One of the established indications for PET/CT scanning is to assess the response of tumor after neoadjuvant chemoradiotherapy or after adjuvant

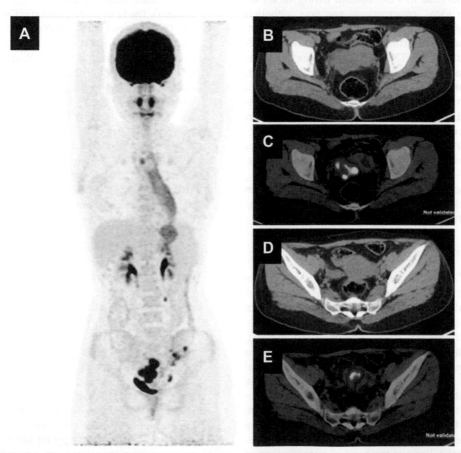

Fig. 5. A 17-year-old woman with known ovarian dysgerminoma, presented with elevated serum alpha fetoprotein levels. Coronal maximum intensity projection PET image with fluorodeoxyglucose (FDG) is shown in (A). Axial FDG PET/computed tomography images reveal a metabolically active solid and cystic lesion in the right adnexa with involvement of fallopian tube (B–E). An associated omental deposit is seen in the left abdomen (A).

chemotherapy. It can predict the functional changes that precede the anatomic changes with high accuracy and, thus, may lead to improved OS in patients with metastatic tumors by altering management. The change in tumor burden is assessed by SUV_{max} on FDG PET/CT scanning, where a substantial decrease after chemoradiation categorizes the patient as a responder to therapy. Using threshold values of SUV_{max} of 3.8% and 65% for percent change, FDG PET scanning could predict pathologic responders in 76% and 86%, respectively $(P<.005)$.[158] In advanced stage ovarian cancer patients (stage III/IV) receiving neo-adjuvant therapy, a significant statistical correlation was observed between the OS of patients and a metabolic tumor response (using a cutoff of percent decrease in SUV_{max} of 20% after the first cycle and 55% after the third cycle), because the OS increased by 15.1 months in responders on FDG PET/CT scanning.[159] In these cases, no correlation was found between the change in CA-125 levels and OS. After radiation therapy, there can be a false increase in FDG uptake owing to an increase in local inflammatory reaction, although there may be some decrease in the tumor burden. This caveat is important to be aware of when evaluating patients on FDG PET/CT scanning postirradiation, and can be mitigated by meticulous history taking, CA-125 level evaluation, using an optimal imaging time of 3 to 6 months after radiation treatment for FDG PET/CT imaging, and anatomic correlation with CT or MR imaging.[160,161] FDG PET/CT scanning can be useful to assess the response of primary tumor to neoadjuvant therapy. FDG PET–derived parameters such as the SUV_{max} and percent change can have a major impact in therapy planning and subsequent follow-up in patients with ovarian cancer.

SUMMARY

FDG PET/CT scanning allows combined for the metabolic and morphologic assessment of tumors, which has led to significant improvements in diagnostic accuracy, resulting in a considerable impact on patient management, initial staging, therapeutic decision making, restaging, response assessment, and prognostication of clinical outcome in patients with gynecologic cancers. The sensitivity and specificity of the modality is superior to that of conventional imaging modalities, although the specificity is often limited by factors such as lesion size and physiologic visceral radiotracer uptake. Various methods of quantification of disease burden have added a new dimension to the usefulness of PET/CT scanning in the evaluation of gynecologic malignancies. Available semiquantitative parameters are useful to determine whether tumors are viable or nonviable, and have been well-correlated with biochemical parameters such as CA-125 and SCC-Ag in various studies. Quantification has been found to be useful in tumor recurrences where other modalities could not identify the latent source of an increase in biochemical parameters in the majority of cases. With the advent of fusion PET imaging with MR imaging, along with new radiotracers and gradual advancements in scanner technologies, PET scanning will continue to play a significant role in the clinical decision making process for patients with these malignancies in the future.

REFERENCES

1. Jemal A, Bray F, Center MM, et al. Global cancer statistics. CA Cancer J Clin 2011;61(2):69–90.
2. Kumar R, Dadparvar S. 18F-fluoro-2-de-oxy-D-glucose-positron emission tomography (PET)/PET-computed tomography in carcinoma of the cervix. Cancer 2007;110(8):1650–3.
3. Gallup D. The Spread and Staging of Cervical Cancer. Glob. libr. women's med 2008. https://doi.org/10.3843/GLOWM.10231 (ISSN: 1756-2228).
4. Iwamoto K, Kigawa J, Minagawa Y, et al. Transvaginal ultrasonographic diagnosis of bladder-wall invasion in patients with cervical cancer. Obstet Gynecol 1994;83(2):217–9.
5. Sun LT, Ning CP, Liu YJ, et al. Is transvaginal elastography useful in pre-operative diagnosis of cervical cancer? Eur J Radiol 2012;81(8):e888–92.
6. Trimble E. Cervical cancer state-of-the-clinical-science meeting on pretreatment evaluation and prognostic factors, September 27e28, 2007: proceedings and recommendations. Gynecol Oncol 2009;114:145–50.
7. Kitajima K, Murakami K, Yamasaki E, et al. Accuracy of integrated FDG-PET/contrast-enhanced CT in detecting pelvic and paraaortic lymph node metastasis in patients with uterine cancer. Eur Radiol 2009;19(6):1529–36.
8. Leblanc E, Gauthier H, Querleu D, et al. Accuracy of 18-fluoro-2-deoxy-D-glucose positron emission tomography in the pretherapeutic detection of occult para-aortic node involvement in patients with a locally advanced cervical carcinoma. Ann Surg Oncol 2011;18(8):2302–9.
9. Ramirez PT, Jhingran A, Macapinlac HA, et al. Laparoscopic extraperitoneal para-aortic lymphadenectomy in locally advanced cervical cancer: a prospective correlation of surgical findings with positron emission tomography/computed tomography findings. Cancer 2011;117(9):1928–34.

10. Kitajima K, Suzuki K, Senda M, et al. Preoperative nodal staging of uterine cancer: is contrast-enhanced PET/CT more accurate than non-enhanced PET/CT or enhanced CT alone? Ann Nucl Med 2011;25(7):511–9.

11. Sheu MH, Chang CY, Wang JH, et al. Preoperative staging of cervical carcinoma with MR imaging: a reappraisal of diagnostic accuracy and pitfalls. Eur Radiol 2001;11(9):1828–33.

12. Bipat S, Glas AS, van der Velden J, et al. Computed tomography and magnetic resonance imaging in staging of uterine cervical carcinoma: a systematic review. Gynecol Oncol 2003;91(1):59–66.

13. Choi HJ, Ju W, Myung SK, et al. Diagnostic performance of computer tomography, magnetic resonance imaging, and positron emission tomography or positron emission tomography/computer tomography for detection of metastatic lymph nodes in patients with cervical cancer: meta-analysis. Cancer Sci 2010;101(6):1471–9.

14. Diddle AW. Carcinoma of the cervix uteri with metastases to the neck. Cancer 1972;29:453–5.

15. Buschbaum H. Extrapelvic lymph node metastases in cervical carcinoma. Am J Obstet Gynecol 1979;133:814–24.

16. Brandt B, Lifshitz S. Scalene node biopsy in advanced carcinoma of the cervix uteri. Cancer 1981;47:1920–1.

17. Tran BN, Grigsby PW, Dehdashti F, et al. Occult supraclavicular lymph node metastasis identified by FDG-PET in patients with carcinoma of the uterine cervix. Gynecol Oncol 2003;90(3):572–6.

18. Lee JH, Kim J, Moon HJ, et al. Supraclavicular lymph nodes detected by 18F-FDG PET/CT in cancer patients: assessment with 18F-FDG PET/CT and sonography. AJR Am J Roentgenol 2012;198(1):187–93.

19. Miller TR, Grigsby PW. Measurement of tumor volume by PET to evaluate prognosis in patients with advanced cervical cancer treated by radiation therapy. Int J Radiat Oncol Biol Phys 2002;53(2):353–9.

20. Pan L, Cheng J, Zhou M, et al. The SUVmax (maximum standardized uptake value for F-18 fluorodeoxyglucose) and serum squamous cell carcinoma antigen (SCC-ag) function as prognostic biomarkers in patients with primary cervical cancer. J Cancer Res Clin Oncol 2012;138(2):239–46.

21. Wright JD, Dehdashti F, Herzog TJ, et al. Preoperative lymph node staging of early-stage cervical carcinoma by [18F]-fluoro-2-deoxy-D-glucose-positron emission tomography. Cancer 2005;104(11):2484–91.

22. Margulies AL, Peres A, Barranger E, et al. Selection of patients with advanced-stage cervical cancer for para-aortic lymphadenectomy in the era of PET/CT. Anticancer Res 2013;33(1):283–6.

23. Kitajima K, Yamasaki E, Kaji Y, et al. Comparison of DWI and PET/CT in evaluation of lymph node metastasis in uterine cancer. World J Radiol 2012;4(5):207–14.

24. Gouy S, Morice P, Narducci F, et al. Nodal-staging surgery for locally advanced cervical cancer in the era of PET. Lancet Oncol 2012;13(5):e212–20.

25. Crivellaro C, Signorelli M, Guerra L, et al. 18F-FDG PET/CT can predict nodal metastases but not recurrence in early stage uterine cervical cancer. Gynecol Oncol 2012;127(1):131–5.

26. Wong TZ, Jones EL, Coleman RE. Positron emission tomography with 2-deoxy-2-[(18)F]fluoro-D-glucose for evaluating local and distant disease in patients with cervical cancer. Mol Imaging Biol 2004;6(1):55–62.

27. Onal C, Oymak E, Findikcioglu A, et al. Isolated mediastinal lymph node false positivity of [18F]-fluorodeoxyglucose-positron emission tomography/computed tomography in patients with cervical cancer. Int J Gynecol Cancer 2013;23(2):337–42.

28. Liu FY, Yen TC, Chen MY, et al. Detection of hematogenous bone metastasis in cervical cancer: 18F-fluorodeoxyglucose-positron emission tomography versus computed tomography and magnetic resonance imaging. Cancer 2009;115(23):5470–80.

29. Akkas BE, Demirel BB, Vural GU. Clinical impact of (1)(8)F-FDG PET/CT in the pretreatment evaluation of patients with locally advanced cervical carcinoma. Nucl Med Commun 2012;33(10):1081–8.

30. Choi HJ, Roh JW, Seo SS, et al. Comparison of the accuracy of magnetic resonance imaging and positron emission tomography/computed tomography in the presurgical detection of lymph node metastases in patients with uterine cervical carcinoma: a prospective study. Cancer 2006;106(4):914–22.

31. Showalter TN, Miller TR, Huettner P, et al. 18F-fluorodeoxyglucose-positron emission tomography and pathologic tumor size in early-stage invasive cervical cancer. Int J Gynecol Cancer 2009;19(8):1412–4.

32. Ciernik IF, Dizendorf E, Baumert BG, et al. Radiation treatment planning with an integrated positron emission and computer tomography (PET/CT): a feasibility study. Int J Radiat Oncol Biol Phys 2003;57(3):853–63.

33. Esthappan J, Chaudhari S, Santanam L, et al. Prospective clinical trial of positron emission tomography/computed tomography image-guided intensity-modulated radiation therapy for cervical carcinoma with positive para-aortic lymph nodes. Int J Radiat Oncol Biol Phys 2008;72(4):1134–9.

34. Lin LL, Mutic S, Low DA, et al. Adaptive brachytherapy treatment planning for cervical cancer using

FDG-PET. Int J Radiat Oncol Biol Phys 2007;67(1): 91–6.

35. Grigsby PW, Siegel BA, Dehdashti F, et al. Post-therapy [18F] fluorodeoxyglucose positron emission tomography in carcinoma of the cervix: response and outcome. J Clin Oncol 2004; 22(11):2167–71.

36. Schwarz JK, Siegel BA, Dehdashti F, et al. Association of posttherapy positron emission tomography with tumor response and survival in cervical carcinoma. JAMA 2007;298(19):2289–95.

37. Mayr NA, Taoka T, Yuh WT, et al. Method and timing of tumor volume measurement for outcome prediction in cervical cancer using magnetic resonance imaging. Int J Radiat Oncol Biol Phys 2002;52(1): 14–22.

38. Boss EA, Massuger LF, Pop LA, et al. Post-radiotherapy contrast enhancement changes in fast dynamic MRI of cervical carcinoma. J Magn Reson Imaging 2001;13(4):600–6.

39. Young H, Baum R, Cremerius U, et al. Measurement of clinical and subclinical tumour response using [18F]-fluorodeoxyglucose and positron emission tomography: review and 1999 EORTC recommendations. European Organization for Research and Treatment of Cancer (EORTC) PET Study Group. Eur J Cancer 1999;35(13):1773–82.

40. Kidd EA, Siegel BA, Dehdashti F, et al. The standardized uptake value for F-18 fluorodeoxyglucose is a sensitive predictive biomarker for cervical cancer treatment response and survival. Cancer 2007; 110(8):1738–44.

41. Amit A, Person O, Keidar Z. FDG PET/CT in monitoring response to treatment in gynecological malignancies. Curr Opin Obstet Gynecol 2013;25(1): 17–22.

42. Kunos C, Radivoyevitch T, Abdul-Karim FW, et al. 18F-fluoro-2-deoxy-D-glucose positron emission tomography standard uptake value ratio as an indicator of cervical cancer chemoradiation therapeutic response. Int J Gynecol Cancer 2011;21(6): 1117–23.

43. Schwarz JK, Lin LL, Siegel BA, et al. 18-F-fluoro-deoxyglucose-positron emission tomography evaluation of early metabolic response during radiation therapy for cervical cancer. Int J Radiat Oncol Biol Phys 2008;72(5):1502–7.

44. Kidd EA, Thomas M, Siegel BA, et al. Changes in cervical cancer FDG uptake during chemoradiation and association with response. Int J Radiat Oncol Biol Phys 2013;85(1):116–22.

45. Lee JE, Huh SJ, Nam H, et al. Early response of patients undergoing concurrent chemoradiotherapy for cervical cancer: a comparison of PET/CT and MRI. Ann Nucl Med 2013;27(1):37–45.

46. Lin LL, Yang Z, Mutic S, et al. FDG-PET imaging for the assessment of physiologic volume response

during radiotherapy in cervix cancer. Int J Radiat Oncol Biol Phys 2006;65(1):177–81.

47. Schwarz JK, Siegel BA, Dehdashti F, et al. Metabolic response on post-therapy FDG-PET predicts patterns of failure after radiotherapy for cervical cancer. Int J Radiat Oncol Biol Phys 2012;83(1): 185–90.

48. Siva S, Herschtal A, Thomas JM, et al. Impact of post-therapy positron emission tomography on prognostic stratification and surveillance after chemoradiotherapy for cervical cancer. Cancer 2011; 117(17):3981–8.

49. Bjurberg M, Kjellén E, Ohlsson T, et al. FDG-PET in cervical cancer: staging, re-staging and follow-up. Acta Obstet Gynecol Scand 2007; 86(11):1385–91.

50. Bodurka-Bevers D, Morris M, Eifel PJ, et al. Post-therapy surveillance of women with cervical cancer: an outcomes analysis. Gynecol Oncol 2000; 78(2):187–93.

51. Chung HH, Jo H, Kang WJ, et al. Clinical impact of integrated PET/CT on the management of suspected cervical cancer recurrence. Gynecol Oncol 2007;104(3):529–34.

52. Mittra E, El-Maghraby T, Rodriguez CA, et al. Efficacy of 18F-FDG PET/CT in the evaluation of patients with recurrent cervical carcinoma. Eur J Nucl Med Mol Imaging 2009;36(12):1952–9.

53. Chung HH, Kim JW, Kang KW, et al. Predictive role of post-treatment [18F]FDG PET/CT in patients with uterine cervical cancer. Eur J Radiol 2012;81(8): e817–22.

54. Chu Y, Zheng A, Wang F, et al. Diagnostic value of 18F-FDG-PET or PET-CT in recurrent cervical cancer: a systematic review and meta-analysis. Nucl Med Commun 2014;35(2):144–50.

55. Bjurberg M, Brun E. Clinical Impact of 2-Deoxy-2-[18F] fluoro-D-Glucose (FDG)–Positron Emission Tomography (PET) on treatment choice in recurrent cancer of the cervix uteri. Int J Gynecol Cancer 2013;23(9):1642–6.

56. Burger IA, Vargas HA, Donati OF, et al. The value of 18F-FDG PET/CT in recurrent gynecologic malignancies prior to pelvic exenteration. Gynecol Oncol 2013;129(3):586–92.

57. Husain A, Akhurst T, Larson S, et al. A prospective study of the accuracy of 18Fluorodeoxyglucose positron emission tomography (18FDG PET) in identifying sites of metastasis prior to pelvic exenteration. Gynecol Oncol 2007;106(1):177–80.

58. Brooks RA, Rader JS, Dehdashti F, et al. Surveillance FDG-PET detection of asymptomatic recurrences in patients with cervical cancer. Gynecol Oncol 2009;112(1):104–9.

59. Chong A, Ha JM, Jeong SY, et al. Clinical usefulness of (18)F-FDG PET/CT in the detection of early recurrence in treated cervical cancer patients with

unexplained elevation of serum tumor markers. Chonnam Med J 2013;49(1):20–6.

60. Chang TC, Law KS, Hong JH, et al. Positron emission tomography for unexplained elevation of serum squamous cell carcinoma antigen levels during follow-up for patients with cervical malignancies: a phase II study. Cancer 2004;101(1):164–71.

61. Waggoner SE. Cervical cancer. Lancet 2003;361(9376):2217–25.

62. Horn LC, Fischer U, Raptis G, et al. Tumor size is of prognostic value in surgically treated FIGO stage II cervical cancer. Gynecol Oncol 2007;107(2):310–5.

63. Werner-Wasik M, Schmid CH, Bornstein L, et al. Prognostic factors for local and distant recurrence in stage I and II cervical carcinoma. Int J Radiat Oncol Biol Phys 1995;32(5):1309–17.

64. Kidd EA, Siegel BA, Dehdashti F, et al. Lymph node staging by positron emission tomography in cervical cancer: relationship to prognosis. J Clin Oncol 2010;28(12):2108–13.

65. Kidd EA, Spencer CR, Huettner PC, et al. Cervical cancer histology and tumor differentiation affect 18F-fluorodeoxyglucose uptake. Cancer 2009;115(15):3548–54.

66. Nakamura K, Okumura Y, Kodama J, et al. The predictive value of measurement of SUVmax and SCC-antigen in patients with pretreatment of primary squamous cell carcinoma of cervix. Gynecol Oncol 2010;119(1):81–6.

67. Yilmaz M, Adli M, Celen Z, et al. FDG PET-CT in cervical cancer: relationship between primary tumor FDG uptake and metastatic potential. Nucl Med Commun 2010;31(6):526–31.

68. Nakamura K, Joja I, Kodama J, et al. Measurement of SUVmax plus ADCmin of the primary tumour is a predictor of prognosis in patients with cervical cancer. Eur J Nucl Med Mol Imaging 2012;39(2):283–90.

69. Chung HH, Nam BH, Kim JW, et al. Preoperative [18F]FDG PET/CT maximum standardized uptake value predicts recurrence of uterine cervical cancer. Eur J Nucl Med Mol Imaging 2010;37(8):1467–73.

70. Xue F, Lin LL, Dehdashti F, et al. F-18 fluorodeoxyglucose uptake in primary cervical cancer as an indicator of prognosis after radiation therapy. Gynecol Oncol 2006;101(1):147–51.

71. Kidd EA1, Siegel BA, Dehdashti F, et al. The standardized uptake value for F-18 fluorodeoxyglucose is a sensitive predictive biomarker for cervical cancer treatment response and survival. Cancer 2007;110(8):1738–44.

72. Lee YY, Choi CH, Kim CJ, et al. The prognostic significance of the SUVmax (maximum standardized uptake value for F-18 fluorodeoxyglucose) of the

cervical tumor in PET imaging for early cervical cancer: preliminary results. Gynecol Oncol 2009;115(1):65–8.

73. Oh D, Lee JE, Huh SJ, et al. Prognostic significance of tumor response as assessed by sequential 18F-fluorodeoxyglucose-positron emission tomography/computed tomography during concurrent chemoradiation therapy for cervical cancer. Int J Radiat Oncol Biol Phys 2013;87(3):549–54.

74. Chung HH, Kim JW, Han KH, et al. Prognostic value of metabolic tumor volume measured by FDG-PET/CT in patients with cervical cancer. Gynecol Oncol 2011;120(2):270–4.

75. Yoo J, Choi JY, Moon SH, et al. Prognostic significance of volume-based metabolic parameters in uterine cervical cancer determined using 18F-fluorodeoxyglucose positron emission tomography. Int J Gynecol Cancer 2012;22(7):1226–33.

76. Maharjan S, Sharma P, Patel CD, et al. Prospective evaluation of qualitative and quantitative (1)(8) F-FDG PET-CT parameters for predicting survival in recurrent carcinoma of the cervix. Nucl Med Commun 2013;34(8):741–8.

77. Yen TC, See LC, Lai CH, et al. Standardized uptake value in para-aortic lymph nodes is a significant prognostic factor in patients with primary advanced squamous cervical cancer. Eur J Nucl Med Mol Imaging 2008;35(3):493–501.

78. Narayan K, Fisher RJ, Bernshaw D, et al. Patterns of failure and prognostic factor analyses in locally advanced cervical cancer patients staged by positron emission tomography and treated with curative intent. Int J Gynecol Cancer 2009;19(5):912–8.

79. Akkas BE, Demirel BB, Dizman A, et al. Do clinical characteristics and metabolic markers detected on positron emission tomography/computerized tomography associate with persistent disease in patients with in-operable cervical cancer? Ann Nucl Med 2013;27(8):756–63.

80. Nakamura K, Joja I, Nagasaka T, et al. Maximum standardized lymph node uptake value could be an important predictor of recurrence and survival in patients with cervical cancer. Eur J Obstet Gynecol Reprod Biol 2014;173:77–82.

81. Chung HH, Cheon GJ, Kang KW, et al. Preoperative PET/CT FDG standardized uptake value of pelvic lymph nodes as a significant prognostic factor in patients with uterine cervical cancer. Eur J Nucl Med Mol Imaging 2014;41(4):674–81.

82. Kidd EA, Siegel BA, Dehdashti F, et al. Pelvic lymph node F-18 fluorodeoxyglucose uptake as a prognostic biomarker in newly diagnosed patients with locally advanced cervical cancer. Cancer 2010;116(6):1469–75.

83. Ho KC, Wang CC, Qiu JT, et al. Identification of prognostic factors in patients with cervical cancer

and supraclavicular lymph node recurrence. Gynecol Oncol 2011;123(2):253–6.

84. Sharma DN, Rath GK, Kumar R, et al. Positron emission tomography scan for predicting clinical outcome of patients with recurrent cervical carcinoma following radiation therapy. J Cancer Res Ther 2012;8(1):23–7.

85. Zhao Q, Feng Y, Mao X, et al. Prognostic value of fluorine-18-fluorodeoxyglucose positron emission tomography or PET-computed tomography in cervical cancer: a meta-analysis. Int J Gynecol Cancer 2013;23(7):1184–90.

86. Jemal A, Siegel R, Ward E, et al. Cancer statistics: 2009. CA Cancer J Clin 2009;59(4):225–49.

87. Jemal A, Siegel R, Ward E, et al. Cancer statistics, 2007. CA Cancer J Clin 2007;57(1):43–66.

88. Benshushan A. Endometrial adenocarcinoma in young patients: evaluation and fertility-preserving treatment. Eur J Obstet Gynecol Reprod Biol 2004;117(2):132–7.

89. Lewin SN, Herzog TJ, BarrenaMedel NI, et al. Comparative performance of the 2009 international Federation of gynecology and obstetrics' staging system for uterine corpus cancer. Obstet Gynecol 2010;116(5):1141.

90. Creasman WT, Odicino F, Maisonneuve P, et al. Carcinoma of the corpus uteri. FIGO 26th Annual Report on the results of treatment in gynecological cancer. Int J Gynaecol Obstet 2006;95(suppl 1): S105.

91. Creasman WT, Morrow CP, Bundy BN, et al. Surgical pathologic spread patterns of endometrial cancer. A gynecologic oncology group study. Cancer 1987;60(8 Suppl.):2035–41.

92. Antonsen SL, Loft A, Fisker R, et al. SUVmax of 18FDG PET/CT as a predictor of high-risk endometrial cancer patients. Gynecol Oncol 2013;129(2): 298–303.

93. Torizuka T, Nakamura F, Takekuma M, et al. FDG PET for the assessment of myometrial infiltration in clinical stage I uterine corpus cancer. Nucl Med Commun 2006;27(6):481–7.

94. Nakamura K, Kodama J, Okumura Y, et al. The SUVmax of 18F-FDG PET correlates with histological grade in endometrial cancer. Int J Gynecol Cancer 2010;20(1):110–5.

95. Lee HJ, Ahn BC, Hong CM, et al. Preoperative risk stratification using (18)F-FDG PET/CT in women with endometrial cancer. Nuklearmedizin 2011; 50(5):204–13.

96. Kitajima K, Kita M, Suzuki K, et al. Prognostic significance of SUVmax (maximum standardized uptake value) measured by [(1)(8)F] FDG PET/CT in endometrial cancer. Eur J Nucl Med Mol Imaging 2012;39(5):840–5.

97. Liu FY, Chao A, Lai CH, et al. Metabolic tumor volume by 18F-FDG PET/CT is prognostic for stage IVB endometrial carcinoma. Gynecol Oncol 2012; 125:566–71.

98. Chung HH, Lee I, Kim HS, et al. Prognostic value of preoperative metabolic tumor volume measured by (18)F-FDG PET/CT and MRI in patients with endometrial cancer. Gynecol Oncol 2013;130:446–51.

99. Ghooshkhanei H, Treglia G, Sabouri G, et al. Risk stratification and prognosis determination using (18)F-FDG PET imaging in N endometrial cancer patients: a systematic review and meta-analysis. Gynecol Oncol 2014;132(3):669–76.

100. Husby JA, Reitan BC, Biermann M, et al. Metabolic tumor volume on 18F-FDG PET/CT improves preoperative identification of high-risk endometrial carcinoma patients. J Nucl Med 2015;56(8): 1191–8.

101. Connor JP, Andrews JI, Anderson B, et al. Computed tomography in endometrial cancer. Obstet Gynecol 2000;95:692–6.

102. Hricak H, Rubinstein LV, Gherman GM, et al. MR imaging evaluation of endometrial cancer: results of an NCI cooperative study. Radiology 1991;179: 829–32.

103. Horowitz NS, Dehdashti F, Herzog TJ, et al. Prospective evaluation of FDG-PET for detecting pelvic and para-aortic lymph node metastasis in uterine corpus cancer. Gynecol Oncol 2004;95(3): 546–51.

104. Suzuki R, Miyagi E, Takahashi N, et al. Validity of positron emission tomography using fluoro-2-deoxyglucose for the preoperative evaluation of endometrial cancer. Int J Gynecol Cancer 2007; 17(4):890–6.

105. Kakhki VR, Shahriari S, Treglia G, et al. Diagnostic performance of fluorine 18 fluorodeoxyglucose positron emission tomography imaging for detection of primary lesion and staging of endometrial cancer patients: systematic review and meta-analysis of the literature. Int J Gynecol Cancer 2013;23(9):1536–43.

106. Kitajima K, Murakami K, Yamasaki E, et al. Accuracy of 18F-FDG PET/CT in detecting pelvic and paraaortic lymph node metastasis in patients with endometrial cancer. AJR Am J Roentgenol 2008; 190(6):1652–8.

107. Shim SH, Kim DY, Lee DY, et al. Metabolic tumour volume and total lesion glycolysis, measured using preoperative 18F-FDG PET/CT, predict the recurrence of endometrial cancer. BJOG 2014;121(9): 1097–106 [discussion:1106].

108. Belhocine T, De Barsy C, Hustinx R, et al. Usefulness of (18)F-FDG PET in the post-therapy surveillance of endometrial carcinoma. Eur J Nucl Med Mol Imaging 2002;29(9):1132–9.

109. Saga T, Higashi T, Ishimori T, et al. Clinical value of FDG-PET in the follow up of post-operative patients

with endometrial cancer. Ann Nucl Med 2003;17(3): 197–203.

110. Kitajima K, Murakami K, Yamasaki E, et al. Performance of 18F-FDG-PET/CT in the diagnosis of recurrent endometrial cancer. Ann Nucl Med 2008;22(2):103–9.

111. Park JY, Kim EN, Kim DY, et al. Clinical impact of positron emission tomography or positron emission tomography/computed tomography in the post-therapy surveillance of endometrial carcinoma: evaluation of 88 patients. Int J Gynecol Cancer 2008;18(6):1332–8.

112. Aabo K, Adams M, Adnitt P, et al. Chemotherapy in advanced ovarian cancer: four systematic meta-analyses of individual patient data from 37 randomized trials. Advanced ovarian cancer trialists' group. Br J Cancer 1998;78(11): 1479–87.

113. Daly MB, Axilbund JE, Buys S, et al. NCCN clinical practice guidelines in oncology. Familial high-risk assessment: breast and ovarian. J Natl Compr Canc Netw 2010;8:562–94.

114. Heintz AP, Odicino F, Maisonneuve P, et al. Carcinoma of the ovary: FIGO 6th annual report on the results of treatment in gynecological cancer. Int J Gynaecol Obstet 2006;95(suppl 1):S161–92.

115. Pentheroudakis G, Pavlidis N. Serous papillary peritoneal carcinoma: unknown primary tumour, ovarian cancer counterpart or a distinct entity?—a systematic review. Crit Rev Oncol Hematol 2010; 75(1):27–42.

116. Kim HJ, Kim JK, Cho KS. CT features of serous surface papillary carcinoma of the ovary. AJR Am J Roentgenol 2004;183(6):1721–4.

117. Mourits MJ, de Bock GH. Managing hereditary ovarian cancer. Maturitas 2009;64(3):172–6.

118. Mironov S, Akin O, Pandit-Taskar N, et al. Ovarian cancer. Radiol Clin North Am 2007;45:149–66.

119. Basu S, Kwee TC, Surti S, et al. Fundamentals of PET and PET/CT imaging. Ann N Y Acad Sci 2011;1228:1–18.

120. Short S, Hoskin P, Wong W. Ovulation and increased FDG uptake on PET: potential for a false positive results. Clin Nucl Med 2005;30:707.

121. Cottrill HM, Fitzcharles EK, Modesitt SC. Positron emission tomography in a premenopausal asymptomatic woman: a case report of increased ovarian uptake in a benign condition. Int J Gynecol Cancer 2005;15:1127–30.

122. Takanami K, Kaneta T, Niikura H, et al. Intense FDG uptake in the ovary with painless torsion. Clin Nucl Med 2007;32:805–6.

123. Ho KC, Ng KK, Yen TC, et al. An ovary in luteal phase mimicking common iliac lymph node metastasis from a primary cutaneous peripheral primitive neuroectodermal tumor as revealed by 18F-FDG PET. Br J Radiol 2005;78:343–5.

124. Bagga S. A corpus luteal cyst masquerading as a lymph node mass on PET/CT scan in a pregnant woman with an anterior mediastinal lymphomatous mass. Clin Nucl Med 2007;32:649–51.

125. Fechel S, Grab D, Nuesle K, et al. Asymmetric adnexal masses: correlation of FDG PET and histopathologic findings. Radiology 2002;223:780–8.

126. Ames J, Blodgett T, Meltzer C. 18F-FDG uptake in an ovary containing a hemorrhagic corpus luteal cyst: false positive PET/CT in a patient with cervical carcinoma. AJR Am J Roentgenol 2005;185: 1057–9.

127. Kim SK, Kang KW, Roh JW, et al. Incidental ovarian 18F-FDG accumulation on PET: correlation with the menstrual cycle. Eur J Nucl Med Mol Imaging 2005;32:757–63.

128. Nishizawa S, Inubushi M, Okada H. Physiological 18F-FDG uptake in the ovaries and uterus of healthy female volunteers. Eur J Nucl Med Mol Imaging 2005;32:549–56.

129. Lerman H, Metser U, Grisaru D, et al. Normal and abnormal 18F-FDG endometrial and ovarian uptake in pre- and postmenopausal patients: assessment by PET/CT. J Nucl Med 2004;45: 266–71.

130. Brooks SE. Preoperative evaluation of patients with suspected ovarian cancer. Gynecol Oncol 1994; 55(3 Pt 2):S80–90.

131. Rieber A, Nussle K, Stohr I, et al. Preoperative diagnosis of ovarian tumors with MR imaging: comparison with transvaginal sonography, positron emission tomography and histologic findings. AJR Am J Roentgenol 2001;177:123–9.

132. Grab D, Flock F, Stöhr I, et al. Classification of asymptomatic adnexal masses by ultrasound, magnetic resonance imaging, and positron emission tomography. Gynecol Oncol 2000;77(3): 454–9.

133. Nam EJ, Yun MJ, Oh YT, et al. Diagnosis and staging of primary ovarian cancer: correlation between PET/CT, Doppler US, and CT or MRI. Gynecol Oncol 2009;116(3):389–94.

134. Castellucci P, Perrone AM, Picchio M. Diagnosticaccuracyof18F-FDG PET/CTincharacterizingovarianlesionsandstagingovariancancer:Correlation with transvaginal ultrasonography, computed tomography, and histology. Nucl Med Commun 2007;28:589–95.

135. Risum S, Høgdall C, Loft A, et al. The diagnostic value of PET/CT for primary ovarian cancer – a prospective study. Gynecol Oncol 2007;105(1):145–9.

136. Subhas N, Patel PV, Pannu HK, et al. Imaging of pelvic malignancies with in-line FDG PET-CT: case examples and common pitfalls of FDG PET. Radiographics 2005;25(4):1031–43.

137. Benedet JL, Bender H, Jones H 3rd, et al. FIGO staging classifications and clinical practice

guidelines in the management of gynecologic cancers. FIGO Committee on Gynecologic Oncology. Int J Gynaecol Obstet 2000;70:209–62.

138. Forstner R, Sala E, Kinkel K, et al. ESUR guidelines: ovarian cancer staging and follow-up. Eur Radiol 2010;20:2773–80.

139. Turlakow A, Yeung HW, Salmon AS, et al. Peritoneal carcinomatosis: role of (18)F-FDG n PET. J Nucl Med 2003;44(9):1407–12.

140. Dromain C, Leboulleux S, Auperin A, et al. Staging of peritoneal carcinomatosis: enhanced CT vs. PET/CT. Abdom Imaging 2008;33:87–93.

141. Risum S, Høgdall C, Loft A, et al. Prediction of suboptimal primary cytoreduction in primary ovarian cancer with combined positron emission tomography/computed tomography – a prospective study. Gynecol Oncol 2008;108(2):265–70.

142. Pfannenberg C, Königsrainer I, Aschoff P, et al. 18F-FDG-PET/CT to select patients with peritoneal carcinomatosis for cytoreductive surgery and hyperthermic intraperitoneal chemotherapy. Ann Surg Oncol 2009;16(5):1295–303.

143. Yang QM, Bando E, Kawamura T, et al. The diagnostic value of PET-CT for peritoneal dissemination of abdominal malignancies. Gan To Kagaku Ryoho 2006;33(12):1817–21.

144. Ledermann JA, Kristeleit RS. Optimal treatment for relapsing ovarian cancer. Ann Oncol 2010; 21(Suppl 7):vii218–22.

145. Niloff JM, Knapp RC, Lavin PT, et al. 125 assay as a predictor of clinical recurrence in epithelial ovarian cancer. Am J Obstet Gynecol 1986;155:56–60.

146. Högberg T, Ka°gedal B. Long-term follow-up of ovarian cancer with monthly determinations of serum CA 125. Gynecol Oncol 1992;46:191–8.

147. Rustin GJ, Vergote I, Eisenhauer E, et al. Gynecological cancer intergroup definitions for response and progression in ovarian cancer clinical trials incorporating RECIST 1.1 and CA 125 agreed by the Gynecological Cancer Intergroup (GCIG). Int J Gynecol Cancer 2011;21:419–23.

148. Potter ME, Moradi M, To AC, et al. Value of serum 125Ca levels: does the result preclude second look? Gynecol Oncol 1989;33(2):201–3.

149. Santillan A, Garg R, Zahurak ML, et al. Risk of epithelial ovarian cancer recurrence in patients with rising serumCA-125 levels within the normal range. J Clin Oncol 2005;23(36):9338–43.

150. Gu P, Pan LL, Wu SQ, et al. CA 125, PET alone, PET–CT, CT and MRI in diagnosing recurrent ovarian carcinoma: a systematic review and meta-analysis. Eur J Radiol 2009;71:164–74.

151. Son H, Khan SM, Rahaman J, et al. Role of FDG PET/CT in staging of recurrent ovarian cancer. Radiographics 2011;31:569–83.

152. Sanli Y, Turkmen C, Bakir B, et al. Diagnostic value of PET/CT is similar to that of conventional MRI and even better for detecting small peritoneal implants in patients with recurrent ovarian cancer. Nucl Med Commun 2012;33(5):509–15.

153. Yuan Y, Gu ZX, Tao XF, et al. Computer tomography, magnetic resonance imaging, and positron emission tomography or positron emission tomography/computer tomography for detection of metastatic lymph nodes in patients with ovarian cancer: a meta-analysis. Eur J Radiol 2012;81(5):1002–6.

154. Risum S, Høgdall C, Markova E, et al. Influenceof2-(18F) fluoro-2- deoxy-D-glucose positron emission tomography/computed tomography on recurrent ovarian cancer diagnosis and on selection of patients for secondary cytoreductive surgery. Int J Gynecol Cancer 2009;19:600–4.

155. Limei Z, Yong C, Yan X, et al. Accuracy of positron emission tomography/computed tomography in the diagnosis and restaging for recurrent ovarian cancer: a meta-analysis. Int J Gynecol Cancer 2013; 23(4):598–607.

156. Fulham MJ, Carter J, Baldey A, et al. The impact of PET-CT in suspected recurrent ovarian cancer: a prospective multi-centre study as part of the Australian PET data collection project. Gynecol Oncol 2009;112:462–8.

157. Garcia-Velloso MJ, Jurado M, Ceamanos C, et al. Diagnostic accuracy of FDG PET in the follow-up of platinum-sensitive epithelial ovarian carcinoma. Eur J Nucl Med Mol Imaging 2007;34:1396–405.

158. Nishiyama Y, Yamamoto Y, Kanenishi K, et al. Monitoring the neoadjuvant therapy response in gynecological cancer patients using FDG PET. Eur J Nucl Med Mol Imaging 2008;35(2):287–95.

159. Avril N, Sassen S, Schmalfeldt B, et al. Prediction of response to neoadjuvant chemotherapy by sequential F-18-fluorodeoxyglucose positron emission tomography in patients with advanced-stage ovarian cancer. J Clin Oncol 2005;23:7445–53.

160. Nakamoto Y, Eisbruch A, Achtyes ED, et al. Prognostic value of positron emission tomography using F-18-fluorodeoxyglucose in patients with cervical cancer undergoing radiotherapy. Gynecol Oncol 2002;84:289–95.

161. Haberkorn U, Strauss LG, Dimitrakopoupou A, et al. PET studies of fluorodeoxyglucose metabolism in patients with recurrent colorectal tumors receiving radiotherapy. J Nucl Med 1991;32: 1485–90.

Emerging Molecular Imaging Techniques in Gynecologic Oncology

Gigin Lin, MD, PhD[a], Chyong-Huey Lai, MD[b],*,
Tzu-Chen Yen, MD, PhD[c]

KEYWORDS

- Cervical cancer • Endometrial cancer • Ovarian cancer • Vulvar cancer • MR imaging
- Molecular imaging • PET • Radiomics

KEY POINTS

- Molecular imaging has played important roles in tumor detection, primary staging, treatment planning, prediction of prognosis, response evaluation, surveillance, and management of recurrence.
- Emerging MR imaging–based technologies include diffusion-weighted imaging, chemical exchange saturation transfer imaging, dynamic contrast enhancement–MR imaging, and magnetic resonance spectroscopy.
- Dynamic nuclear polarization increases signal by more than 10,000-fold for stable isotope carbon-13–enriched compounds on MR imaging.
- ^{18}F-fluorodeoxyglucose–PET provides semiquantitative functional readouts: standardized uptake value maximum, total lesion glycolysis, and metabolic tumor volume.
- Radiomics converts high-throughput extraction of quantitative imaging features into mineable data by machine-learning tools and will evolve rapidly for decision support in the near future.

INTRODUCTION

Molecular imaging in oncology refers to in vivo spatial and temporal analysis of the key biomolecules representing the cancer phenotype. Tumor heterogeneity is not only attributed to genetic alteration but also an adaptation to the tumor microenvironment. The anatomy of the female pelvis contains delicate structures, and many oncologic lesions are better demonstrated using molecular imaging tools. The most prominent example, the Warburg effect, explains how glycolysis confers a significant growth advantage by producing lactate as oxidative fuel, sparing glucose for the more anoxic cells in the center of the tumor.[1] Because tumor heterogeneity and its adaptations to microenvironment are important factors that could affect the effectiveness of cancer treatment, the ability to image and spatially map the heterogeneity of metabolism within a tumor will be beneficial for planning the treatment regime in gynecologic oncology.[2]

Advances in MR imaging techniques have enabled noninvasive assessment of structural,

Disclosure Statement: No conflicts of interest to disclose.
[a] Department of Medical Imaging and Intervention, Chang Gung Memorial Hospital, Chang Gung University College of Medicine, 5 Fu-Shin Street, Kueishan, Taoyuan 333, Taiwan; [b] Division of Gynecologic Oncology, Department of Obstetrics and Gynecology, Chang Gung Memorial Hospital, Chang Gung University College of Medicine, 5 Fu-Shin Street, Kueishan, Taoyuan 333, Taiwan; [c] Department of Nuclear Medicine, Chang Gung Memorial Hospital, Chang Gung University College of Medicine, 5 Fu-Shin Street, Kueishan, Taoyuan 333, Taiwan
* Corresponding author.
E-mail address: sh46erry@ms6.hinet.net

PET Clin 13 (2018) 289–299
https://doi.org/10.1016/j.cpet.2017.11.011

functional, and metabolic phenotypes of cancer on a variety of scales. The complex relaxation mechanisms of nuclear spins provide unique and convertible tissue contrasts, offering abundant parameters that can be extracted from a single acquisition to provide general structural data, functional pathophysiologic data, and various heterogeneity-based metrics in the tumor. Moreover, it is critical to understand each data acquisition and reconstruction scheme for proper image analysis and valid assessment of associated metabolic parameters. The most prominent applications include diffusion-weighted imaging (DWI),[3] chemical exchange saturation transfer (CEST) imaging,[4] dynamic contrast enhancement (DCE)–MR imaging,[5] and magnetic resonance spectroscopy (MRS).[6] The latest addition to the MR imaging armamentarium is the dynamic nuclear polarization (DNP), which could increase signal more than 10,000-fold for stable isotope carbon-13 (^{13}C) -enriched compounds.[7] These imaging modalities could provide markers for tumor diagnosis, prognosis, and treatment response, as well as insights into cancer biology and factors that promote tumor growth.

PET detects pairs of gamma rays emitted indirectly by specifically labeled radionuclide tracers, to provide functional or metabolic information in various disease scenarios.[2] ^{18}F-fluorodeoxyglucose (FDG) PET is by far the most widely used imaging technique to study glucose uptake in tumors in vivo. The semiquantitative imaging parameters of the tumor, for example, standardized uptake value maximum (SUV_{max}), total lesion glycolysis (TLG), and metabolic tumor volume (MTV), are used in daily oncology practice.[2] In addition to FDG, ^{11}C-choline[8] and 3′-deoxy-3′-^{18}F-fluorothymidine (FLT)[9] have been used to assess the diagnosis and treatment response in patients with cancer, with many other PET radiotracers under development on the pipeline.

A novel analysis approach, radiomics, refers to the extraction and analysis of large amounts of quantitative imaging features with high throughput from computed tomography (CT), PET, or MR imaging.[10] Radiomics data are mineable information that can be used to build descriptive and predictive models relating image phenotypes and to provide valuable diagnostic, prognostic, or predictive information.[10]

The purpose of this review is to summarize the literature pertaining to emerging techniques in MR imaging and PET, as well as new radiomics analyses, that hold translatable potential for gynecologic oncology in the clinic.

MR IMAGING
Diffusion-Weighted Imaging Measurements Reflecting Tumor Microstructure

DWI is an MR imaging method that is sensitive to the Brownian motion of water molecules. Because most cancer types demonstrate an increased cellularity than the adjacent normal tissue, tumors are highlighted on DWI and can be measured quantitatively on the apparent diffusion coefficient (ADC) map. Newer DWI techniques, such as computed DWI resulting in higher b values, could potentially increase diagnostic specificity by improving the suppression of signal from normal tissues that may mimic disease.[3] The ADC values may provide additional information about tumor microstructure with potential relevance for staging and prediction of aggressive disease. For example, low ADC values of endometrial cancers are associated with deep myometrial invasion, cervical involvement, and lymph node metastases, and in patients with high-grade endometrioid subtype.[11] Furthermore, ADC minimum significantly predicts a reduced disease-free survival,[11] suggesting that tumor ADC measurements may potentially aid in risk stratification when selecting patients for treatment. Whole-body DWI for the staging of patients with suspected ovarian cancer was reported superior to CT or F18-FDG/CT, with a 94% accuracy rate for primary tumor characterization and 91% accuracy for peritoneal staging.[12]

Chemical Exchange Saturation Transfer Imaging

CEST imaging selectively saturates exogenous or endogenous compounds containing either exchangeable protons or molecules, detected indirectly through the water signal with enhanced sensitivity.[4] The extracellular pH (pH_e) decrease correlates with tumor proliferation, invasion, metastasis, and chemoresistance, which can be detected by CEST. CEST MR imaging has been used to achieve pH_e mapping of the cancer microenvironment by in vitro studies on hepatoma cell lines and in vivo in an MMTV-Erbb2 transgenic mouse breast cancer model.[13] CEST imaging was capable of differentiating radiation necrosis from tumor progression in brain metastases, superior to the conventional amide proton transfer imaging.[14] An emerging technique, acidoCEST-MR imaging, uses an exogenous compound, iopromide, to assess in vivo pH_e more accurately as compared with ^{31}P MRS.[15] Because of its sensitivity to motion artifact, there has not yet been application of this technique in gynecology oncology.

Dynamic Contrast Enhancement–MR Imaging Parameters Reflecting Tumor Microvasculature

DCE–MR imaging is a method that makes use of an intravenous gadolinium-based contrast agent that is blocked by the tight junction of the normal blood vessel, but which leaks out through neovascularization in the tumor. DCE–MR imaging quantitative assessment of tissue perfusion and vascular permeability enables characterization of tumor microvasculature and the angiogenic profile of tumor tissues in vivo.[5] Recent findings suggest that DCE–MR imaging tumor parameters correlate with clinical and histologic phenotypes in endometrial cancer.[16] DCE–MR imaging might help to understand how tumor hypoxia leads to tumor growth and metastatic spread, which promote tumor progression and resistance to therapy in endometrial cancer.[17]

MR Imaging with Lymph Node–Specific Contrast Agent

Ultrasmall superparamagnetic iron oxide (USPIO) is a lymph node–specific MR imaging contrast agent that has been shown to improve the detection of nodal metastasis in endometrial and cervical cancer. The reported sensitivity of USPIO-enhanced MR imaging was 91% to 100%, with specificity of 87% to 94%, and accuracy of 88% to 95%.[18] Unfortunately, the implementation of USPIO in the clinic has been postponed by the manufacturer pending further validation.

Magnetic Resonance Spectroscopy

Most clinical MR scanners have sequences for ^{1}H-MRS measurements, which can semiquantitatively measure chemical composition in a selected region of interest.[6] MRS has provided a valuable adjunct to conventional MR imaging in the assessment of various tumors in the brain, prostate gland, and breast.[17] A recent study found that the choline-to-water ratio increased with increasing tumor stage and large tumor size in endometrial cancer.[19] Furthermore, choline-to-noise ratio is reportedly significantly higher in the more aggressive type 2 endometrial cancers than in type 1 endometrial cancers.[20] An altered choline profile in endometrial cancer tissue has also been validated using high-resolution nuclear magnetic resonance techniques,[21] confirming the central role of choline in the metabolic derangements in endometrial cancer. The increase in the total choline content is also detected in ovarian cancer cell lines[22] and in clinical ovarian tumors.[23] In addition to choline, MRS has been used to depict the elevated lipid resonance levels in cervical cancers, which can predict the poor prognostic human papilloma virus genotypes and persistent disease following chemoradiation therapy. Further larger-scale studies with longer follow-up times are warranted to validate the initial MRS findings.[24]

Dynamic Nuclear Polarization

DNP is a novel MRS technique that uses specialized hyperpolarization to enhance the MR signal over 10,000-fold for stable isotope ^{13}C-enriched compounds.[7] Hyperpolarized [1-^{13}C]pyruvate is the most widely studied DNP tracer, based on the real-time flux of pyruvate-to-lactate conversion in various preclinical models.[25–30] Hyperpolarized [1-^{13}C]pyruvate has demonstrated increased lactate labeling in tumors[25] and decreased metabolism to bicarbonate,[26] indicating suppressed pyruvate flux into mitochondria. The metabolic fate of pyruvate into the mitochondria has also been explored with hyperpolarized [2-^{13}C]pyruvate in a preclinical glioma model.[31] In addition to pyruvate, hyperpolarized bicarbonate ($H^{13}CO_3^-$) can probe pH_e,[32] [1,4-$^{13}C_2$]fumarate for necrotic cell death,[7] and [1-^{13}C]dehydroascorbate for redox status.[33] Glutamine addiction, another phenotype in bioenergetics often found in multiple cancer models that are less glycolytic, can also be assessed with hyperpolarized ^{13}C substrates.[34,35] The first clinical trial of DNP-MRS has recently demonstrated the use of hyperpolarized [1-^{13}C]pyruvate to examine prostate cancer metabolism in humans[36] and sheds light on the possible translation of this exciting technology into clinical applications. The preclinical and clinical applications of DNP were actively developed and are summarized in **Table 1**. Many clinical trials are actively being carried out to evaluate the utility of hyperpolarized [1-^{13}C]pyruvate in patients with cervical, breast, prostate gland, and brain malignancies, with a total of 357 subjects planned in 12 trials registered at the clinicaltrial.gov registry (accessed 26 July 2017).

PET
^{18}F-Fluorodeoxyglucose PET/Computed Tomographic Applications for Endometrial Cancer

The potential value of FDG PET in predicting clinical and histologic tumor characteristics in endometrial cancer has been explored.[37–39] Tumor SUV_{max} is the most frequently reported PET parameter. SUV_{max} represents the value of the voxel with the highest SUV within the drawn volume of interest putatively representing tumor tissue.[37] TLG is derived from SUV_{mean} and MTV, representing a measure of total viable tumor cells

Table 1
Summary of applications of dynamic nuclear polarization tracers

	Tracer	Readout	Target	Cancer	Treatment	Endpoint	Status	Reference
1	[1-¹³C]Pyruvate	[1-¹³C]Lactate	Pyruvate dehydrogenase (PDH)-mediated flux	Prostate	Not applicable (NA)	Detection	Human	Nelson et al,[36] 2013
2	[1-¹³C]Pyruvate	[1-¹³C]Lactate, [1-¹³C]Alanine	PDH flux	Prostate	NA	Detection	Preclinical	Albers et al,[25] 2008
3	[1-¹³C]Pyruvate	[1-¹³C]Lactate, [1-¹³C]Bicarbonate	PDH flux	Brain	Dichloroacetate	Monitor response	Preclinical	Park et al,[26] 2013
4	[1-¹³C]Pyruvate	[1-¹³C]Lactate	Apoptosis	Lymphoma	Etoposide	Monitor response	Preclinical	Day et al,[27] 2007
5	[1-¹³C]Pyruvate	[1-¹³C]Lactate	Autophagy	Colon	Dichloroacetate	Monitor response	Preclinical	Lin et al,[28] 2014
6	[1-¹³C]Pyruvate	[1-¹³C]Lactate	Carbonic anhydrase IX	Brain	Everolimus	Monitor response	Preclinical	Chaumeil et al,[29] 2012
7	[1-¹³C]Pyruvate	[1-¹³C]Lactate, [1-¹³C]Bicarbonate	Readjustment of the metabolic balance	Brain	VEGF	Monitor response	Preclinical	Park et al,[30] 2016
8	[2-¹³C]Pyruvate	[2-¹³C]Lactate, [5-¹³C]Glutamate, [1-¹³C]Acetyl-carnitine	Pyruvate into the mitochondria	Brain	Dichloroacetate	Monitor response	Preclinical	Park et al,[31] 2016
9	[1-¹³C]Bicarbonate (HCO₃⁻)	[1-¹³C]HCO₃⁻, [1-¹³C]CO₂	Extracellular pH	Lymphoma	NA	Detection	Preclinical	Gallagher et al,[32] 2008
10	[1,4-¹³C₂]Fumarate	[1,4-¹³C₂]Malate	Necrotic cell death	Lymphoma	Etoposide	Monitor response	Preclinical	Gallagher et al,[7] 2009
11	[1-¹³C]Dehydroascorbate	[1-¹³C]Vitamin C	Redox [NADP⁺]/[NADPH]	Prostate	NA	Detection	Preclinical	Keshari et al,[33] 2011
12	[5-¹³C]Glutamine	[5-¹³C]Pyroglutamate, [5-¹³C]Glutamate	Glutamine metabolism	Liver	Gemcitabine, etoposide	Monitor response	Preclinical	Cabella et al,[34] 2013
13	[5-¹³C]Glutamine	[5-¹³C]Pyroglutamate, [5-¹³C]Glutamate	Glutaminolysis	Prostate	Resveratrol, sulforaphane	Monitor response	Preclinical	Canape et al,[35] 2015

within the tumor, and is increasingly reported in studies on endometrial cancers.[37–39] Increased tumor SUV$_{max}$, SUV$_{mean}$, MTV, and TLG are reported to predict poor prognostic factors, such as deep myometrial invasion, cervical stromal invasion, and lymph node metastases. However, the proposed cutoffs for these parameters to identify high-risk patients have a relatively wide range in the literature: for SUV$_{max}$ >9 to 18, for MTV >9 to 30 mL, and for TLG >56 to 70 g.[37–39] Further studies are warranted to validate and better standardize metabolic imaging parameters, including optimized thresholds for risk stratification for potential clinical use.

^{18}F-Fluorodeoxyglucose PET/Computed Tomographic Applications for Cervical and Vulvar Cancers

In the initial pretreatment planning of cervical cancer, PET can be used in correlation with pelvic MR imaging to determine the initial extent of disease. For example, the high resolution of small field-of-view (FOV) MR imaging can be used to assess for the presence of parametrial invasion, whereas whole-body PET can be used to detect distant metastatic disease. The small FOV is also adaptable to the clinical question. PET may detect nodes not sufficiently enlarged to be detectable by MR imaging or CT,[40] and adding a fused MR imaging to the PET/CT examination increases sensitivity.[41] Using MR imaging rather than CT can resolve the location of PET-detected lesions not easily seen on CT or make subtle lesions more evident, and MR imaging itself may help assess for the presence of local invasion. It may also avoid confusing physiologic accumulations of radiotracer, such as in the urine, in a ureter, or in a functional ovary that may mimic disease.[42] Studies of PET/CT for vulvar cancer, however, have shown variable sensitivity.[43,44] There is also evidence that false-positive nodal or distant metastatic PET findings may be common in vulvar cancer, where MR imaging and CT may be more useful.[45]

Novel PET Radiotracers

^{18}F-FLT, a thymidine analogue, is used to image cell proliferation by PET.[9] FLT uptake measures thymidine kinase 1 activity that is upregulated in the S phase of the cell cycle and is correlated with proliferation marker Ki67 positivity as measured by immunohistochemistry.[46] FLT PET has also been used noninvasively to predict and assess treatment response in ovarian cancer xenografts treated with carboplatin and paclitaxel, belinostat, and APO866.[47] FLT PET showed an early but transient response, whereas FDG PET showed a late and prolonged response.[47] It has demonstrated that FLT PET can be used to assess response in platinum-resistant ovarian cancer in tumor xenografts in mice.[48] Moreover, FLT PET can be used to monitor early treatment response of cisplatin-resistant ovarian tumors by targeting the mammalian target of rapamycin inhibitors.[49] ^{11}C-methionine (MET) has been applied to assess amino acid transport and metabolism in tumors.[50] Malignant tumors accumulated MET, whereas benign lesions and borderline-malignant tumors did not.[50]

Radiolabeled nitroimidazole derivatives such as ^{18}F-fluoroazomycinarabinofuranoside are PET radiotracers that can be used to detect hypoxia in cancer cells, because hypoxia in tumors is an important predictor of chemotherapy response.[51] ^{64}Cu-DOTAtrastuzumab PET has value for monitoring treatment response in human ovarian cancers implanted in mice that were treated with 17-dimethylaminoethylamino-17 demethoxygeldanamycin, because HER2-overexpressing tumors may be resistant to chemotherapy and endocrine therapy.[52] ^{11}C-labeled Sel-tagged affibody PET is helpful in selecting cell surface receptors in HER2 expression in SKOV3 xenografts.[53] ^{18}F-NOTA-ZHER2:2395 affibody PET may be useful in the future to select patients for HER2-targeted therapy.[54] ^{89}Zr-bevacizumab PET could be used to evaluate early treatment response to everolimus on vascular endothelial growth factor (VEGF)-A secretion in an ovarian cancer xenograft model, potentially providing an early biomarker for antiangiogenic treatment effects in ovarian cancer.[55] The ^{64}Cu-labeled anti-CA125 monoclonal antibody has been evaluated for specific targets for immunotherapy in preclinical ovarian SKOV3 and OVCAR3 models.[56] Despite the success in other cancers, the use of ^{11}C-choline PET has rarely applied to ovarian cancers with limited results.[8] Deuterium-substituted ^{18}F-fluoromethyl-[1,2-^{2}H$_4$]-choline is a recently developed stable radiotracer that overcomes the short physical half-life of ^{11}C and seems to be a promising tool for choline metabolism imaging for tumors with high choline level such as ovarian cancer.[57]

Novel PET radiotracers developed to assess the diagnosis and treatment response of patients with gynecology malignances are summarized in **Table 2**.

Applications of PET/MR Imaging in Gynecologic Cancers

The recently introduced hybrid PET/MR imaging combines the major strengths of MR imaging,

Table 2
Summary of PET radiotracers other than ^{18}F-fluorodeoxyglucose

	Tracer	Target	Cancer	Treatment	Endpoint	Status	Reference
1	^{18}F-FLT	Proliferation	Lung	NA	Detection	Human	Buck et al,[9] 2003
2	^{18}F-FLT	Proliferation	Ovary	Carboplatin and paclitaxel, belinostat, and APO866	Monitor response	Preclinical	Munk Jensen et al,[47] 2013
3	^{18}F-FLT	Proliferation	Ovary	AKT inhibitor, API-2 (resensitized platinum-resistant tumors to cisplatin)	Monitor response	Preclinical	Perumal et al,[48] 2012
4	^{18}F-FLT	Proliferation	Ovary	Mammalian target of rapamycin inhibitors	Monitor response	Preclinical	Aide et al,[49] 2010
5	^{18}F-FLT	Thymidine kinase 1	Melanoma, colon	Mitogenic extracellular kinase 1/2 inhibitor: PD0325901	Monitor response	Preclinical	Leyton et al,[46] 2008
6	^{11}C-Methionine	Amino acid transport and metabolism	Ovary	Doxorubicin combined with UIC2 anti-Pgp monoclonal antibody and cyclosporine A	Monitor response	Preclinical	Trencsenyi et al,[51] 2014
7	^{18}F-fluoroazomycinarabinofuranoside	Hypoxia	Ovary	Doxorubicin combined with UIC2 anti-Pgp monoclonal antibody and cyclosporine A	Monitor response	Preclinical	Trencsenyi et al,[51] 2014
8	^{64}Cu-DOTAtrastuzumab	HER2	Ovary	17-Dimethylaminoetthylamino-17 demethoxygeldanamycin	Monitor response	Preclinical	Niu et al,[52] 2009
9	^{18}F-NOTA-ZHER2:2395 affibody	HER2	Ovary	NA	Detection	Preclinical	Heskamp et al,[54] 2012
10	^{11}C-labeled Sel-tagged affibody	HER2	Ovary	NA	Detection	Preclinical	Wallberg et al,[53] 2012
11	[89]Zr-bevacizumab	VEGF	Ovary	Everolimus	Monitor response	Preclinical	van der Bilt et al,[55] 2012
12	^{64}Cu-labeled anti-CA125 monoclonal antibody	CA125	Ovary	NA	Detection	Preclinical	Sharma et al,[56] 2014
13	^{11}C-Choline	Choline metabolism	Ovary	NA	Detection	Human	Torizuka et al,[8] 2003
14	Deuterium-substituted ^{18}F-fluoromethyl-[1,2-[2]H$_4$]-choline	Choline metabolism	Melanoma, colon	NA	Detection	Preclinical	Witney et al,[57] 2012

including multiplanar image acquisition, superior soft tissue contrast, and functional imaging capability through specialized techniques, with those of PET. MR imaging is better at assessing tumor size and local changes, such as stromal invasion and parametrial involvement, whereas PET is better at detecting metastases to lymph nodes and bone marrow. MR imaging is also better at assessing liver metastases because of better soft tissue contrast and the moderate background physiologic liver uptake of FDG.[58] The radiation exposure from PET/MR imaging was reported to be up to 80% less than that of PET/CT.[59] PET/MR imaging can also be used to plan radiation therapy for cervical cancer and is superior to PET/CT regarding delineation of the primary tumor.[60] Although tumor volume discrepancies were observed between T2-weighted MR imaging–gross tumor volume (GTV) (manually contoured) and PET-GTV (auto-contoured by 40% SUV threshold),[61] strong volume concordances between FDG PET and T2-weighted MR imaging and DWI were also reported.[62] Detailed contouring of the radiation field can be aided by careful delineation of the primary tumor and the inclusion of metastatic nodes.[63] PET may detect additional nodes too small to be diagnosed as malignant by MR imaging and is 90% to 95% sensitive for detection of pelvic and para-aortic nodes in advanced disease.[63] Changes in uptake on PET during therapy[64] as well as after treatment[65] have been shown to have prognostic value, and so PET/MR imaging can also be used to assess response. PET/CT is thought to be optimal to detect suspected tumor recurrences, with MR imaging being very useful to localize them. MR imaging also has the potential to avoid image artifacts from the bony pelvis.[66] MR imaging can aid in the detection of small-volume tumor recurrences, whereas the PET component can find small tumor recurrences throughout the whole body. PET is sensitive in detecting both locoregional and distant tumor recurrence.[67] The soft tissue contrast of MR imaging is of particular use in separating radiation changes from tumor recurrence. A recent study suggested that both PET/CT and PET/MR imaging have a high diagnostic value for recurrent malignancies of the female pelvis, whereas PET/MR imaging may be superior for separating benign and malignant lesions.[68] In another recent study, the lesion-based diagnostic accuracy for the detection of recurrent lesions showed no statistically significant difference between PET/CT and PET/MR imaging.[69] More evidence is needed to validate the appropriate applications for PET/MR imaging in gynecology oncology.

Radiomics

Radiomics is a novel imaging analysis approach, converting high-throughput extraction of quantitative imaging features into mineable data that are subsequently analyzed for decision support.[70] The central hypothesis of radiomics is that these libraries of quantitative individual voxel-based variables are more robust in association with various clinical endpoints compared with the conventional qualitative radiologic, histopathologic, and clinical data. Radiomics data can be enhanced by adding existing prognostic tools.[71] Radiomics offers immense potential for integrating other -omics data and hence draws attention in the oncologic audience.[72] A common radiomics approach, texture analysis, is an image analysis based on the spatial arrangement of intensities in a volume of interest. The use of texture analysis for quantification of intratumor uptake heterogeneity has received increasing attention in the past few years, including gynecologic malignancies.[73] An early attempt has demonstrated radiomics features from baseline FDG PET images could predict local recurrence of locally advanced cervical cancer better than SUV_{max}.[74] Quantitative texture-based heterogeneity metrics of CT may predict outcomes in patients with ovarian cancers.[75] Using texture feature analysis comparing pretherapy and posttherapy CT images yielded higher prediction accuracy in predicting ovarian cancer response to chemotherapy.[76] Machine-learning analysis of MR imaging radiomics has been shown to improve the performance in clinical prostate and breast cancer.[77,78] The variability and robustness of PET/CT image radiomics in advanced reconstruction settings are feature dependent, and radiomics features with low coefficients of variation can be considered appropriate variables for reproducible tumor quantification in multicenter studies.[79] However, comparison of literature results is difficult due to the heterogeneity of studies and lack of standardization. Therefore, a plea for standardization and recommendations/guidelines has been made to enable the field to move forward, because progress as a field requires pooling of results.[80] Because the radiomics approach is designed to extract data from standard-of-care images, the future efforts of radiomics would vigorously validate the evidence on vast imaging databases.

SUMMARY

In summary, molecular imaging (mainly PET and MR imaging) has played important roles in gynecologic oncology, for tumor detection, primary staging, treatment planning, prediction of prognosis, as well as response evaluation, surveillance, and the management of recurrence. Emerging MR-based technologies, including DWI, CEST, DCE–MR imaging, MRS, and DNP, as well as FDG PET and many novel PET radiotracers, will continuously improve practices. In combination with radiomics analysis, a new era of decision-making in personalized medicine and precisely guided radiation treatment planning or real-time surgical interventions is being entered into, which will directly impact patient survival. No single imaging tool will universally apply to different tumor types. Prospective trials with well-defined endpoints are encouraged to evaluate the multiple facets of these emerging imaging tools in the management of gynecologic malignancies.

REFERENCES

1. Lin G, Chung YL. Current opportunities and challenges of magnetic resonance spectroscopy, positron emission tomography, and mass spectrometry imaging for mapping cancer metabolism in vivo. Biomed Res Int 2014;2014:625095.
2. Lai CH, Lin G, Yen TC, et al. Molecular imaging in the management of gynecologic malignancies. Gynecol Oncol 2014;135(1):156–62.
3. Blackledge MD, Leach MO, Collins DJ, et al. Computed diffusion-weighted MR imaging may improve tumor detection. Radiology 2011;261(2):573–81.
4. van Zijl PC, Yadav NN. Chemical exchange saturation transfer (CEST): what is in a name and what isn't? Magn Reson Med 2011;65(4):927–48.
5. Leach MO, Morgan B, Tofts PS, et al. Imaging vascular function for early stage clinical trials using dynamic contrast-enhanced magnetic resonance imaging. Eur Radiol 2012;22(7):1451–64.
6. Glunde K, Bhujwalla ZM. Metabolic tumor imaging using magnetic resonance spectroscopy. Semin Oncol 2011;38(1):26–41.
7. Gallagher FA, Kettunen MI, Hu DE, et al. Production of hyperpolarized [1,4-13C2]malate from [1,4-13C2] fumarate is a marker of cell necrosis and treatment response in tumors. Proc Natl Acad Sci U S A 2009;106(47):19801–6.
8. Torizuka T, Kanno T, Futatsubashi M, et al. Imaging of gynecologic tumors: comparison of (11)C-choline PET with (18)F-FDG PET. J Nucl Med 2003;44(7):1051–6.
9. Buck AK, Halter G, Schirrmeister H, et al. Imaging proliferation in lung tumors with PET: 18F-FLT versus 18F-FDG. J Nucl Med 2003;44(9):1426–31.
10. Kumar V, Gu Y, Basu S, et al. Radiomics: the process and the challenges. Magn Reson Imaging 2012;30(9):1234–48.
11. Nakamura K, Imafuku N, Nishida T, et al. Measurement of the minimum apparent diffusion coefficient (ADCmin) of the primary tumor and CA125 are predictive of disease recurrence for patients with endometrial cancer. Gynecol Oncol 2012;124(2):335–9.
12. Michielsen K, Vergote I, Op de Beeck K, et al. Whole-body MRI with diffusion-weighted sequence for staging of patients with suspected ovarian cancer: a clinical feasibility study in comparison to CT and FDG-PET/CT. Eur Radiol 2014;24(4):889–901.
13. Chen M, Chen C, Shen Z, et al. Extracellular pH is a biomarker enabling detection of breast cancer and liver cancer using CEST MRI. Oncotarget 2017;8(28):45759–67.
14. Mehrabian H, Desmond KL, Soliman H, et al. Differentiation between radiation necrosis and tumor progression using chemical exchange saturation transfer. Clin Cancer Res 2017;23(14):3667–75.
15. Chen LQ, Howison CM, Jeffery JJ, et al. Evaluations of extracellular pH within in vivo tumors using acidoCEST MRI. Magn Reson Med 2014;72(5):1408–17.
16. Haldorsen IS, Stefansson I, Gruner R, et al. Increased microvascular proliferation is negatively correlated to tumour blood flow and is associated with unfavourable outcome in endometrial carcinomas. Br J Cancer 2014;110(1):107–14.
17. Harry VN, Semple SI, Parkin DE, et al. Use of new imaging techniques to predict tumour response to therapy. Lancet Oncol 2010;11(1):92–102.
18. Rockall AG, Sohaib SA, Harisinghani MG, et al. Diagnostic performance of nanoparticle-enhanced magnetic resonance imaging in the diagnosis of lymph node metastases in patients with endometrial and cervical cancer. J Clin Oncol 2005;23(12):2813–21.
19. Zhang J, Cai S, Li C, et al. Can magnetic resonance spectroscopy differentiate endometrial cancer? Eur Radiol 2014;24(10):2552–60.
20. Han X, Kang J, Zhang J, et al. Can the signal-to-noise ratio of choline in magnetic resonance spectroscopy reflect the aggressiveness of endometrial cancer? Acad Radiol 2015;22(4):453–9.
21. Trousil S, Lee P, Pinato DJ, et al. Alterations of choline phospholipid metabolism in endometrial cancer are caused by choline kinase alpha overexpression and a hyperactivated deacylation pathway. Cancer Res 2014;74(23):6867–77.
22. Iorio E, Ricci A, Bagnoli M, et al. Activation of phosphatidylcholine cycle enzymes in human epithelial ovarian cancer cells. Cancer Res 2010;70(5):2126–35.
23. Esseridou A, Di Leo G, Sconfienza LM, et al. In vivo detection of choline in ovarian tumors using 3D magnetic resonance spectroscopy. Invest Radiol 2011;46(6):377–82.
24. Lin G, Lai CH, Tsai SY, et al. 1 H MR spectroscopy in cervical carcinoma using external phase array body

coil at 3.0 Tesla: prediction of poor prognostic human papillomavirus genotypes. J Magn Reson Imaging 2017;45(3):899–907.

25. Albers MJ, Bok R, Chen AP, et al. Hyperpolarized 13C lactate, pyruvate, and alanine: noninvasive biomarkers for prostate cancer detection and grading. Cancer Res 2008;68(20):8607–15.

26. Park JM, Recht LD, Josan S, et al. Metabolic response of glioma to dichloroacetate measured in vivo by hyperpolarized (13)C magnetic resonance spectroscopic imaging. Neuro Oncol 2013;15(4): 433–41.

27. Day SE, Kettunen MI, Gallagher FA, et al. Detecting tumor response to treatment using hyperpolarized 13C magnetic resonance imaging and spectroscopy. Nat Med 2007;13(11):1382–7.

28. Lin G, Hill DK, Andrejeva G, et al. Dichloroacetate induces autophagy in colorectal cancer cells and tumours. Br J Cancer 2014;111(2):375–85.

29. Chaumeil MM, Ozawa T, Park I, et al. Hyperpolarized 13C MR spectroscopic imaging can be used to monitor Everolimus treatment in vivo in an orthotopic rodent model of glioblastoma. Neuroimage 2012; 59(1):193–201.

30. Park JM, Spielman DM, Josan S, et al. Hyperpolarized (13)C-lactate to (13)C-bicarbonate ratio as a biomarker for monitoring the acute response of anti-vascular endothelial growth factor (anti-VEGF) treatment. NMR Biomed 2016;29(5):650–9.

31. Park JM, Josan S, Jang T, et al. Volumetric spiral chemical shift imaging of hyperpolarized [2-(13) c] pyruvate in a rat c6 glioma model. Magn Reson Med 2016;75(3):973–84.

32. Gallagher FA, Kettunen MI, Day SE, et al. Magnetic resonance imaging of pH in vivo using hyperpolarized 13C-labelled bicarbonate. Nature 2008;453(7197):940–3.

33. Keshari KR, Kurhanewicz J, Bok R, et al. Hyperpolarized 13C dehydroascorbate as an endogenous redox sensor for in vivo metabolic imaging. Proc Natl Acad Sci U S A 2011; 108(46):18606–11.

34. Cabella C, Karlsson M, Canape C, et al. In vivo and in vitro liver cancer metabolism observed with hyperpolarized [5-(13)C]glutamine. J Magn Reson 2013; 232:45–52.

35. Canape C, Catanzaro G, Terreno E, et al. Probing treatment response of glutaminolytic prostate cancer cells to natural drugs with hyperpolarized [5-(13) C]glutamine. Magn Reson Med 2015;73(6): 2296–305.

36. Nelson SJ, Kurhanewicz J, Vigneron DB, et al. Metabolic imaging of patients with prostate cancer using hyperpolarized [1-(1)(3)C]pyruvate. Sci Transl Med 2013;5(198):198ra108.

37. Husby JA, Reitan BC, Biermann M, et al. Metabolic tumor volume on 18F-FDG PET/CT improves preoperative identification of high-risk endometrial carcinoma patients. J Nucl Med 2015;56(8):1191–8.

38. Kitajima K, Suenaga Y, Ueno Y, et al. Preoperative risk stratification using metabolic parameters of (18)F-FDG PET/CT in patients with endometrial cancer. Eur J Nucl Med Mol Imaging 2015;42(8): 1268–75.

39. Shim SH, Kim DY, Lee DY, et al. Metabolic tumour volume and total lesion glycolysis, measured using preoperative 18F-FDG PET/CT, predict the recurrence of endometrial cancer. BJOG 2014;121(9): 1097–106 [discussion: 1106].

40. Choi HJ, Ju W, Myung SK, et al. Diagnostic performance of computer tomography, magnetic resonance imaging, and positron emission tomography or positron emission tomography/computer tomography for detection of metastatic lymph nodes in patients with cervical cancer: meta-analysis. Cancer Sci 2010;101(6):1471–9.

41. Kim SK, Choi HJ, Park SY, et al. Additional value of MR/PET fusion compared with PET/CT in the detection of lymph node metastases in cervical cancer patients. Eur J Cancer 2009;45(12):2103–9.

42. Bagade S, Fowler KJ, Schwarz JK, et al. PET/MRI evaluation of gynecologic malignancies and prostate cancer. Semin Nucl Med 2015;45(4): 293–303.

43. Dolanbay M, Ozcelik B, Abdulrezzak U, et al. F-18 fluoro-D-glucose (FDG)-positron emission tomography (PET)/computed tomography (CT) in planning of surgery and sentinel lymph node screening in vulvar cancers. Arch Gynecol Obstet 2016;293(6): 1319–24.

44. Kamran MW, O'Toole F, Meghen K, et al. Whole-body [18F]fluoro-2-deoxyglucose positron emission tomography scan as combined PET-CT staging prior to planned radical vulvectomy and inguinofemoral lymphadenectomy for squamous vulvar cancer: a correlation with groin node metastasis. Eur J Gynaecol Oncol 2014;35(3):230–5.

45. Lin G, Chen CY, Liu FY, et al. Computed tomography, magnetic resonance imaging and FDG positron emission tomography in the management of vulvar malignancies. Eur Radiol 2015;25(5):1267–78.

46. Leyton J, Smith G, Lees M, et al. Noninvasive imaging of cell proliferation following mitogenic extracellular kinase inhibition by PD0325901. Mol Cancer Ther 2008;7(9):3112–21.

47. Munk Jensen M, Erichsen KD, Bjorkling F, et al. Imaging of treatment response to the combination of carboplatin and paclitaxel in human ovarian cancer xenograft tumors in mice using FDG and FLT PET. PLoS One 2013;8(12):e85126.

48. Perumal M, Stronach EA, Gabra H, et al. Evaluation of 2-deoxy-2-[18F]fluoro-D-glucose- and 3'-deoxy-3'-[18F]fluorothymidine-positron emission tomography as biomarkers of therapy response

in platinum-resistant ovarian cancer. Mol Imaging Biol 2012;14(6):753–61.

49. Aide N, Kinross K, Cullinane C, et al. 18F-FLT PET as a surrogate marker of drug efficacy during mTOR inhibition by everolimus in a preclinical cisplatin-resistant ovarian tumor model. J Nucl Med 2010; 51(10):1559–64.

50. Risum S, Loft A, Hogdall C, et al. Standardized FDG uptake as a prognostic variable and as a predictor of incomplete cytoreduction in primary advanced ovarian cancer. Acta Oncol 2011;50(3): 415–9.

51. Trencsenyi G, Marian T, Lajtos I, et al. 18FDG, [18F]FLT, [18F]FAZA, and 11C-methionine are suitable tracers for the diagnosis and in vivo follow-up of the efficacy of chemotherapy by miniPET in both multidrug resistant and sensitive human gynecologic tumor xenografts. Biomed Res Int 2014;2014: 787365.

52. Niu G, Li Z, Cao Q, et al. Monitoring therapeutic response of human ovarian cancer to 17-DMAG by noninvasive PET Imaging with (64)Cu-DOTA-trastuzumab. Eur J Nucl Med Mol Imaging 2009;36(9): 1510–9.

53. Wallberg H, Grafstrom J, Cheng Q, et al. HER2-positive tumors imaged within 1 hour using a site-specifically 11C-labeled Sel-tagged affibody molecule. J Nucl Med 2012;53(9):1446–53.

54. Heskamp S, Laverman P, Rosik D, et al. Imaging of human epidermal growth factor receptor type 2 expression with 18F-labeled affibody molecule ZHER2:2395 in a mouse model for ovarian cancer. J Nucl Med 2012;53(1):146–53.

55. van der Bilt AR, Terwisscha van Scheltinga AG, Timmer-Bosscha H, et al. Measurement of tumor VEGF-A levels with 89Zr-bevacizumab PET as an early biomarker for the antiangiogenic effect of everolimus treatment in an ovarian cancer xenograft model. Clin Cancer Res 2012;18(22):6306–14.

56. Sharma SK, Wuest M, Wang M, et al. Immuno-PET of epithelial ovarian cancer: harnessing the potential of CA125 for non-invasive imaging. EJNMMI Res 2014; 4(1):60.

57. Witney TH, Alam IS, Turton DR, et al. Evaluation of deuterated 18F- and 11C-labeled choline analogs for cancer detection by positron emission tomography. Clin Cancer Res 2012;18(4):1063–72.

58. Lee SI, Catalano OA, Dehdashti F. Evaluation of gynecologic cancer with MR imaging, 18F-FDG PET/CT, and PET/MR imaging. J Nucl Med 2015;56(3): 436–43.

59. Hirsch FW, Sattler B, Sorge I, et al. PET/MR in children. Initial clinical experience in paediatric oncology using an integrated PET/MR scanner. Pediatr Radiol 2013;43(7):860–75.

60. Queiroz MA, Kubik-Huch RA, Hauser N, et al. PET/MRI and PET/CT in advanced gynaecological

tumours: initial experience and comparison. Eur Radiol 2015;25(8):2222–30.

61. Zhang S, Xin J, Guo Q, et al. Comparison of tumor volume between PET and MRI in cervical cancer with hybrid PET/MR. Int J Gynecol Cancer 2014; 24(4):744–50.

62. Sun H, Xin J, Zhang S, et al. Anatomical and functional volume concordance between FDG PET, and T2 and diffusion-weighted MRI for cervical cancer: a hybrid PET/MR study. Eur J Nucl Med Mol Imaging 2014;41(5):898–905.

63. Speirs CK, Grigsby PW, Huang J, et al. PET-based radiation therapy planning. PET Clin 2015;10(1): 27–44.

64. Kidd EA, Thomas M, Siegel BA, et al. Changes in cervical cancer FDG uptake during chemoradiation and association with response. Int J Radiat Oncol Biol Phys 2013;85(1):116–22.

65. Schwarz JK, Siegel BA, Dehdashti F, et al. Association of posttherapy positron emission tomography with tumor response and survival in cervical carcinoma. JAMA 2007;298(19):2289–95.

66. Partovi S, Kohan A, Rubbert C, et al. Clinical oncologic applications of PET/MRI: a new horizon. Am J Nucl Med Mol Imaging 2014;4(2): 202–12.

67. Chu Y, Zheng A, Wang F, et al. Diagnostic value of 18F-FDG-PET or PET-CT in recurrent cervical cancer: a systematic review and meta-analysis. Nucl Med Commun 2014;35(2):144–50.

68. Beiderwellen K, Grueneisen J, Ruhlmann V, et al. [(18)F]FDG PET/MRI vs. PET/CT for whole-body staging in patients with recurrent malignancies of the female pelvis: initial results. Eur J Nucl Med Mol Imaging 2015;42(1):56–65.

69. Grueneisen J, Schaarschmidt BM, Heubner M, et al. Implementation of FAST-PET/MRI for whole-body staging of female patients with recurrent pelvic malignancies: a comparison to PET/CT. Eur J Radiol 2015;84(11):2097–102.

70. Gillies RJ, Kinahan PE, Hricak H. Radiomics: images are more than pictures, they are data. Radiology 2016;278(2):563–77.

71. Verma V, Simone CB 2nd, Krishnan S, et al. The rise of radiomics and implications for oncologic management. J Natl Cancer Inst 2017;109(7).

72. Hatt M, Tixier F, Visvikis D, et al. Radiomics in PET/CT: more than meets the eye? J Nucl Med 2017; 58(3):365–6.

73. Lai CH. Measuring tumor metabolic heterogeneity on positron emission tomography: utility in cervical cancer. J Gynecol Oncol 2016;27(2):e12.

74. Reuze S, Orlhac F, Chargari C, et al. Prediction of cervical cancer recurrence using textural features extracted from 18F-FDG PET images acquired with different scanners. Oncotarget 2017;8(26): 43169–79.

75. Vargas HA, Veeraraghavan H, Micco M, et al. A novel representation of inter-site tumour heterogeneity from pre-treatment computed tomography textures classifies ovarian cancers by clinical outcome. Eur Radiol 2017;27(9):3991–4001.

76. Danala G, Thai T, Gunderson CC, et al. Applying quantitative CT image feature analysis to predict response of ovarian cancer patients to chemotherapy. Acad Radiol 2017;24(10):1233–9.

77. Wang J, Wu CJ, Bao ML, et al. Machine learning-based analysis of MR radiomics can help to improve the diagnostic performance of PI-RADS v2 in clinically relevant prostate cancer. Eur Radiol 2017. https://doi.org/10.1007/s00330-017-4800-5.

78. Braman NM, Etsami M, Prasanna P, et al. Intratumoral and peritumoral radiomics for the pretreatment prediction of pathological complete response to neoadjuvant chemotherapy based on breast DCE-MRI. Breast Cancer Res 2017;19(1):57.

79. Shiri I, Rahmim A, Ghaffarian P, et al. The impact of image reconstruction settings on 18F-FDG PET radiomic features: multi-scanner phantom and patient studies. Eur Radiol 2017. https://doi.org/10.1007/s00330-017-4859-z.

80. Hatt M, Tixier F, Pierce L, et al. Characterization of PET/CT images using texture analysis: the past, the present… any future? Eur J Nucl Med Mol Imaging 2017;44(1):151–65.

Moving?

Make sure your subscription moves with you!

To notify us of your new address, find your **Clinics Account Number** (located on your mailing label above your name), and contact customer service at:

Email: journalscustomerservice-usa@elsevier.com

800-654-2452 (subscribers in the U.S. & Canada)
314-447-8871 (subscribers outside of the U.S. & Canada)

Fax number: 314-447-8029

Elsevier Health Sciences Division
Subscription Customer Service
3251 Riverport Lane
Maryland Heights, MO 63043

*To ensure uninterrupted delivery of your subscription, please notify us at least 4 weeks in advance of move.

Printed and bound by CPI Group (UK) Ltd, Croydon, CR0 4YY

03/10/2024

01040298-0020